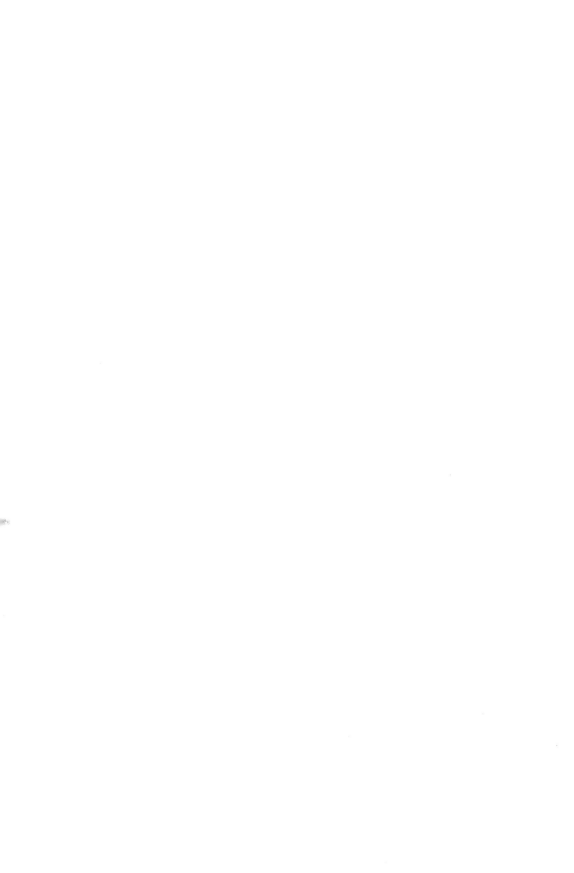

Biomechanics of Normal and Pathological Human Articulating Joints

NATO ASI Series

Advanced Science Institutes Series

A Series presenting the results of activities sponsored by the NATO Science Committee, which aims at the dissemination of advanced scientific and technological knowledge, with a view to strengthening links between scientific communities.

The Series is published by an international board of publishers in conjunction with the NATO Scientific Affairs Division

A	Life Sciences	Plenum Publishing Corporation
B	Physics	London and New York
C	Mathematical and Physical Sciences	D. Reidel Publishing Company Dordrecht and Boston
D	Behavioural and Social Sciences	Martinus Nijhoff Publishers Dordrecht/Boston/Lancaster
E	Applied Sciences	
F	Computer and Systems Sciences	Springer-Verlag Berlin/Heidelberg/New York
G	Ecological Sciences	

Series E: Applied Sciences – No. 93

Biomechanics of Normal and Pathological Human Articulating Joints

edited by

Necip Berme
Dept. of Mechanical Engineering
The Ohio State University
Columbus, Ohio, USA

Ali E. Engin
Dept. of Engineering Mechanics
The Ohio State University
Columbus, Ohio, USA

Kelo M. Correia da Silva
Gulbenkian Institute of Science
Oeiras, Portugal

1985 **Martinus Nijhoff Publishers**
Dordrecht / Boston / Lancaster
Published in cooperation with NATO Scientific Affairs Division

Proceedings of the NATO Advanced Study Institute on Biomechanics of Normal and Pathological Human Articulating Joints, Estoril, Portugal, 20 June–1 July, 1983

ISBN 90-247-3164-X (this volume)
ISBN 90-247-2689-1 (series)

Distributors for the United States and Canada: Kluwer Boston, Inc., 190 Old Derby Street, Hingham, MA 02043, USA

Distributors for the UK and Ireland: Kluwer Academic Publishers, MTP Press Ltd, Falcon House, Queen Square, Lancaster LA1 1RN, UK

Distributors for all other countries: Kluwer Academic Publishers Group, Distribution Center, P.O. Box 322, 3300 AH Dordrecht, The Netherlands

TABLE OF CONTENTS

PREFACE

The widespread occurrence of the various forms of arthritis not only results in a great waste of manpower, but also causes immeasurable pain and suffering for the patients. Due to the limited understanding of its etiology, the currently available treatments are directed at the effects of the disease rather than its causes. The solutions available to the clinician at the advanced stages of arthritis are frequently surgical and include prosthetic replacement arthroplasty. Many advances have been made in the last decade in the basic understanding of the kinematics and kinetics of anatomical joints, as well as in the technology of joint replacement. The NATO Advanced Study Institute held in Portugal during June 20-July 1, 1983 addressed these topics and provided instruction on the advances in biomechanics of diarthrodial joints. The proceedings of this Institute are presented in this volume.

Many different areas of specialization contribute to the field of joint biomechanics. Due to the complexity of each individual topic, it was not attempted here to present a complete treatise of each of these areas. Each chapter typically gives a review and a flavor of the subject matter, as well as discussing the state-of-the-art advances in general or in specific research areas. Some of the chapters, such as those on lubrication and muscle mechanics, are more mathematically oriented than the others. Nevertheless, the reader with a non-engineering background, I trust, would still find most of the book informative and easy to read. On the other hand, the engineering expert will benefit from the chapter on clinical review, as well as from those that are not in his immediate field of expertise.

I would like to thank my co-editors Dr. K. M. Correia da Silva and Professor A. E. Engin for their contributions in organizing the Advanced Study Institute, as well as for their input in shaping the scientific program. I would also like to thank the lecturers of the Institute for their presentations, and particularly for their contributions to this book. Finally, special thanks go to my family for their support, understanding and patience throughout the time it took me to give uniformity to this volume.

Necip Berme

CLINICAL ASPECTS OF HUMAN ARTICULATING JOINTS

J.C. Mulier

Department of Orthopaedic Surgery,
University Hospital, 3041 Pellenberg, Belgium

1.   INTRODUCTION

A human synovial joint has two essential characteristics: its stability and its mobility which are both provided by a complicated system of structures. If damaged, most of the tissues making up a joint have the possibility to repair themselves. In more differentiated cells this function is less pronounced. Of all the structures making up a joint, cartilage is the most vulnerable tissue and the least able to repair itself. Practically all serious acute or chronic joint damage ends with damage of the cartilage. Although cartilage is able to grow and resist wear very well under normal circumstances, it looses its function as soon as excessive damage or wear occurs.

In most cases deterioration of joint cartilage starts with a mixture of causes. For the sake of clarity the causes will be discussed under two headings: a) pure mechanical causes, and b) structural causes. In practice this separation exists only rarely.

1.1 Mechanical Causes of Joint Degeneration

Osteoarthritis (OA) is the term used for description of degeneration or destruction of joints by mechanical reasons. It is a slow progressive disorder, usually starting with very little pain. The course of osteoarthritis is variable and unpredictable since the factors causing it are so multiple and variable. In some rare occurrences it becomes stationary. This happens in the case after osteotomy for instance. Only about 5% of untreated patients with osteoarthritis remain pain free. In osteoarthritis we always find two pathological processes:

a) Deterioration and detachment of the weight bearing
   surface.
b) Proliferation of new osteoarticular tissue at the margins
   and beneath the detached joint surface.

Most clinicians agree that: a) Under abnormally high
mechanical pressures osteoarthritis begins as a focal fibrillation
of the joint cartilage that leads to secondary remodeling of the
bony components of the joint. Fibrillation may remain silent for a
long period, but eventually cartilage will respond with gradual
wear.   Particles loosen and act as deteriorating factors.
b) Osteoarthritis can also be caused by changes in stiffness of
subchondral bone. Cracks occurring in the bone as typically seen
in aseptic necrosis of the head of the femur lead to partial
overloading. Stress peaks in the cartilage cause fissures in the
bone with subsequent loosening and deterioration.

The structural disintegration of the osteoarticular cartilage
and its abrasion leads to the loss of the subchondral tissue of the
articular surface. This causes proliferative phenomena including
the formation of new cartilage at the surface and at the edges of
the osteoarthritic joint.   Characteristically degradation of
cartilage is focal. It is therefore likely that degradation
results from short range enzymes released by affected chondrocytes
in their immediate neighborhood.   The nature of the mechanical
signal for the chondrocytes to digest their own matrix is unknown.

Remodeling of bone is the alteration of the internal and
external architecture of the skeleton dictated by Wolff's law in
response to variation in mechanical loading (1). It involves
removal of bony tissue at certain points and laying down bone
tissue elsewhere.

Cartilaginous repair is biologically possible by:
a) Replication of articular chondrocytes.
b) Metaplasia (change of a cell of a certain type into a cell
   of another type) of granulation tissue that proliferates
   in the subchondral bone marrow and at the margins of the
   joint surface.

The traditional teaching that chondrocytes are incapable of
mitotic division has been disproven by cell culture studies.
Clusters of chondrocytes in fibrillated cartilage represent clones
of newly proliferated cells. But a degree of chondrolysis seems to
be a necessary condition for growth of these cells.

It is not known why cartilage becomes mineralized at the lower
layers and where it has been destroyed. It becomes mineralized
however, under certain pathological conditions. The osteogenesis-

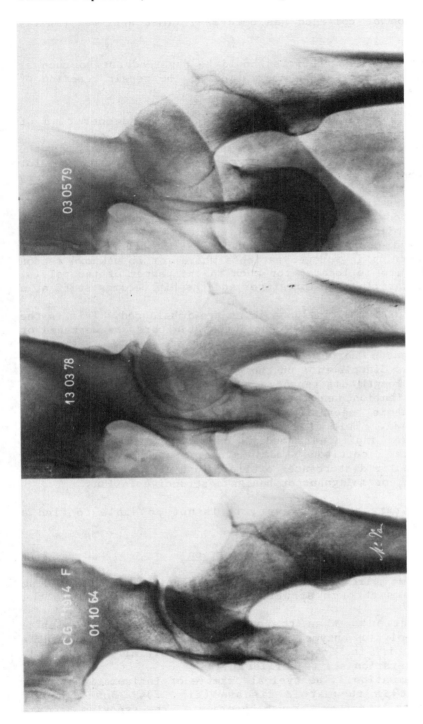

Fig. 1 Evolution of the left side of a mild bilateral dysplastic hip disease. 01 10 64: Normal left hip at 40 years of age; 13 03 78: Slight limp; 03 05 79: Rapid destruction of cartilage.

inducing action of collagen has been many times affirmed empiri-
cally.

In summary, osteoarthritis should be regarded not so much as
an inability but more as an aberration of the repair reaction of
osteoarticular tissue.

There are a number of reasons for early degeneration of
cartilage which include the following:
   a) The shape of the joint components is abnormal and the
      stress in focal zones is too high. This is the case, for
      example, in dysplasia of the hip, which is a very
      complicated situation depending of the shape of the joint,
      muscles forces, location in space of the joint, weight of
      the body, activities and so on. Fig. 1 depicts evolution
      of a mild bilateral dysplastic hip disease. Protrusion is
      looked upon as another mechanical disorder of the hip
      occurring in younger patients where for an unknown reason
      the hip is located too much to the center of the pelvis.
      The cartilage disintegrates and the hip becomes stiff at a
      very early age.
   b) The muscles acting on a joint are imbalanced. This is the
      case in poliomyelitis where the abductors are weakened or
      in spasticity where the adductors are spastic. In those
      instances cartilage degenerates because of changes in
      stress distribution on the joint surfaces.
   c) Leg length discrepancy. This causes asymmetric weight
      distribution, and therefore alters joint forces.
   d) Ischaemic necrosis of bone below the cartilaginous
      surface. This disease has been seen more frequently in
      younger individuals and is caused by different factors:
      general cortisone administration, ethylism, trauma,
      metabolic disturbances of lipids and gout.
   e) Cysts, or malignant or benign destructive lesions.

In some rare cases however, it is not possible to find a
clearcut reason for osteoarthritis.

1.2 Structural Causes of Joint Degeneration

Under some circumstances the deterioration of the gliding
surfaces occurs through structural causes. These include the
following:
   a) Infection: When there is pus in the joint with a
      proteolytic enzyme the proteoglycans will deteriorate.
      Even if the cartilage is only partially destroyed,
      degeneration starts earlier.
   b) Inflammation: The typical example of inflammation of the
      joint is rheumatoid disease (Fig. 2). Bone becomes
      generally softer through hyperaemia, the synovium becomes

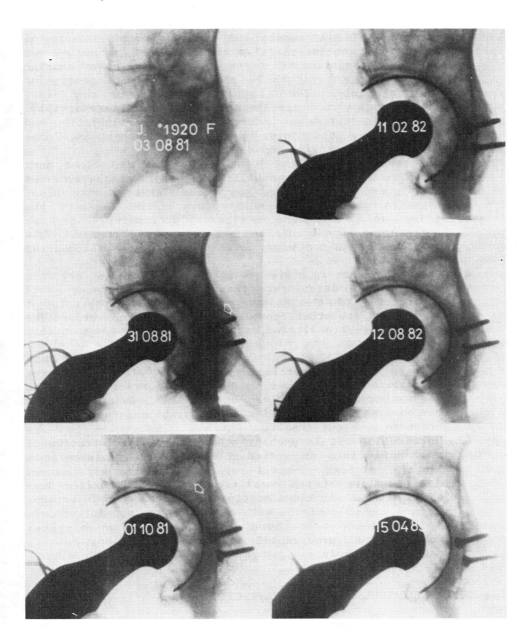

Fig. 2 Inflammatory joint destruction: Bilateral total destruction of the medial acetabular wall by Rheumatoid disease. The
right hip is shown. The medial part of the head was preserved at
surgery. Gradual remodelling of the autogenous bone graft. Compare 01 10 81 with 15 04 83.

thickened and hypertrophic and secretes abnormal components. The ligaments and muscles weaken because of
disuse. A special reactive tissue called "pannus" grows
both on the surface and below the cartilage layer causing
the cartilage layer to be shut off from its nourishing
synovial fluid. There is higher pressure in the joint,
and gradually the cartilage disintegrates irreversibly.
When all cartilage on both sides of the articulation has
disappeared, the joint may fuse together and bone
substance may replace the cartilage.

c) Hemarthrosis: When a joint is filled with blood many
    times as happens in hemophilic patients first the synovium
    and later the cartilage may become stained with blood
    pigments. Fibrous tissue may form at the edges of the
    joint and limit the motion. Osteoporosis of the
    surrounding bone occurs and the joint deteriorates. This
    happens also in a disease called hypertrophic villonodular
    synovitis.

d) Chemical: Gout is a disease in which deposits of crystals
    of uric acid deteriorate the cartilage and cause early
    destruction of the joint. Pyrophosphate arthrosis or
    ochronosis are other examples. The mechanical properties
    of cartilage are altered, and it becomes more susceptible
    to destruction.

e) Denervation: When a joint is deprived from its pain
    signals through neurological disease, either local or
    generalized, it becomes worn out by overactivity. The
    ligamentous insertions may be torn off, muscle activity
    may be exaggerated, fluid may accumulate and the joint may
    start to wear out itself.

f) Corticoids: It is probable that local administration of
    corticoids into an articulation causes diminished pain
    signals through removal of inflammation or causes
    deterioration of the cartilage itself. In earlier days
    when this was not known multiple intraarticular injections
    were given to patients with inflammatory, not infectious,
    joint disease. In those patients the joint surfaces
    deteriorated very rapidly to a degree comparable to
    neurological joints.

2.   DIAGNOSTIC TOOLS IN CLINICAL PRACTICE

2.1 Biological Techniques

Many biological techniques are used in clinical practice.
From the examination of products contained in blood, urine and
joint fluid for instance, we can arrive at a diagnosis of a
disease. Some of these examinations are carried out on a routine

basis.   Only those techniques which are important for orthopedic bone and joint affections will be discussed here.

    a) Calcium and phosphorus levels in the bloodserum are important to study the uptake and breakdown of bone.   The balance of calcium has to be positive.

    b) Alkaline phosphatases of bloodserum are increased with intensified activity of osteoblasts, as in osteomalacia, fracture healing and Paget's disease.

    c) The sendimentation rate, or the speed with which the red blood cells sink in a test tube, is increased in infections and rheumatoid disease because of changes in protein contents of the serum.

    d) The urine is examined for calcium and phosphorus excretion.

    e) Biochemistry of joint fluids is also carried out and helps us to decide whether an inflammatory or an infectious reaction exists.

2.2   Physical Visualization Techniques

    2.2.1   X-Rays: At the present time radiography is still the most useful tool for the examination of bones and joints. It is a simple, fast and accurate technique.

Subtraction radiography is a method used to enhance the visualization of contrast studies, particularly when there is considerable overlying of bone or soft tissue. A diapositive mask is made from a plain radiograph and superimposed over the contrast radiograph. A subtraction radiograph is produced from these two. This method is used in arthrography or arteriography.

Stereo radiography can also be used to see a three-dimensional picture of the joint.

    2.2.2   Computerized Axial Tomography (CAT): This technique has brought a new dimension to the study of joints. Not only can we see the bone structure in slices of any directions and whatever dimensions, but we can also see the cartilage layers, the muscles, the arteries, the tendons, etc. It has been possible to physically reconstruct bones using these scan pictures, and at present we are trying to reproduce a blueprint of the shape of the femoral shaft using a computer-assisted design.

At the present time there are certain limitations to detail in the CAT scan. When metal is present, the scatter of the metal prevents taking pictures of good quality which makes a CAT scan not useful to follow the evolution of the bone with a metal prosthesis.

    2.2.3   Arthroscopy: Arthroscopy is a technique by which the examiner looks directly into joint cavities. A special large

needle is introduced; and through another needle, fluid or gas is
injected to distend the joint cavities. Light is supplied by fiber
optics. The picture can also be reproduced on a monitor screen,
with a video camera in the optical system. The best optical
quality is obtained with a system composed of articulating prisms
with practically no loss of sharpness or light intensity.
Arthroscopy is not only useful for viewing, but also operations can
be performed with special fine instruments introduced through these
needles under direct vision of the surgeon.

2.2.4 Arthrography: In arthrography an opaque fluid,
sometimes together with air, is injected into the joint space
allowing us to see the different radiolucent structures such as
cartilaginous menisci of the knee joint. It is used to detect
loosening of implanted materials.

2.2.5 Arteriography: In arteriography the large arteries
are injected with a contrast medium to visualize the smaller
arteries. This can be useful, for example, to study the
vascularization of the femoral head. In some cases a selective
arteriography is carried out. That is, a small catheter is
inserted through a puncture in the vessel and moved forward to a
given point where a specific artery must be visualized. It is also
possible to embolize or occlude arteries at a distance, for
instance, when uncontrollable bleeding of a deep vessel occurs.
Phlebography or lymphography uses the same technique for veins or
lymph vessels to detect obstructions.

2.2.6 Isotope scans: Radioactive tracers are injected into
a vein. These substances have a special affinity for some
structures. For instance, iodium molecules are captured by the
thyroid gland. Strontium, gallium or technetium are captured in
the same way a calcium would be in the bone cells. In this way a
fuzzy picture is obtained of the location of a higher absorption of
these molecules. A bone scan is usually positive when there is
higher metabolism in a region. Because bone breakdown is always
accompanied by some new bone formation, the isotope scans are not
only typical for new bone formation but also for all increased
metabolism of bone.

2.2.7 Nuclear magnetic resonance is an image forming
technique based on the magnetic properties of matter. This
technique allows differentiation of different kinds of tissue. An
example is the picture obtained of the cruciate ligaments with this
technique. Also tumors can be better differentiated because of
different water contents.

2.3　Clinical Examination

To take care of the problems of the disturbed function of joints, and usually of the pain caused by malfunctioning joints, is an art; and requires more than technical ability. Through years of education, orthopedic surgeons have to be able to assess the patient's problems, put them in the proper perspective, select the best individual treatment and carry it out. In complicated cases, this can be a formidable task.

It is necessary to start any assessment of the patient's problems with an anamnesis. By questions and answers the doctor tries to obtain an insight into the patient's difficulties. The most important problems bringing an orthopedic patient into the doctor's office are: a) fear of becoming crippled, b) pain, and c) reduced function.

Usually and fortunately patients come to the doctor for joint disorders well in time, and in at least half of the cases any treatment is postponed for many months after the first visit. This is very useful for the orthopedic surgeon, because it allows him to follow the evolution of the disease and to have the time to know the patient better. This helps him to make a better decision in the choice of treatment. In doubtful cases the patient is put on a waiting list for a few months. This has generally a beneficial effect for the patient. Something is being done positively about his disease, he feels more secure and can arrive at a better decision about the necessity of the intervention.

During the anamnesis many questions must be asked before a clear picture of the patient's problem is obtained:
a) Is there night pain? Night pain is usually due to an inflammatory factor.
b) Is the pain only present with activity? The mechanical factor is more important.
c) What is the intensity and character of the pain?
d) Where is the pain: For hip disease it is quite common that the pain is only situated in the knee joint.
e) Is the patient spontaneously using a cane or crutch?
f) Is the patient unable to leave his home?
g) What about the walking distance?
h) Can he raise from a chair without help, and can he tie his shoe laces?
i) Can he lift something from the floor?

The answers allow the surgeon to obtain some insight not only into the physical abilities but also into the degree of pain. This interview is important because it is the beginning of a cooperation between doctor and patient and starts a relationship of confidence.

After the anamnesis, it is customary to analyze the patient's function by a clinical examination of the joints in a passive and active way. The study of the gait pattern is most useful, and the study of the passive motion, which means the mobility checked by the examiner while the patient relaxes, is also important. It is the only way that an accurate opinion can be made of the limitation of motion by muscle spasms produced by the pain.

3.   THE TREATMENT OF PATHOLOGICAL JOINTS BY
      PRESERVATION OF PRIMARY COMPONENTS

3.1 Medical Treatment

It is customary that in any patient suffering from pain the treatment starts by medical treatment. Pain suppressive drugs are used. These drugs can be divided into two: those which act independently of the nature of the disease process to relieve symptoms, and those which act on some aspect of the disease process itself. The former are "non-specific" or symptomatic remedies and include analgesic and anti-inflammatory drugs. Anti-inflammatory drugs not only relieve pain, but also cause a reduction in the duration of severity of stiffness in the morning or after sitting, a reduction in the number of tender joints, a reduction in the swelling of the joints and a reduction in joint temperature. Specific drugs are used in gout, septic conditions, Paget's disease.

However, since these drugs have side effects, prolongation of medical treatment during years can lead to serious complications with lesions to the gastrointestinal tract such as peptic ulcer, gastroenteritis, proctitis, rectal bleeding, perforation and hemorrhages of the esophagus, stomach, duodenum or small intestine. Symptoms of the central nervous system such as headache, dizziness, vertigo, etc., are communicated. Hematological compliations, including leucopenia, aplastic anemia, hemolytic anemia are seldom but sometimes fatal.

In many cases however, continuous medical therapy is necessary. This is the case in gout where a treatment against increased uric acid has to be continued for life to arrest the disease in the affected joints and to protect the non-affected ones.

Cortisone as medical treatment is used in some generalized rheumatic diseases, but carries the risk of necrosis of the femoral head if administered in a dose of 20 mg a day during a period exceeding two weeks and can cause degeneration of cartilage when injected.

3.2 Physical Treatment

Heat or cold application, ultrasound and other forms of physiotherapy have only a limited application. Exercises are carried out, sometimes with increased clinical symptoms. There is a question whether the patient with osteoarthritis should be told to limit his activities. In general this does not affect the symptoms very much, and it may well be that activity and motion of an osteoarthritis joint improves its function. In general, patients are told not to limit their activity except when this increases their pain to a great extent. The use of canes or crutches on the contrary must be stimulated. For some joints an immobilizing orthosis is possible. For example, the knee joint can be held in a straight position with a hinged brace. For the hip, however, orthoses are usually impractical.

3.3 Surgical Treatment

Many different surgical procedures have been carried out in the past. None of them, however, had an effectiveness of more than 60% to 70%. In most of these procedures the rationale is to relieve pressure at the joint surfaces.

3.3.1 Tenotomies: The simplest procedures are those where the joint pressure is relieved by cutting some of the tight muscle insertions. The adductor tendons of the hip, for example, can be cut very easily since they are superficially located. The result is temporary but sometimes very gratifying since it brings the joint into a better load-carrying position, and since it relieves a painful spasm.

In the fifties a German surgeon, Voss, carried this further and performed what he called a hanging hip operation. Not only the adductors but also the abductors and flexors were cut. The results were unpredictable but some cases were improved for many years. In all cases where similar operations are carried out it is necessary before surgery is undertaken to check under anesthesia whether joint mobility allows a change of the position of the joint itself.

3.3.2 Tendon transplants. Tendinous insertions have been transplanted. This is especially interesting in the case of the greater trochanter where some of the forces can be influenced by its position. One can transplant the trochanter more distally or more laterally and change the lever arm thus affecting pressure in the joint itself. The patella is a bone where the different lengths of the tendinous insertions are very important to keep it in line with the femoral groove and rerouting of tendons can have a very beneficial effect on preventing dislocation and even diminishing the valgus stress on the knee.

3.3.3   Osteotomy.   When cutting or rerouting soft tissues is not sufficient, changing the position of the joint surfaces itself through osteotomy is the next logical step (Fig.3). This can be done at the distal or proximal side of the joint. Special calculations have to be made to make sure that the weight carrying bone surface after the osteotomy is larger to spread the weight over a larger area. In the hip joint this is less predictable in cases where a valgus osteotomy seems to be in order than when a varus osteotomy is needed for better coverage of the head.

In the knee valgisation osteotomies carry a better prognosis than in the hip. A good result may last for 20 years and longer. Another indication of osteotomy in the hip is the flexion osteotomy of the head of the femur in the case of aseptic necrosis to turn the   non-affected   cartilage   under   the   supporting   dome   of   the acetabulum.

3.3.4   Arthrodesis.   Arthrodesis, or stiffening a joint, is biomechanically not a sound procedure in the case of the hip. The diminished mobility of the hip joint must be compensated by the mobility of the lumbar spine and through the knee joint. However, the result as pain reliever for the hip joint is good. Unfortunately 10 to 15 years later many arthrodeses of the hip have to be converted again in an arthroplasty because of pain in the back or the knee. A fibrous arthrodesis, as was found after extensive joint destruction as in tuberculosis, where some degree of motion persists, can last much longer. Although a stiff knee joint is a cumbersome affection, because patients have difficulties to adjust to low chairs especially in rows and because the visible abnormality of the gait pattern is usually more obvious than with a stiff hip, important side effects on other articulations do not seem to exist. Even with two stiff knees function is quite possible if the hips are normally movable.

3.3.5   Interposition arthroplasties.   One type of interposition arthroplasties still in use today is the cup arthroplasty. In younger patients with aseptic necrosis of the femoral head where the cartilage at the femoral side is coming loose because of necrosis and collapse of the underlying bone, this procedure is carried out with success. Normal cartilage at the acetabular side and an exactly fitting cup in the acetabulum is necessary. A large smooth gliding surface in contact with the remaining articular surface is thus created. The feeling of stability this carries to the patient and which is one of the physiological factors for success in total hip replacement, is not quite the same as for completely fixed total hip implants but comes close to it. Patients   operated   with   the   conventional   interposition   Smith Peterson cups (a reshaping of the two joint surfaces) never had this feeling of total stability and walked usually with external support.

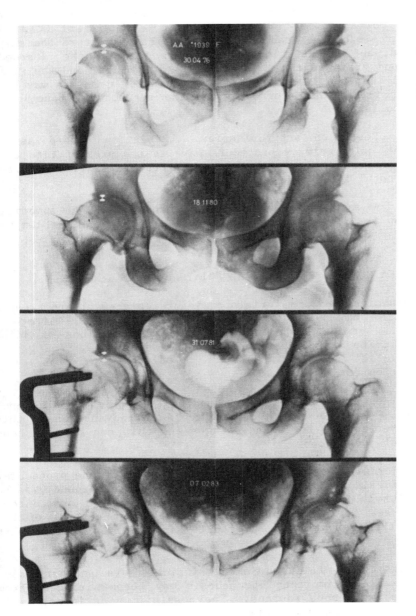

Fig. 3 Typical evolution of degenerative arthritis treated with osteotomy. Gradual deterioration of cartilage at the right side from 1976 to 1980. Osteotomy on 19.11.1980. Six months later reappearance of the joint space. In the meantime, deterioration of the cartilage at the opposite hip.

3.3.6 ´ Bone grafts. A very biological procedure is to support the triangle of bone at the apex of the femoral head where danger for collapse exists by a bone graft (Phemister) (2). In partial necrosis of the head this procedure can safeguard the shape of the head, and degeneration of the whole joint can be retarded. A strong bone graft is taken using the whole fibula, and the graft is inserted from the lateral side into the head in such a way that it supports the triangle of bone and the subchondral bone under danger of collapse.

3.3.7 Resection arthroplasties. Resection arthroplasties (Girdlestone) as a primary procedure have at the present time only historical interest. It is, however, a procedure still used after failure of total implants.

3.38 Low angulation osteotomies (Schanz), although sometimes with lasting results are no longer in use. Their main problem was the valgus stress created at the knee.

4. THE TREATMENT OF PATHOLOGICAL JOINTS BY REPLACEMENT

Biomechanics and biomaterials of joint replacement are treated elsewhere in this book. Here discussion will be limited to clinical and surgical aspects, including complications of joint replacement. The hip joint will be used as an example.

4.1 Indication for Hip Replacement

The screening of patients is based on the "primum non nocere" principle. The surgeon trys to weigh off the advantages of this major intervention to its disadvantages and this can only be done on individual judgment.

The major disadvantage is the mortality risk of the procedure. Even under ideal circumstances the mortality figures around 0.5% to 1% which fits it into a category of dangerous surgical procedures. All the causes for this mortality are not under control of the surgeon at the present time. Mortality is for the greatest part due to fatal embolies.

Possibility of failure through infection is another major disadvantage. Any implanted prosthesis may become infected from endogenous or exogenous sources. The possibility of infection is under some control and lies between 0.5 − 5%.

Loosening of a prosthesis is another cause for failure. Some factors as the weight of the patient or his size may influence early loosening and may be under some control. Loosening occurs in

5% of the patients after 10 years and increases by 1% every year. The age of the patient is a factor one has to consider.

The morbidity for a primary operation at the time of surgery is two to three weeks hospitalization and two-three weeks reconvalescence. For secondary operations the morbidity may be as long as six months.

Economical considerations are different according to the social system of the country.

An indefinite annual follow-up seems to be necessary in order to predict complication and correct them in time.

The advantages of the operation are the 97% good result rate in primary cases and 75% rate good results in secondary cases. Function can be compared very favorably with the normal situation allowing the patient an almost normal lifestyle.

4.2   Complications

Although it has never before been possible to implant definitively such a large piece of material in the human body with such consistently good results, complications with THR (and other hip surgery) are still numerous.

It was the foresight of Charnley not only to solve the problems of the prosthesis itself, but to attack at the same time concomitant problems. Small breaks in technique can be the cause for poor results. Here we will survey some of the surgical problems of primary and secondary implant surgery.

4.2.1   Early complications:
a) Anesthesia itself is not a special danger whether it be general or spinal. Hypotensive anesthesia under low blood pressure requires special experience but diminishes blood loss. However, special attention must be drawn to the fall in blood pressure when cement is inserted and monomer released in the bloodstream. Sudden collapse and death has followed the absorption of monomer in exceptional cases.
b) Acute early infection is the second problem. In the primary cases the incidence of infection is very low. Today it is accepted that most infections originate during surgery by penetration of bacteria into the wound. Rarely an early infection is carried by the bloodstream from the urinary tract or gall bladder into the wound. We talk about an early infection when the wound breaks open with a discharge of pus. An early infection may be superficial or deep. When superficial and treated with competence,

the deep tissues and the prosthesis may be saved. When deep from the onset, the outcome is usually poor. Infections can remain unrecognized by administration of antibiotics. Early infections are monitored by taking bacteriological samples during the surgery. The findings of these cultures correspond well with the agents and appropriate antibiotic therapy may be started at once.

c) Postoperative fat emboli occur in the few days that follow surgery but there does not seem to be a higher incidence than with other bone surgery. The incidence is higher in knee prosthesis than in hip prosthesis.

d) Dislocations occur often immediately after surgery when the patient is under anesthesia with his muscles still relaxed.

e) Thrombophlebitis is an obstruction of the deep pelvic iliac veins or some of the other veins of the leg. Due to the trauma to the inner walls of these vessels when manipulating the hip joint, a thrombus or clot is formed during surgery. These deep vessels may become completely or partially obstructed. If completely obstructed, a painful swelling of the limb occurs which is called thrombophlebitis. From these complete or partial thrombi, fragments may free themselves and obstruct the veins of the lung causing partially obstructed lung tissue which is called an infarct. A lung infarct may cause a reflex fatal cardiac arrest which is the greatest danger in hip surgery. The incidence of fatal emboli is 1% - 0.5%. The incidence of non-fatal thrombo-embolism in the veins is more than 50%. It seems that the incidence of non-fatal emboli in the lungs is about 35%. Up to the present time, the diagnosis of thrombophlebitis and lung infarcts is based on clinical observations. There are technical possibilities, however, to discover those complications more objectively (phlebography, lungscans, Doppler effect, blood flow impedance).

4.2.2   Late complications:

a) Instability. The patient has a feeling of giving away when the two components slip partially with respect to each other in certain body conditions. Usually this is due to mal-positioning of the trochanter (visible) or the abductor muscles (invisible).

b) Fixed deformities and lengthened limb. The hip is usually in an abnormal position of flexion and adduction before surgery and unless special precautions are taken some muscles may remain in shortened position. Especially the adductor muscles and flexor muscles may cause a problem. When these are shortened their insertions must be cut during or after surgery. Lengthening of a limb during surgery causes pain or discomfort.

c) New bone formation. Myositis ossificans with ankylosis is mostly due to mechanical damage to the soft tissues. The joint can become blocked by new bone production in the muscle masses around it.

d) Loosening of the implants. Whether fixed or not with cement, loosening of either component has been the problem inherent to any joint replacement. Most of the efforts now are directed to improve on the loosening of the implanted joints.

e) Late infection. After a problem-free period of a few months, but often in patients who exhibited a small temporary drainage of the wound, or a hematoma or an intercurring infection (bladder, bowel, gall bladder); pain in the operated hip reappears, especially during rest. The sedimentation rate remains elevated and sometimes, but not always, X-Rays show signs of loosening. In a much later state these signs of loosening are almost constant. In many cases the continued administration of antibiotics masks the infection, and sometimes there is a periodicity in the symptoms (as in chronic osteomyelitis). Aspirations are sometimes carried out for diagnosis. Antibiotics are administered to find out whether they influence the pain. When the sedimentation rate remains more elevated than its preoperative level, the diagnosis of a low grade infection is almost certain. In some cases spontaneous abscedation, fistulization and continuous drainage occur.

f) Late dislocation. Late dislocations occur after a few weeks, a few months or even years. Usually the trochanter is avulsed, and the hip is dislocated posteriorly. The cause is a movement of external rotation and adduction.

4.3 Special Problems

4.3.1 Bilateral and multiple lesions. Osteoarthritis is very often a disease affecting many joints at the same time. In about one third of the cases osteoarthritis of the hip is bilateral. Bilateral hip disease impairs very much the functional possibilities of the patient, and operation is needed at an earlier stage. In the period that Smith-Peterson cups were carried out, it was admitted that a fairly good result could be obtained for unilateral disease while no good results were obtained for bilateral disease. A bilateral functioning hip operation is one of the best tests for the quality of the surgical procedure.

4.3.2 Hip and knee disease. Because of the abnormal position of the hip in osteoarthritis or congenital dislocation of the hip the knee is very often abnormally loaded. For instance, with adduction contracture of the femur, the knee is pushed into valgus overloading the lateral compartment. The same happens to a greater extent when the hip is ankylosed and the patient uses the mobility of his knee to walk. Bilateral hip disease puts an enormous strain on the knee, and the patient's complaints are sometimes more related to the knees than to the hip joints.

4.3.3   Influence of back disease. During gait and in sitting position, hip flexion is combined with flexion in the lumbar spine. Stiffness of the hip joint and a flexion contracture put a great strain on the lower back region. Patients with an arthrodesed hip are suffering so much from this overloading of the spine that an arthroplasty of the hip must often be carried out.

4.3.4   Osteoporosis. When the calcified tissue starts to diminish in mass and in quality, the resistance of our supporting skeleton diminishes, and microscopic fatigue cracks occur in the bone. This happens frequently in the vertebral bodies. In older, osteoporotic patients the vertebral body collapses under the pressure of the soft but elastic intervertebral disc. In the hip fatigue fractures may occur but this is rare. Nevertheless, osteoporosis is more important in rheumatoid arthritis where the soft bone causes the implanted cup to protrude through the pelvic wall, and where insufficient bone is present for holding a prosthesis in the shaft.

4.3.5   Tumors. A tumorous lesion, whether primary or secondary may invade the hip joint or the surrounding structures. In that case a replacement by an alien supporting structure or an amputation of the limb are the only possibilities.

5.   LESSONS LEARNED FROM EXPERIENCE AND LONG–TERM
     FOLLOW–UP OF PATIENTS WITH IMPLANTS

5.1 Study of Secondary Operations

5.1.1   The late results of the Moore prosthesis. In the fifties many hip joints were replaced by a Moore prosthesis not only in patients with a fractured femoral neck, for which this prosthesis was originally designed, but also in patients with degenerative arthritis. Generally it was found that if the cartilage of the acetabulum was intact, as in young adults with aseptic necrosis or after a fracture, a long useful result could be expected. We have seen patients with a follow–up of a Moore prosthesis where the problems arose only after 20 years of use. In all other cases with degenerated cartilage of the acetabulum, poor long–term results have to be expected because of gradual but continuous bone destruction.

Pain is absent in the beginning and the destruction can take enormous proportions before clinical symptoms arise. A cavity as big as a whole femoral head may wear away at the pelvis. At the side of the prosthesis however follow-up shows that the straight stem is well supported especially in younger patients where it was implanted in a thick and heavy cortex. Reaming had to be done in these cases to accommodate the 10 mm stem. This supports the theory that the cementless stems implanted today may well remain sufficiently stable to allow long-term excellent results. In the proximal part of the stem of a Moore prosthesis, cavities allow bone ingrowth and indeed bone grows into these cavities. While this bone bridge is a stabilizing factor in patients with a thick shaft and a well fitting stem, it can act as a pivot point and cause wear of the bone at the distal part of the prosthetic stem in a later stage. It can be said that the problem of a Moore prosthesis in younger patients is not in the prosthetic fixation in the femur but in the acetabulum. When the stem was too small to accommodate a large femoral canal as was usually the case in older patients; the position was unstable from the start, and sinking occurred from the onset with destruction of the calcar and of the proximal part of the shaft.

5.1.2   The late results of the cup arthroplasties. Cup arthroplasties were never carried out as commonly as total replacements today. The initial and late problems were manifold. In patients where a unilateral stable hip joint could be obtained, the result was gratifying especially for pain relief. As taught by Smith-Peterson, the implanted cup was usually very large and protruding through the inner pelvic wall of the acetabulum. Because of the large surface and the wide distribution of stresses, further protrusion did not occur. The cup moved very little in the acetabulum. Because of the wearing off of the femoral head sometimes up to the base of the neck, a large supporting surface was obtained and this larger area became stable. New fibrocartilage or dense sclerotic bone covered this area; and since there was no complete ankylosis, the remaining mobility was sufficient if only one hip was affected. Studies from cases of former cup arthroplasties show that a cup fixed in the acetabulum can remain very stable even with only a thin layer of bone. The formation of these sockets in cup arthroplasties show that a thin but strong layer of cortical bone can be formed when stresses are evenly distributed on a large surface. Further destruction of the acetabulum does not occur if the cup is stable. Cup arthroplasties are a proof that a non-cemented cup could produce long lasting results if a stable fixation is obtained.

5.1.3   The late results of replacement arthroplasties. Usually a revision is carried out for loose components. When only one component is loose, we have an opportunity to examine in vivo the long-standing result of cement fixation of the other component. The acetabular component as well as the femoral component may remain extremely well fixed. The best examples are those where the distal part of the prosthesis is broken. In those cases the distal part of the prosthesis was very well fixed while the proximal part was mobile causing stress in the metal. Even after 10 years of use it is not possible to detect the slightest motion of the cement where it has been well imbedded in the cortical shaft.

5.1.4 Late removal of plates and screws. Also other implanted materials can be extremely well fixed to the host bone. Plates and screws can be fixed without any visible sign of corrosion and with bone growing over them. Growth changes of the bone itself prove that weight is carried through the plate. The reasons for stability or loosening of similar implants are not always obvious.

5.1.5 Wear studies of removed cups. The assumption that a cup wears out 0.1 mm per year is probably correct. When wear is found it is eccentric and occurs towards the anterior and proximal side. When the cup has been empty for some time as in cases where a dislocation has occurred, the cavity loses its round shape; and as we can see on removed cups, it becomes oval shaped. A thin walled metal Smith Peterson cup may break through fatigue after many years. A polyethylene cup wears very little, but there have been cases of broken polyethylene cups.

5.1.6 Fractures of femoral components. From fractures of the prosthesis we learn that high stresses occur at a level situated in the upper 5 to 7 cm of the proximal shaft. From fractures of the neck of the femur in surface replacements we learn that important stresses pass through the region of the anatomical femoral neck.

5.1.7 Wear of acetabular bone. It is evident that the highest stresses are at the roof of the acetabulum when we see the follow-up X-Rays of patients where the acetabular roof is wearing off. This applies to dysplastic hips as well as to hips with a Moore or total joint prosthesis. Indeed the head moves almost vertically upward in the pelvis, except in protrusion cases. But even in these cases there is also displacement in the vertical direction. From this study it appears that all cortical bone at the roof of the acetabulum must be preserved carefully.

5.1.8 Trochanter fixation. From studying the loosening of the trochanter when fixed with wires, we learn that the forces from the abductor mechanism are high; and since there is some loading of the wire accompanying every cycle, fatigue of the vertical wires occurs always first. It shows also that in cases where the trochanter is implanted at a lower position, the percentage of breakage of wires is much higher proving that the site of the insertion is important for the forces produced.

5.1.9   Study of the position of the acetabular cup. For some time in the past, the so-called Johnston cups were used. These cups were oval shaped with an eccentric hole. They were placed in oval shaped acetabula with the hole directed medially. In many of these cases, the cup loosened and turned around on its eccentric axis indicating that important twisting moments occurred in the cup.

For this reason, any substitute for a normal hip should be implanted with its center of rotation as close as possible to the normal center. Furthermore, gait studies should be able to prove that under those circumstances a gait must be produced which resembles the normal gait as closely as possible. Under those circumstances also, wear on a new joint located in the position of the normal head is probably the lowest possible.

5.2   Study of General Factors in Follow-up of the Patients

The activity level and the weight of the patient is of importance on fatigue fractures and on loosening. In practically all cases where two or even three subsequent femoral components broke, the patient's mass was over 90-100 kg. There is a limit of the size of stem we can accommodate in an anatomical femur. For wear, no figures are available yet. For fractures of the metal shaft, figures prove the assumption that overweight carries the risk of a fracture (3).

From gait studies on a force plate before and after implantation of the prosthesis, it is clear that part of the weight can be taken over to the cane or the crutch if correctly used.

Leg length discrepancies of less than 1 cm were never thought to be of any importance by the clinician before. Recently it has become clear that a 2 cm difference may cause degenerative arthritis of the hip and thus also wear of the implanted joint.

6.   IMPROVEMENTS IN SURGICAL TECHNIQUES DURING THE LAST DECADE

6.1   Introduction

The period of 1962 to 1972 must be considered the experimental period for total hip surgery. From 1972 to 1982 many problems were understood better and some statistics were available. While some people tried to work in different directions (surface cups, ceramic cups, cementless fixation) others have tried to improve the existing techniques.

6.1.1   Planning and control of the environment.   Under ideal circumstances the hospital where implant surgery is carried out should devote at least part of its facilities to this kind of surgery.   There should be a team of implant surgery, there should be clean wards or clean rooms without so-called resistant "hospital contaminants", there should be technicians trained for the purpose and special surgical facilities.   To master all problems and to decrease the financial burden of all the special requirements, the number of patients should be high enough to allow replacement surgery to be carried out on a routine basis.

6.1.2   Aseptic and antiseptic technique.   There are three possible sources for infection:
   a)   The environment contaminated with infected particles when people have been in a room for some time.
   b)   The surgical personnel shedding contaminated particles.
   c)   The patient carrying particles and microbes on his skin and around the surgical area (anus, bladder).

Many precautions are taken: The patients are screened on any superficial or deep source of infection before surgery, and the sedimentation rate which after surgery will be an index for low grade infection is always taken before surgery.   Before surgery bacterial cultures are taken of the patient's skin and urine which may give a clue on the causal germ if an infection occurs afterwards.   Every patient is given an injection of a broad spectrum antibiotic before surgery so as to imbibe his tissues with chemicals that immediately prevent the growth of bacteria.   During surgery and after surgery many more bacterial cultures of the wound and of any discharged fluid are taken routinely to make sure any possible contamination is at least recognized.   Cement in which penetration of blood is obviously not possible is impregnated with slowly dissolving antibiotics.   The air in the operating room is filtered, and a laminar flow system must be available if one wants to reduce the danger of circulating contaminated particles further. The surgical team should be completely covered to avoid any direct or indirect contact of the wound with the particles it is continuously shedding.   The permeable cloth of surgical suits should be covered with impermeable paper, and rubber gloves should be covered with cotton gloves to avoid punctures.   Working under these conditions of almost complete antisepsis and asepsis we still find positive cultures in one of 10 cases.   These usually are from the skin of the patient when it is uncovered for stitching up the wound.   If results of positive cultures return after surgery, the patient is given immediately appropriate antibiotics postoperative until the sedimentation rate is normalized.   On patients where all cultures are negative, no more antibiotics are given after surgery in order not to upset their immunological defense system.

6.1.3 Surgical approach. The surgical approach to the hip and the knee joint is important. One of the problems with the hip joint is the need to osteotomize the trochanter of the hip if a sufficiently large view is needed on both components of the hip. In that case the osteotomized trochanter has to be fixed again. This fixation creates problems in about 2% of the cases. In primary cases, anterior muscle insertions can be cut from the trochanter in order to avoid section of the trochanter. Most surgeons admit that the best possible approach for meeting any complicated problem is the transtrochanteric approach from the lateral side. An anterior approach is rarely used. A posterior approach is preferred by some surgeons. There are advantages to any of these techniques. The patient is either in supine position or on the side. Better techniques exist today for fixing the great trochanter, in which a smaller proportion of the trochanters come loose. A foolproof technique does not exist and further research for better fixation is necessary. The general idea for any incision should include that a well closed deep layer of fascia isolates the deeper structures from the fat and skin where infection is more common. In that way a superficial infection may remain forever isolated from the deeper structures. The first incision should always be made with the possibility in mind that a revision could be necessary later through the same lengthened approach (to avoid skin sloughs).

6.1.4 Bone stock. At the acetabular side bone stock can be a problem in protrusive hips and hips where the original cup became loose. In clinical practice there is certainly a difference between the acetabulum consisting of strong and overgrown hard bone of osteoarthritis patients and soft and brittle cancellous bone of patients with rheumatoid arthritis or osteoporosis. This is clearly reflected in the fact that an implant in strong bone remains more stable. Form this experience the tendency has arisen to remove as little bone as possible medially and none of the cortical bone of the roof of the acetabulum. Deepening of the acetabulum in a horizontal manner is necessary since the cup has to be covered by bone also on the lateral side. Deepening vertically is never necessary.

The same principle applies to the femoral shaft. If at any time a prosthesis has to be removed to perform a Girdlestone operation, the length of the remaining bone is one of the great problems. For this reason, it is common sense not to resect more of the femoral neck than strictly necessary. The shortest possible prosthetic neck which does not impinge against the acetabulum is the best. Technically it is much easier to resect a large piece of the neck and insert a prosthesis with a longer neck since more working room is then provided and in those cases removal of the trochanter is not necessary. The ideal situation would be to put a small joint inside the area provided by the original femoral head.

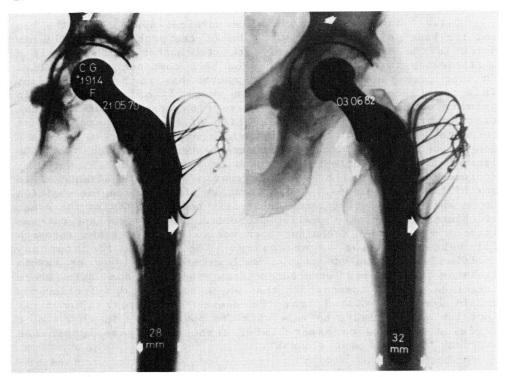

Fig 4   Excellent result of a THR performed in 1979.   Perfectly
fitting stem in a narrow femoral canal.   Compare X-Ray of 1982 and
observe: a) Remodelling of bone at the calcar, b) increased width
of the cortex (4 mm) at the tip, and c) no lining around the cup.

In that case all structures retain their original location and the
least fibrous tissue is needed to wall off the new joint.   All
structures including the capsule can remain intact.   The calcar is
very stong bone and will be able to support an appreciable part of
the pressure of the prosthesis.   Reaming of the canal is never
pushed further than is necessary to remove the loose spongious bone
inside the medullary canal.   Cortical bone should never be removed.

    6.1.5   Size of implanted material.   It is easier to produce a
more uniform layer of cement under equal pressure around a cup or
the shaft of a prosthesis when the cup or shaft fits the size of
the cavity.   Different sizes of both components are thus required
to accommodate all possible cavities.   From year to year more and
more different sizes are produced by manufacturers.   The optimal
length for a standard prosthetic shaft is not known, but correct
insertion of longer shafts is more difficult than shorter shafts.
The shaft should be long enough to stabilize in the heavy cortical
region of the middle portion of the femoral shaft.

6.1.6 Toxicity of the monomer. During anesthesia, precautions should be taken to measure central venous pressure in order to recognize immediately the fall of blood pressure caused by the monomer in the cement. Everything should be ready to combat cardiac arrest (defibrillation). A surplus of oxygen should be given during the periods of introduction of cement. The cavities should be impregnated with adrenalin, diminishing the absorption of monomer.

6.1.7 Pressurization of cement. When the techniques for inserting the cement were improved, better original stabilization of prostheses was obtained. In the early days, lots of cancellous bone were left inside the shaft of the femur, cement was placed inside the canal in the marrow cavity, and then the prosthesis was inserted. Spontaneous pressurization of cement occurred only in those cases where the femoral cavity was narrow and the prosthesis relatively large (Fig. 4). In those cases, often a periosteal reaction is seen showing more load taken up by the bone of the shaft at the level of the lower part of the prosthesis. In about 50% of the early cases, a fracture of the cement below the tip of the prosthesis occurred early and proved that some settling of prosthesis took place in early stages.

It has also become common practice to place a cement plug or a bone plug into the femoral shaft in order to improve pressurization of the cement which is now introduced with a cement gun. Further pressurization may be obtained with special instruments developed by Harris. At the side of the acetabulum, pressurization is reached by cutting flanges of a cup developed by Charnley as equal as possible to the cavity of the acetabulum with only a space of a few mm for extrusion of the cement. Multiple small 3 mm diameter holes just deep enough for good penetration of cement are holding the cement. If the circumference of the cup is closed during the introduction of the cup, a sufficient pressure can be obtained for introduction of the cement into these small holes. The flange of the Charnley cup seems to be an advantage. Other systems to improve pressurization of the cement are also used by Harris and Ling.

6.1.8 Prevention of hematomas. Hematomas or blood collections under the skin or around the prosthesis where immunological or antibiotic defense is much lower must be avoided at all cost. For this reason aspiration tubes are placed in the deep and superficial layers of the wound and coagulation of all bleeding vessels during surgery is performed very carefully. Draining of the wound is monitored daily and as long as there is some draining of blood or serous material, no anticoagulants are administered since they could increase the drainage.

6.1.9 Prevention of emboli (anticoagulation). When a wound is completely dry for four days, anticoagulants are given to prevent fatal emboli for the risk period which lasts about six weeks or longer if the patient has been longer recumbent. This delay is because of the danger of infection if hematomas are caused by immediate postoperative anticoagulation.

6.1.10 Postoperative care. Ten days of bedrest has been our practice for many years, the idea being that it is better for the deep tissues to heal with less scar and fibrous tissue just as the skin heals better without extremes of motion. There is less danger of hematoma formation, and the patient is more comfortable. In complicated cases, where dislocation is threatening, immobilization in a short hip spica made of a thin layer of plastic material is very comfortable and allows the patient to get up sooner. Even after two or three months of this type of immobilization, full mobility is quickly regained even in the cases where the procedure was performed after undoing an arthrodesis of the hip joint. In cases where a real danger of postoperative dislocation is present as after a large resection, it is certainly wiser to immobilize the whole leg with a hip spica to prevent rotation until all soft tissues are healed rather than take the risk of dislocation. In such cases, however, the patient is allowed to stand up daily within the cast as early as possible on a tilting table. Walking with a walker, crutches or without any support is encouraged as soon as the patient is allowed out of bed. Passive motion is discouraged. Special positioning in bed to avoid adduction and flexion is necessary. To avoid adduction, an abduction pillow is used. To avoid flexion, the patient is placed in prone position twice or three times a day with a sandbag under the knee and with a bag on top of the buttocks so that complete passive extension of the hip is obtained before the sectioned tissues become shorter in a position of flexion.

6.1.11 Follow-up and gait studies. During the follow-up, several factors have to be studied. Infection? Does the sedimentation rate return to normal? Pain or stiffness? Mostly due to overexercising or overlengthening or a flexion or adduction contracture. In some cases secondary sectioning of the adductor tendons is necessary. Irradiating pain in back and leg (sciatic pain) is usually due to positioning in prone position. After bilateral hip surgery performed in one session, some precautions have to be taken. Since these hips are usually very stiff before surgery, special attention to mobility has to be given if we want the patient to give up his "knee walking" gait to which he has been used to before. The length of the two extremities has to be carefully adjusted in order not to overload one of the hips. Gait studies may help the patient to improve the quality of his gait.

6.2 Improvements in Surgical Tools
     During the Last Five Years

    6.2.1 Headlights. Since working in deep cavities is
required most of the time, a spotlight fixed to a band around the
forehead is of great help for improving sight. This allows
particular control by direct vision if the cavity of the femoral
canal is sufficiently reamed and cleaned of debris. Since it is
necessary to look into the shaft of the femur, it is also necessary
for the operating table to be raised higher than normally made
possible by conventional tables.

    6.2.2 Use of X-Ray pictures and intensified fluoroscopy.
X-Rays are taken routinely during surgery especially to check the
position of the cup and the length of the prosthesis before it is
fixed with cement. A special table was constructed keeping the
axis of the X-Ray tube parallel to the plate holding device. Some
surgeons use intensified fluoroscopy during surgery especially for
revision cases to monitor the position of the drill inside the
femoral canal while reaming.

    6.2.3 Better drills and motors. High speed or low speed
electric and pneumatic drills facilitate removal of bone and
especially of cement in revision cases. Special reamers for
shaping the acetabulum have been devised and work extremely well.
Speed of 70,000 rpm and special bits for drilling through cobalt
chrome alloy are necessary and are now available. Different
guiding tools are on the market.

    6.2.4 Tools for cleaning, debriding and drying tissues.
When it became clear that better cementing techniques were
necessary, tools for debriding cavities mechanically with rotating
brushes and cleaning cavities with water jets were made. The
principle is usually an eccentric wheel rotating against a flexible
tube through which water is fed. Special absorbing sponges are
also used for drying the bone tissues before inserting the cement.

    6.2.5 Making molds of cavities. In order to improve on the
size of prosthetic stems, we make a mold of the cavity during
surgery, the idea being that sooner or later a computer guided
copying machine might make a prosthesis on exact measurement.

    6.2.6 Deep frozen homografts. The femoral heads of patients
operated upon are saved as a material used to fill up large
cavities, especially for revisions. This bone is selected from
patients who are otherwise healthy, and these grafts can be saved
for many months at $-80\ ^{\circ}C$. They can be tooled during surgery to
any shape and easily fixed with screws in the receiving cavity.

6.2.7   Modular prosthesis.   In order to increase the number
of sizes and shapes of protheses, there is a tendency to produce
modular prostheses where different lengths and sizes of shafts can
be adjusted to different neck lengths and head diameters.   A system
is also being developed to adjust the length of the stem of tumor-
prothesis with prefabricated increments.   By this system we could
adjust the length of the prosthesis during surgery.

6.2.8   Cementless fixation.   Many types of prostheses allow
cementless fixation.   For the cup it is either a metal cup with a
HDP liner and a large thread on the outside of a plastic cup fixed
with two pegs and screws.   There is also an aluminum oxide ceramic
screw-in-type of cup.   On the side of the prosthesis the femoral
cavity is adjusted with special gages and a three point fixation is
obtained in the canal.   A micro- or macro-porous coating is
supposed to allow bone ingrowth into the prosthesis.

6.2.9   Improved mixing of the cement may improve its
qualities.   Mechanical mixing has proven to remove more air of the
mixture and diminish its porosity.   In manually introduced cement
many folds are seen.   If more liquid cement is introduced with a
syringe, these folds are less pronounced.   Further research on
cementing technique is needed.

6.2.10   T.V. cameras.   The latest improvement is a very small
I.C. television camera weighing only 30 grams, fixed to the
headband of the surgeon and allowing him to record everything the
surgeon is seeing and anything he does, for retrieval later,
especially in problem cases.

6.2.11   Biological bone glue.   "Fibrinkleber" is a product
derived from human blood.   It is being used recently in Germany to
mix with small bone fragments to make a paste which fixes small
fragments of bone.   Blood vessels can grow through this paste.   It
is used mostly with cementless prostheses.

6.2.12   Through use of the "cell saver" an automated device
permitting the re-use of the patient's own red blood cells, it has
become possible to save up to 8 pints of blood during revision
surgery.   This system may also decrease some of the problems
arising from incompatible donor blood.

7.   REVISION SURGERY FOR LOOSENING OF IMPLANTS

7.1   Introduction

As soon as the first total implants had failed, the need arose
to find techniques for revisions.   The first revisions carried out
by Charnley in some of the 300 cases with Teflon cups opened the

way to these techniques. In those cases an enormous mass of amorphous material was found around the cups. An infiltrating, not infected, cold abscess filled up a large space around loose cups. A few years later, loose or broken metal stems had to be removed, and these hips had to be revised as well.

At the present time, the best obtainable fixation can be compared to the biological fixation of our teeth which are fixed to our bones through a layer of special fibers. As we see daily when we remove plates, screws or any implants, bone will under certain physical conditions increase its holding grip on the implant, but once it loosens its grip the opposite effect seems to take place, and osteoclasts start to do their job of removing the unwanted implant by breaking away all tissues around it.

The initial mechanism is far from understood, but the consequences are quite visible. Just like a non-union of a fracture, it is probably a one way reaction; and once a fibrous tissue layer has formed, the process of secure bone fixation will not start again of its own. It is probable that very close initial contact of the implant with the bone is necessary before any fibrous tissues have formed. The signal telling the cells to remove everything around the implant seems to be a conglomerate of very small particles of foreign material. This we find when acrylic or nylon or polyethylene wears away in an artificial joint. When the fragment is large enough as a whole cup together with its cement mantle, we find only fibrous tissue reaction. Solid bone is replaced by a layer of fibrous tissue; but as soon as a certain number of very small particles are present, another reaction sets in.

7.2 Diagnosis of Loose Implants

Since the diagnosis of a loose implant is usually made from X-Ray pictures (Fig. 5), pain is not the most important symptom in its detection. This is one of the reasons why all patients operated upon must be screened by X-Rays at least once a year. In the early days of implant surgery, it was seen that cement broke 1 cm or so under the tip of the prosthesis. Many people thought it was of no importance. We know now, however, that this early fracture of the cement under the tip of a prosthesis meant a "settling" of the prosthesis in most cases. The trabecles of bone in the marrow cavity which were not removed as we do now, broke away and another stable position was obtained. This gave rise to the idea of the prosthesis of Ling which allowed such stabilization because of its shape. Any crack in the cement of the femoral canal is now considered a sign of motion of the cement. When the cement at the proximal part of the prosthesis is broken, it is a sign that the prosthesis moves into valgus or varus; and this was most clearly seen in prostheses bending because of material failure. An increasing cavity was seen between the back of the stem and the cement. Fragmentation of crumbling cement is more difficult to see since there are no clear visible lines when there are multiple cracks.

Resorption of the calcar is not always a sign of loosening since it may occur with perfect fixation of the prosthetic stem.

A lining increasing in width in the course of time between the shaft and the cement is one of the better signs of loosening. The only definite sign of loosening, however, is subsidence. When a prosthesis shows motion on sequential X-Rays from its original position relative to some bony landmarks, it is a certain sign of loosening. Nevertheless, as said before, a new stable position may be reached; and clinical symptoms may never occur.

To diagnose the initial loosening of a cup is more difficult than it is of a stem. The cup is not metallic, and its circum-ference not so well visualized. The cup is under compression, and a lining between it or its cement mantle may gradually disappear because the cup sinks further into the softened bone. So it is only its relative position to some landmarks, sometimes its varus or valgus shifting (rotation), that points to gross loosening. For this reason, the metallic markers included in the cup and radio-opaque cement are important.

Arthrography means the injection of a radio-opaque fluid in the articulation. This dye can penetrate between the cement mantle and the cup or the prosthesis. Sometimes, however, especially in aseptic cases when the fissure is very small, an arthrography is negative. For instance, a cup may be loose and still pressed in the acetabular roof.

7.3   Technique

The technique for replacement of loose implants is difficult. There is a double problem—the remaining cement must be removed and enough solid bone must be left for fixation of the new prosthesis.

The skin incision is the first problem. A very large exposure is needed. Sometimes the scars of the first incisions do not allow a sufficiently large incision for the revision surgery because of the danger of devascularization of part of the skin with danger of sloughs. In those cases a preliminary skin incision six weeks before the definitive surgery is necessary to improve on the blood supply.

Removal of the cup is usually no serious problem since it is soft material and can be nibbled away if necessary. In some cases the cup is split in two or three fragments in order not to damage

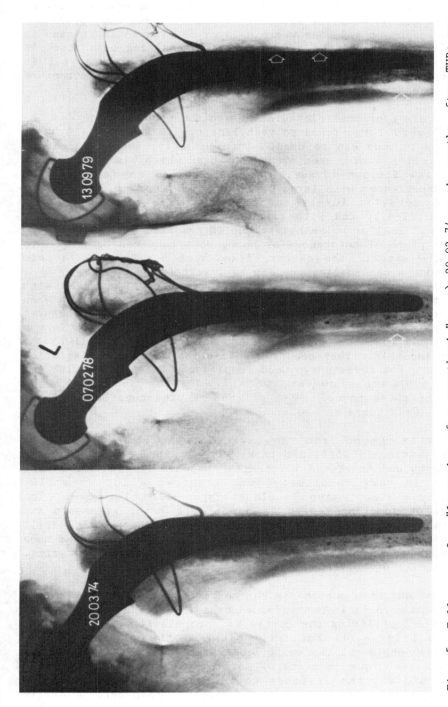

Fig. 5 Follow-up of a "loosening of a prosthesis": a) 20.03.74 - six months after THR; no abnormalities, b) 07.02.78 - first signs of widening of the lining between cement and bone, and c) 13.09.79 - progressive widening and accumulation of debris.

the underlying bone stock. In most cases it can be removed intact. Usually the cement is still attached to the cup, and the separation lies between cement and bone where a layer of granulation tissue is found. Replacement of the cup is easy if remaining bone stock is sufficient. Unfortunately, this is usually not the case; but in some instances the bone under the cup becomes denser in structure and stable enough for a new one.

There are four possible solutions to the problem:
a) A very large round polyethylene cup is inserted. A 55 to 60 mm cup can be used. Unfortunately, such a large cup creates a vast area around the head which has to be filled with fibrous tissue, and dislocations may occur. The experiences with large oval cups were poor.
b) A metallic insert can be fixed with screws directed vertically and with cement. In this cemented insert a next smaller polyethylene cup is cemented again.
c) A piece of autogenous or homogenous bone can be shaped to the size of the cavity, fixed with screws, and in this bone a new smaller cup can be inserted.
d) A large screw-in type cup without cement and even with added bone fragments is another possible solution. When the original acetabular wall consists of well structured bone, initially good stability is obtained, but it is not known what the future of these cementless cups will be.
It is not impossible that cementless fixation will be the solution in the future for revisions. Good results can be obtained with any of these systems. However, we know nothing about the late follow-up of these cases. Most of the cemented cups become loose only after 10-15 years of use.

Removing cement from the cavity of the femoral shaft is usually an extremely difficult task. Usually the cement is fixed in some parts and fractured in others. Especially removing a ring of cement is very complicated and requires a lot of skill. Specifically a cement stop is almost impossible to remove. The difficulty of removing cement is one of the major arguments its proponents use in favor of using cementless implants. Any drill has a tendency to deviate and to cut rather through the softer bone than through the harder cement. When splitting the cement ring, there is danger of splitting the cortex as well.

When a long stem prosthesis has to be removed, the problem may become unsurmountable in non-infected cases. Cutting holes through the cortex and splitting the cortex is a possibility. However, in some cases later a fracture will occur as the result of these holes. Some people cut the shaft lengthwise and fix it with bands. My personal technique consists of cutting off the trochanter very low. In this way the distance to the bottom of the cement is shortened and its removal is easier. Special fast cutting drills may be used (Midas Rex). The use of a headlight is absolutely necessary to visualize the femoral cavity.

The secondary implant needs a heavier, wider and longer stem in these cases. As the femoral cavity is sometimes very oddly shaped and has an anterior bowing, many different models of revision prostheses are manufactured. Still it is nearly impossible to find a suitable prosthesis in many cases. A special problem is the anterior bowing of the femoral shaft for which practically no provision is made.

7.4 Long-Term Results

Interesting statistical data are given by Schneider (4). While in the 109 primary cases operated upon between 1961 and 1967, 50 reoperations were necessary; this number dropped to 17.5% of the cases operated upon between 1967-1978.

In a series between 1967-1978 when only the cup was replaced, there were 63% good results and 13% poor results. For the prostheses, these figures become 72% and 15%. For both, they are 69% good and 20% bad. In a later series (1977-1980) where Schneider used metallic inserts, there were 83 good results and 4 poor results in 91 cases. The same author also inserts metallic plates in the cement to fill up the cavity and to reinforce the cement layer. The follow-up, however, is much too short. It is clear that results of secondary procedures will never equal those of a first implant.

8. REVISION SURGERY FOR INFECTION OF IMPLANTS

8.1 Diagnosis of Infected Implants

How many implants get infected? This is a difficult question to answer. We must first have a good definition of infection. The problem is that even in infected cases because of administration of antibiotics, it is sometimes difficult to find bacteria when a culture is taken, and up to eight cultures of a wound may remain negative. The fact that no bacteria are found in the tissues during surgery is certainly no proof of the absence of infection.

Since the sedimentation rate is accelerated in practically all cases where an infection is present, we have accepted that standard. We compare the patient's sedimentation rate before surgery with the sedimentation rate after surgery and find that within a period of three to nine months it normalizes in non-infected cases. In this way we can make a decision about non-infected cases. Reoperations are a predisposing factor for infection. Surgery takes longer, and the scar tissue is more prone to infection since it contains less blood supply. The danger after reoperation is estimated to be three times as high as in primary cases.

8.1.1   Acute early infections are extremely rare and mostly we talk about chronic early infection. The sedimentation rate never comes down to its preoperative level, and the patient is not completely pain free. Often there was a hematoma or some oozing from the wound. Usually chronic infection is only diagnosed after one year.

8.1.2   Late infections. After a period where everything seems to be normal, and sometimes even 10 years after surgery, the infection may flare up. In some cases we find the same bacteria as during the first procedure. Metastic infection has been seen, but late metastic infection is very rare.

Usually it is diffidult to make a diagnosis of any infected implant.
a)   The pain is frequently more severe than with loosening alone, and is also present at night.
b)   There is an elevated sedimentation rate of the red blood cells and often a history of a good result followed by pain after some months.
c)   The X-Ray signs may not differ very much from those in simple sterile loosening, but the signs are more pronounced and generalized. There is more bone absorption. Furthermore, cloaca or holes are seen in spaces where pus can collect. There is also a periosteal reaction around the shaft.
d)   The fluid obtained at aspiration may in some cases give positive cultures. Many different bacteria may be found, and they are usually not very aggressive, difficult to culture and often not sensitive to antibiotics.

8.2 Bacteriological Considerations

In the beginning it was thought that an implant could never survive in the presence of an infection. We were thinking in terms of "infection--no infection" "black or white". Later it became clear that with implant surgery we dealt with many cases of "low grade infection"--"gray". Because antibiotics were very often administered, the bacteria were weakened and some sub-infection persisted. Usually it was not the infection itself but the loosening of the prosthesis which was responsible for the reoperation. It was as if a symbiosis existed in the body between the infected implant and the tissues around it. As a matter of fact, this is seen in other bone infections as well, where a large fragment of dead bone can remain dormant as a sequestrum during many years. In those cases the implant is encapsulated by fibrous

tissue and almost walled off from its neighborhood. Later it
became clear that even in infected cases a reoperation was possible
when the immunological resistance of the body was increased with
antibiotics. Before attacking any infected implant now, the
patient is given powerful broad-spectrum antibiotics for many
weeks. Only then surgery is performed and followed by injections
of antibiotics and oral antibiotics for very long periods or
forever, hoping that in this way the implant may become stable and
well fixed. The results are rewarding. In 70% of these
reoperations for infection, results are good. Some questions of
antibiotic cement remain. Although the addition of antibiotics
diminishes the strength of the cement about 5%, an area where
antibiotics penetrate with much difficulty is impregnated with
these antibiotics during many months in bacteriostatic doses. In
the meantime, healing of soft tissues and bone can take place.
From the bacteria recovered during secondary surgery the results
can be predicted as some are known worse than others. Pseudomonas
are among the worse and staphylococcus aureus among the best if
their culture is sensitive to antibiotics.

8.3 Technique for Replacement of Infected Prosthetic Components

The technique for replacement of a prosthesis is essentially
similar in non-infected and infected cases. It is easier to remove
the prosthesis and the cement in infected cases because the
infection has a tendency to loosen all foreign material. On the
other hand, a thorough removal of all the infected tissue is
necessary for good results. Bone is much softer in infected cases
and much more care must be exerted not to damage the acetabular
wall on the cortex of the femur. Special long stem prostheses to
obtain fixation in intact bone are necessary, and much thicker
stems than commonly used should be available. Some authors advise
revisions in two sessions. First, the prosthesis is completely
removed, and in a second operation a new prosthesis is inserted.

8.4 Early and Late Results

Early results in infected cases are good if antibiotic
protection is possible. Late results are generally good in 70%
after the first revision and 50% after the second revision. Nobody
knows what the future of these cases will be. The idea to use
non-cemented prostheses in revision cases is valid since their
eventual removal will be much easier if there is recurrence.
Patients prefer by far the situation after a revision than the
results of a Girdlestone procedure when the hip is left without a
joint. All the problems of antibiotherapy before and after surgery
and the very long revalidation period are very well accepted by
patients who once had a temporarily well functioning total hip
replacement.

REFERENCES

1.   Wolff, J. Zur Knochenwachstuur Frage. Archiv. Path. Anat.
     Physiol. 61 (1874), 417.
2.   Phemister, D.B. Treatment of the Necrotic Head of the Femur
     in Adults. J.B.J.S. 31 A (1949), 55.
3.   Charnley, J. Low Friction Arthroplasty of the Hip. Springer
     Verlag, (1979).
4.   Schneider, R. Die Totalprothese der Hufte, Hans Huber, Bern,
     (1982).

BIBLIOGRAPHY

1.   Black, J. and Sholtes V. Biomaterial Aspect of Surface
     Replacement Arthroplasty of the Hip. Orth. Clin. of North Am.
     (1982) 709.
2.   Bourke, D. L. et al. Methylmethacrylate and the Cardiovas-
     cular System. Anesth. Rev. 4 (1977) 17.
3.   Carlson, R.S. Erythrocyte Sedimentation Rate in Infected and
     Non-Infected Hip Arthroplasty. Acta Orthop. Scand. 49 (1978)
     287.
4.   Dambacher, M.A. Praktische Osteology. Thieme Verlage 1982.
5.   Elson, R.A. Ads Calduell. Revision Arthroplasty.
6.   Ficat, P.J. Arlet .Ischemie et necrose osseuse. Masson 1979.
7.   Mears. Materials and Orthopaedic Surgery. Williams L. and
     Wilkins, 1979.
8.   Oh and Harris. Design Concepts Indications and Surgical
     Technicque for Use of the Protrusio Shell. Clin. Orth. (1975)
     1962.
9.   Salter. Textbook of Disorders and Injuries of the
     Musculoskeletal System. Williams and Wilkins 1970.
10. Swanson, S.A.V., Freeman, M.A.R. Die wissenschaftlichen
     Grundlagen des Gelenkersatzes. Springer Verlag Berlin,
     Heidelbert, New York, 1979.
11. Willert, H.G., Semlitsch, M. Reaction of the Articular
     Capsule to Plastic and Metallic Wear Products from Joint
     Endoprostheses. Sultzer Technical Review, 1975.
12. Wroblenski, B.M. ESR and Polymethyl Metacrylate. J. R. Coll.
     Swig. Eding. 19 (1974) 182.

CONSIDERATIONS IN JOINT REPLACEMENT

J.P. Paul

Bioengineering Unit, University of Strathclyde
Glasgow, Scotland, U.K.

Joint replacement in the human may be undertaken for several reasons: pain and its associated loss of function, tumors in the skeletal structure confined to the region of the joint and trauma. Surgery to remove tumors may involve resection of more bony material than is general in joint replacement surgery.

The question of joint replacement to alleviate loss of function is difficult to discuss, since function is usually limited by pain. Generally, with joint replacement surgery the effective functional range of joint movements is increased and the ability to transfer loads within the restricted range previously limited by pain is sufficient to give a very satisfactory degree of rehabilitation. The question of how much joint replacement to aim for in rehabilitation is open to controversy. The current television programs relating to "bionic man" suggest that physical performance of the athletic normal individual might be enhanced by appropriate surgery. To date, no indication of this is present in literature, although ligamentous replacement for appropriate athletes is undertaken by specialist centers in North America. No suggestion has been seen however that their performance with synthetic ligaments is an improvement on their previous performance.

For joint replacements, the selection of relevant material is critical. Obvious factors such as absence of toxicity and carcinogenicity of the material will be looked at early in the design process but, in particular, the matter of carcinogenicity may be related to the shape of the test sample and not solely to the material characteristics. Similarly, both of these factors have to be reviewed in respect of the implant after several years of implantation. A major point is that there is likely to be wear of the materials producing particles of small size and, therefore, large surface area per unit mass. The characteristics of these may be quite different from the characteristics of the bulk material, and appropriate tests by cell culture and animal implantation should be undertaken as part of the routing series of tests for material assessment for this purpose. Materials also must be assessed for their own intrinsic strength, since the restraints of the anatomical sizes will frequently mean that the stress levels corresponding to normal functional loads will be high, so that yield strength and fatigue strength under the adverse conditions of the biological environment should be fully assessed. Similarly, the rate of wear of the materials under cyclical loads frequently involving only boundary lubrication or even more adverse conditions should be considered. In this respect also, because of the low velocities of these sliding surfaces and the comparatively rapid rate of increase of the joint loads during loading cycles, direct contact of the materials may occur without the benefit of surface lubrication.

In respect of the characteristics of the materials, attention should be paid particularly to plastics materials due to the possibility of major changes in their characteristics due to leaching of constituent materials. Many plastics include, as well as the basic polymers, additives in the form of plasticizers, stabilizers, anti-oxidants, fillers, etc., and, particularly with high density polyethylene, traces are found corresponding to small particles of dust or other derivatives from manufacturing processes. These latter may be of considerable hardness and prejudice the wear characteristics.

Mention is made in other chapters of the intensity of loading to which these implanted materials may be subjected and the volume of material which can be used is frequently limited by anatomical constraints, since for example, there is a limit to the cross section of the metallic stem which can be put into a medullary cavity. Similarly, all of the anatomical space may not be available, since the niceties of the surgical procedure in respect of the presence of vessels and nerve trunks may inhibit the maneuvers that the surgeon would wish to undertake in the implantation.

A major consideration in the design of the implant will be the fact that, because its form is different from the natural joint it replaces, there will be constraints on the range of movement which can be allowed. For instance, in the hip joint, contact between the neck of a prosthetic implant and the acetabular component will be the limiting factor in the range of joint movement, as opposed to the tension in the capsular ligaments in the natural case. Alternatively, bone spurs or scar tissue may present similar limitations at the hip joint. Remaining bone cement is of course a hazard to any joint replacement, and good surgical practice takes particular care to remove such material. With regard to complex joints, such as the knee, the selective movements in the normal anatomy may not be matched by the joint replacement. The kinematics of the tibia relative to the femur in a normal situation is controlled by ligaments and the kinematics of the joint replacement may be constrained by axes and rigid links. In general these will match approximately for a restricted range of movement: but as the range of movement is extended so the remaining ligamentous structure will tend to inhibit the range of movement of the prosthetic implant, or overload the implant/bone interface.

A major consideration in the design of any joint replacement should also be the possibility of a salvage procedure in the event of the failure of the implant for whatever cause. Desirably, there should be the chance of another joint replacement with a procedure of choice in the event of a second failure. Fusion may be a solution but many knee joint replacements involve too much resection of bone to allow a reasonable remaining leg length; and fusion at the knee or at the hip involves a considerable reduction in mobility for a patient for whom there may be a prospect in restriction in joint function in the other joints in any case. Fortunately, for failed hip surgery there is the possibility of special custom made replacements of enhanced dimensions or the Girdlestone procedure. The latter involves removal of the femoral neck and retention of the femur relative to the pelvis by scar tissue remaining from previous surgery. The locomotion capability of patients following this procedure has been demonstrated to be surprisingly good (1).

Generally the patient will hope for good cosmetic results from the surgery; this could either be in respect of equality of leg length or improved gait or such minor considerations as the absence of solid protrusions at the skin in the hip region. These can sometimes be of sufficient discomfort to prevent sleeping on the affected side.

It is of interest to look at the expectations of the patient and the surgeon from joint replacement surgery of this kind, and Tables 1 and 2 are drawn from Burton and Wright (2). Interesting factors are the range of expectation of the patient and the even greater range of the expectation of the surgeon from the procedure.

	Significant Level
1. The unfulfilled group (UFE) had more previous admissions to hospital prior to the operation	$p < 0.05$
2. UFE group had a greater 'feeling' of deformity (eg. leg shorter/hip sticking out)	$p < 0.01$
3. UFE group had greater feeling of disappointment in the success of the operation	$p < 0.001$
4. UFE group were more unhappy about the information given prior to the operation	$p < 0.05$
5. UFE group were less optimistic about the future	$p < 0.01$
6. UFE group had less desire to have the operation again if necessary	$p < 0.05$
7. UFE group had greater reliance on help from the family or outside sources although there was no significant difference between the two groups on the amount of help available	$p < 0.05$
8. UFE group ere less positive in their attitude toward their general health	$p < 0.05$

Table 1   Significant distinguishing factors between fulfilled and unfulfilled expectations (from Ref. 2).

	Expectation	Time After Operation
1.	Getting out of bed and putting full weight on the limb	2 – 14 days
2.	Discarding walking aids	6 – 26 weeks
3.	Length of time in hospital	2 – 6 weeks (if alone) 2 – 4 weeks (if not alone)
4.	Period as outpatient	Not at all – life
5.	Exercises upon going home	None – supervised
6.	Possible life of arthroplasty	5 – 30 years
7.	Resume employment/housework	3 weeks – 1 year
8.	Resume sexual activities	3 weeks – 6 months
9.	Resume golf/dancing	6 weeks – 1 year
10.	Resume gardening	1 month – 1 year
11.	Starting a family	3 weeks – 1 year
12.	Bathing normally	2 weeks – 12 weeks
13.	Giving instructions on sitting in chairs or lying on beds	Not necessary – essential
14.	Pain – 6 months after operation	None at all – aching
15.	Walking – 6 months after operation	1/2 a mile – Unlimited
16.	Deformity – 6 months after operation	None – 1" discrepancy
17.	Discomfort – 6 months after operation	None – mild tenderness

Table 2   Surgeons' range of expectations for patients undergoing total hip replacement (from Ref. 2)

REFERENCES

1.   Brown, T.R.M., Paul, J.P., Kelly, I.G., and Hamblen, D.L.
     Biomechanical Assessment of Patients Treated by Joint Surgery.
     J. Biomed. Engng. 3 (1981) 297 - 304.
2.   Burton, K.E., and Wright, V. The 'Total Solution' for Total
     Hip Replacement Surgery. J. Med. Engng. and Technology.
     4:4 (1980) 183 - 185.

SIGNIFICANCE OF MATHEMATICAL MODELING

J.P. Paul and N. Berme*

Bioengineering Unit, University of Strathclyde
Glasgow, Scotland
*Department of Mechanical Engineering, The Ohio State University
Columbus, Ohio 43210, U.S.A.

1.   INTRODUCTION

Biomechanical analysis of the function of the human body can allow the acquisition of information leading to the external loads and the displacement of the segments of the body during various functions. In fact, a considerable volume of data exists relating to walking in a straight line at uniform speed on a level surface. The questions of why the human person walks in the way he does is one which has exercised those formulating mathematical models and, although there is a large volume of experimental data, the mathematical models have found great difficulty in predicting this. If they cannot predict what has already been measured, they cannot predict what has not been measured, which is the principal use of this kind of model. If these basic parameters can be modelled, then the modelling can extend to the derived quantities which are obtainable from the experimental measurements, namely, the load actions transmitted between body segments, or intersegmental loading. This terminology of intersegmental loading is deliberately utilized to indicate the resultant loads transmitted, for instance, between the thigh and the shank rather than the frequently used but confusing terminology "knee force and moment". The term "knee joint force" is generally reserved for the loading transmitted at the articulating surfaces of the knee and not for the resultant transmitted between the calf and the thigh. Even the comparatively planar exercise of walking in a straight line develops load actions in three dimensions and, therefore, the resultant intersegmental loads are generally described in terms of three mutually perpendicular components of force and the three corresponding moments about the reference axes.

2.   INTERSEGMENTAL LOADING

Intersegmental loading has been determined experimentally by several investigators, Bresler and Frankel (1), Paul (2,3), Morrison (4), Cappozzo et al. (5) and many others. Most of these investigations were three dimensional and referred to level walking, although some included tests on ramps and stairs in addition. Nubar and Contini undertook an analysis to look at the optimal position of the leg in static function using the criterion of minimizing the "muscular effort" (6). They undertook a two dimensional analysis and defined muscular effort as $\Sigma M^2 dt$, where M is a moment in flexion or extension and dt implies summation over a defined time period. Raising the moment to the power 2 effectively prevented problems in dealing with positive or negative values. Beckett and Chang analyzed in two dimensions level walking with the forward velocity of the trunk assumed constant (7). They also assumed that the flexion extension moment at the hip approximated to a square wave and prescribed a trajectory for the foot. Chow and Jacobson extended this analysis but set up a cost function defined as a constant factor multiplied by the square of the hip moment plus another constant factor times the square of the moment at the knee (8). By minimization of this cost function, they came to conclusions about the relative values of these moments. Similarly, McGhee et al. utilized measured displacements from kinematic studies in the same way as Beckett and Chang but they also assumed values for ground to foot force components of simplified form in order to model the walking action (9). Because of the simplicity of the assumptions made by these authors, their model predictions for limb configuration during gait and for relevant loading actions do not match the complex three dimensional parameters which characterize human performance. Correspondingly, therefore, they cannot fulfill one of the aims in this type of work, that is prediction of the load actions in nonstandard activities or the prediction of the optimal gait for individuals suffering from pathologies restricting their performance. In these circumstances it might be hoped that analyses of these kinds could predict the optimal form of gait to protect the body part with the functional deficit and avoid overloading of the remaining parts.

3.   JOINT FORCES

In a different category altogether are the systems of analysis aimed at interpreting which of the anatomical structures transmit the intersegmental loads defined by the previous investigators. The problem here is that, in respect of rotational movements, there are invariably more muscles suitably disposed to transmit the loading than there are equations which would allow solution. For instance, if a section of the leg is taken through the hip joint, there are some 21 muscles having an action tending to produce three dimensional rotation of the lower extremity relative to the trunk. There are basically only three moment equations available and, to obtain a solution, gross simplifications of the anatomical system may be necessary. If force equilibrium is to be the only physical basis of the equations an early example of this is Inman, who analyzed the load at the hip joint during stationary one legged standing (10). The situation is well known and illustrated in Fig. 1. The center of mass of the body must be over the supporting foot and therefore the trunk and attachments must be prevented from tilting at the supporting hip joint by the action of relevant muscles. These were assumed to be gluteus medius, gluteus minimus and gluteus maximus, and their share of the overall load was determined by consideration of their relative volumes. With appropriate measurements of this, a single resultant force was set up in terms of position and line of action of resultant and a two dimensional analysis allowed the computation of the force at the hip joint which was reported as 2.4 times body weight. It was indicated that this varied corresponding to the angle of tilt of the trunk, and this factor was looked into in more detail by McLeish and Charnley (11). Paul (2), Morrison (4) and Paul and Poulson (12) considered the corresponding situations in three dimensions presenting in level walking. The philosophy of these authors was to consider the direction of moment developed by the ground forces and the appropriate gravitational and inertial actions acting on the limb segments. In the light of this, the muscles appropriate to transmission of this loading were identified. As far as the hip joint was concerned these were treated in groups comprising muscles whose lines of action relative to the joint in question were adjacent and whose phasic activity interpreted by EMG recordings was similar. These six groups comprised two in flexion, two in extension and one each in adduction and abduction. The flexion and extension groups were differentiated by consideration of whether they were "one joint" or "two joint" muscles. It was recognized that, although muscles were nominally designated by their principal action when the subject is in the standard anatomical position, nevertheless, functionally, each muscle group would be associated with more than one rotational action. At the knee joint, the differentiation has to be made between gastrocnemius and the hamstrings muscles. The assumption was made of minimal antagonistic activity and, for Paul and Morrison, the data was considered as it referred to the hip joint or to the knee joint in order to obtain the minimum possible values for the loading. Paul and Poulson attempted to consider minimization of the sum of the forces at the knee and hip joint as being a more realistic target.

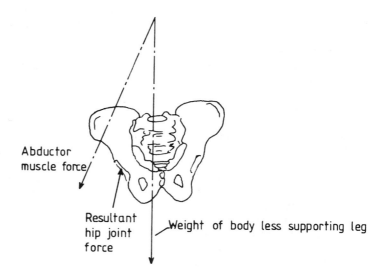

Fig. 1   Simplified force system on the pelvis for standing on one leg.

        Seireg and Arvikar (13, 14), considered the whole leg and defined a cost function U where:

$$U = \sum (F + r\,M + kR_i)$$

F was defined as the force in a particular muscle. M as the moment transmitted by a joint not under the control of muscle action, and R_i was the joint reaction.

        The intersegment force actions were defined from analysis of walking, with certain assumptions with regard to the external loads, and a minimization procedure undertaken for the cost function U to obtain the force in each muscle separately. Crowninshield et al. recognized one of the deficiencies of the analysis of Seireg and Arvikar, namely that the model tended to predict unreasonably high forces in a restricted number of muscles instead of allowing for load sharing (15). To take account of this, they predicted that the muscle force per unit physiological cross sectional area would be the same for all active muscles and that this quantity would be less than a value specified from physiological measurements. They then minimized the summation of the forces in all the muscles. This method was applied to a three dimensional analysis of walking.

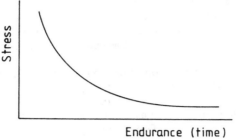

Fig. 2 Muscle stress F/A relationship to endurance time (from Ref. 17).

There is always controversy over the functions, if any, which are optimized during repetitive body movements. Some protagonists claim that since, eventually, walking produces tiredness, energy or rate of energy consumption, should be the factor whose minimization defines the gait trajectories adopted. Others have stipulated that tiredness in the muscle is a response to excessive forces developed by muscles and that the sum or weighted sum of the forces in the muscles is the relevant factor. Others again, particularly considering the patient with joint disease, feel that the resultant forces transmitted at the articulating joints with appropriate weightings, should give the relevant result, and there is no experimental work to allow a definitive decision on this matter.

Hardt decided to minimize the muscle energy output and, after consideration of various factors, defined a cost function to be determined by the instantaneous length of a muscle, its rate of contraction and its physiological cross sectional area (16). He also included the stipulation that the force in the muscle should be less than a limit based on a physiological cross sectional area.

One of the more recent analyses of this kind has been reported by Crowninshield and Brand (17) and they cite, as shown in Fig. 2, a muscle stress/endurance relationship indicating that the endurance time for a given physiological muscle stress is given by the equation $T = (F/A)^{-3}$, where T is the endurance time, F the muscle force and A the physiological cross sectional area. They therefore say that, in normal function, the neuromuscular control system will adjust the loading on particular muscles to allow the factor F/A to some power to be the criterion of load sharing, and they therefore minimize a function involving this F/A term to power three to predict the load sharing.

The ultimate test of any model, be it physical or mathematical, is measurement of its predictions. The models cited,
relating to intersegment loading, have been compared to the
measured dynamics of walking and found to have been relatively
coarse approximations. Such comparisons for the muscle and joint
loads pose very considerable experimental and ethical difficulties.

Rydell undertook tests on two patients following traumatic
fracture of the proximal femur (18). He treated them with an
Austin-Moore type hip prosthesis which had been specially prepared
with electrical resistance strain gages mounted on its internal
structure with leads carried from the cavity to a connection box
which was covered during initial surgery. Some six months later a
minor incision was made in the leg of the patient and the connection box was withdrawn to allow a series of tests in relevant
activities. The force transducer allowed measurements of the three
components of force and the bending moments on the neck of the
femur of the implanted device. In one case it allowed measurement
of the torque on the neck also. When this data is compared to the
predictions from normal subjects Rydell's data are seen to be
considerably smaller, even when interpreted normalized for body
mass. The clue to the discrepancy is that, although Rydell quoted
his test subjects as walking rapidly, they were in fact walking at
the speed designated as "slow" for most tests on normal subjects.
With this proviso, the data as shown in Fig. 3 appeared to
correspond quite closely.

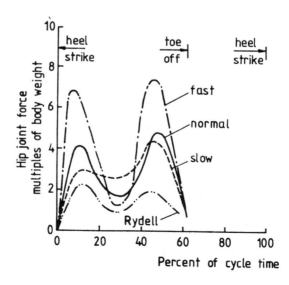

Fig. 3 Variation of hip joint force with time for level walking by
young healthy subjects at various speeds compared with data from
Rydell (18).

Carlson et al. (19) and Burstein (20) produced designs for hip prostheses and knee joint prostheses respectively with radio-telemetry for data acquisition. As far as is known at the present time these devices have not been implanted into living persons. In recent times there has been one other piece of experimentation of relevance, and that is the work of English and Kilvington (21), in which a special type of proximal femoral replacement was modified to measure one component of the hip joint force with the data acquisition being by radio telemetry. Data were acquired on a restricted number of patients but unfortunately this information was not correlated with data acquired from force plate and displacement analysis.

Barbenel from a simplified analysis of the function of the muscles of the jaw in relation to EMG concluded that no optimization was apparent in the load sharing which was present (22). For the walking activity the phasic pattern of myoelectric activity is frequently used as the only means whereby the model analysis can be assessed. Unfortunately, many of the models include the phasic EMG activity as one of their criteria and, therefore, they would be expected to indicate muscle loading inconformity to this. Paul (3) pointed out the discrepancies between reported values of phasic activity from different authors, and Crowninshield and Brand (17) are very definite that EMG data can be used to validate models only if it has been obtained from the test subject whose dynamics are being investigated and modelled. Intersubject differences and the differences between the same subject on different days negate any reasonable comparisons in a wider sense. It should also be noted that the various authors of reports on phasic EMG patterns differ in their interpretations of when a muscle is active and not, and frequently are not particularly clear in their description of this vital criterion.

As a consequence of all the factors cited here, modelling of human mechanical function must be considered as an idealization as yet not fully supported by real data. It continues in the hope that solutions will be formulated to allow the elucidation of the very complex phenomena associated with body movement and, hopefully, the formulation of optimization techniques for the treatment of patients.

REFERENCES

1. Bresler, B. and Frankel, J.P. The Forces and Moments in the Leg During Level Walking. Trans. Am. Soc. Mech. Eng. 72, (1950) 27 - 36. (Paper No. 48-A-62).

2. Paul, J.P. Forces Transmitted by Joints in the Human Body. Proc. Inst. Mech. Eng. <u>3J</u> (1967) 8 - 15.
3. Paul, J.P. Comparison of EMG Signals from Leg Muscles with Corresponding Force Actions Calculated from Walkpath Measurements. Proc. Conf. Human Locomotor Engineering. Inst. Mech. Eng. London (1971) 16 - 26.
4. Morrison, J.B. Bioengineering Analysis of Force Actions Transmitted by the Knee Joint. Biomed. Engng. 3, (1968) 164 - 170.
5. Cappozzo, A., Leo, T. and Pedotti, A. A General Computing Method for the Analysis of Human Locomotion. Istituto di Automatica, Universita di Roma (1973).
6. Nubar, Y. and Contini, R. A Minimal Principle in Biomechanics. Bulletin of Mathematical Biophysics <u>23</u>, (1961) 377.
7. Beckett, R.B., Chang, K. An Evaluation of the Kinematics of Gait by Minimum Energy. J. Biomechanics 1:(1968) 147 - 159.
8. Chow, C.K. and Jacobsen, D.H. Studies of Human Locomotion via Optimal Programming. U.S. Govt. Office of Naval Research Contract N00014-67-A-0298-006 NR-372-012. Technical Report No. 617 (1970).
9. McGhee, R.B., Koozekanani, S.H., Gupta, S., and Cheng, T.S. Automatic Estimation of Joint Forces and Moments in Human Locomotion from Television Data. Proc. IV IFAC Symp. "Identification and Parameter Estimation" USSR (1976).
10. Inman, V.T. Functional Aspects of the Abductor Muscles of the Hip. JBJS <u>39</u> 3, (1947) 607.
11. McLeish, R.D., and Charnley, J. Abduction Forces in the One-Legged Stance. J. Biomechanics 3 (1970) 191 - 200.
12. Paul, J.P., Poulson, J. The Analysis of Forces Transmitted by Joints in the Human Body. Proc. of 5th International Conference on Experimental Stress Analysis, Udine, Italy. (1974) CISM Udine 3.34 - 3.42.
13. Seireg, A. and Arvikar, R.J. A Mathematical Model for Evaluation of Forces in Lower Extremities of the Musculo-Skeletal System. J. Biomechanics 6 (1973) 313 - 326.
14. Seirig, A. and Arvikar, R.J. The Prediction of Muscular Load Sharing and Joint Forces in the Lower Extremities During Walking. J. Biomechanics, 8:(1975) 89 - 102.
15. Crowninshield, R.D., Johnston, R.C., Andrews, J.G. and Brand, R.A. A Biomechanical Investigation of the Human Hip. J. Biomechanics, 11(1) (1978), 75 - 85.
16. Hardt, D.E. A Minimum Energy Solution for Muscle Force Control During Walking. PhD Thesis, MIT, Boston, Mass. (1978).
17. Crowninshield, R.D. and Brand, R.A. A Physiologically Based Criterion of Muscle Force Prediction in Locomotion. J. Biomechanics 14 (1981) 793 - 801.
18. Rydell, N. Forces Acting on the Femoral Head Prosthesis. Acta Orthop. Scand. Suppl. 88 (1966).

19. Carlson, C.E., Mann, R.W. and Harris, W.H. A Radio Telemetry Device for Monitoring Cartilage Surface Pressures in the Human Hip. Trans. IEEE, BME-21, (1974) 257 - 264.
20. Burstein, A. Personal Communication (1974).
21. English, T.A. and Kilvington, J. A Direct Telemetric Method for Measuring Hip Load in "Orthopaedic Engineering". Harris, J.D. and Copeland, K. Eds. Biological Engineering Society, London (1978) 198 - 201.
22. Barbenel, J.C. The Application of Optimisation Methods for the Calculation of Joint and Muscle Forces. Engineering in Medicine ₁2(1) (1983) 29 - 33.

EXPERIMENTAL TECHNIQUES, DATA ACQUISITION AND REDUCTION

A. Cappozzo

Laboratory of Biomechanics – Istituto di Fisiologia Umana
Universita degli Studi "La Sapienza"
00185 Roma – Italy

1.   INTRODUCTION

The investigation of the biomechanics of articulating joints requires the following basic knowledge: a) the resultant force actions transmitted across an imaginary surface which separates the two adjacent body segments (intersegmental force and couple vectors), and b) the relative motion between the opposing bones.

As will become apparent in other parts of this book, from this knowledge and soft tissue anatomical and functional information one may proceed to the determination of internal loads (ligament tension, muscular forces, forces transmitted through the joint contact area and relevant stress distribution) occurring during physical exercise.   This is achieved using analytical mechanics and modeling.

Intersegmental forces and couples cannot be measured. However, they can be calculated using measurable quantities and analytical mechanics.   This is achieved through the following sequence of operations:
a) development of a mechanical model of the human body or a relevant part of it,
b) selection of the model parameters (inertia parameters),
c) selection of a set of quantities (variables) that completely describe the mechanical behavior of the model and that are measurable on a living subject while executing the physical exercise under investigation (kinematic quantities),
d) identification of the mathematical equations which permit the calculation of the intersegmental actions using the measured quantities as input variables and the model parameters (solution of the inverse problem of dynamics),

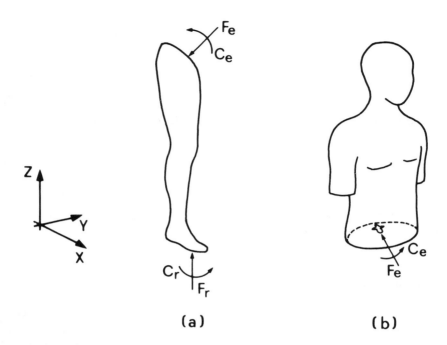

Fig. 1 Free-body diagram of the lower limb (a), and of the upper body (b) (inertia actions not shown).

    e) experimental assessment of these quantities and parameters,
    f) calculation of the intersegmental forces and couples.

    For mathematical tractability, this approach requires the use of simplifying assumptions about the mechanical structure and behavior of the human body. Thus, the accuracy of the analytical predictions depends not only on the quality of the input data, but also on the validity of these simplifying assumptions. In general it is necessary to validate the predicted quantities by comparing them or other related quantities with empirical observations in a number of selected cases.

    A by-product of the above procedure is a quantitative description of the relative motion between body segments. However, since the degree of approximation carried by an investigation procedure depends on the final aim, this description is not as accurate as it should be for pursuing objectives other than that described above. If a refined three-dimensional (3-D) description of joint kinematics is required, then ad hoc experimental and analytical techniques must be used.

The major purpose of the present chapter is to illustrate the experimental and analytical methods used for the prediction of intersegmental actions. For completeness, reference will also be made to the techniques specifically used for the assessment of joint kinematics. However, more details concerning this latter topic are provided in other parts of this book.

2.   THE MECHANICAL MODEL AND THE RELEVANT DYNAMIC EQUATIONS

As is always the case, the mechanical stereotype which allows for a cost-effective optimization of solution to the problem is to be sought. In the present context this stereotype is the rigid body. The human body is divided into segments, each of which is considered a rigid body. The ensemble of these rigid segments constitutes the mechanical model. Joints may be included within individual segments when occasionally characterized by a negligible amount of motion.

In order to make the intersegmental forces and couples explicit, and thus to be able to calculate them using analytical mechanics, the procedure of "cutting" is applied. The body is divided into two parts by an imaginary plane passing through the joint under investigation. All physical connections of one part with the other are then represented by forces and couples. These are assumed to maintain both body parts in the same dynamical state they had before their imaginary separation. The intersegmental actions are the resultants of all of these forces and couples reduced to a point chosen according to some circumstantial criterion.

Of the two separated body parts only one is to be taken into consideration for the analysis. The choice is based upon practical convenience. If a lower or upper limb joint is under investigation, then the distal portion of the limb is to be chosen. If a torso joint is analysed, then the part of the body superior to the cut is preferable in most circumstances (Fig. 1).

The body portion taken into consideration may have physical interactions with the environment. If this is the case, then this interaction is represented using resultant (external reaction) forces and couples. An example is given in Fig. 1a where the interaction between foot and ground during the stance phase of walking is represented by a resultant force and couple (ground reaction). Gravitational forces also belong to this category. Other examples are given by the drag forces associated with the fluid through which the human body moves. All of these force actions are usually referred to as external forces and couples.

At this stage we have a mechanical model made of a linkage of physically-united rigid segments, the mechanical interactions of which with surrounding bodies are represented by forces and couples. This is the free-body diagram of the portion of the human body under investigation (Fig. 1). In order to proceed with the analysis of the mechanics of the model, other properties must be associated with it. These may be divided into positional and inertial properties.

The positional properties convey the information needed to locate, at any instant in time, the position of any point in a segment relative to an arbitrarily chosen reference observer. This is achieved by defining a local coordinate system (x, y, z) fixed to the segment and a global coordinate system (X, Y, Z) fixed to the observer. Given the position vector p of any point in the local coordinate system (l.c.s.), the relevant position vector P in the global coordinate system (g.c.s.) is given by

$$\underline{P} = [A]\,\underline{p} + \underline{P}_0 \tag{1}$$

where [A] is the rotation matrix and $\underline{P}_0$ is the position vector of the l.c.s. origin relative to the g.c.s. The columns of matrix [A] are the direction cosines of the l.c.s. axes with respect to g.c.s. axes. Hence, the definition of the instantaneous position of the moving segment relative to the fixed observer reduces to determining the position vector $\underline{P}_0$ and rotation matrix [A], which therefore become the mechanical model positional properties.

The inertial properties associated with each model segment are represented by the following parameters of the relevant body segment:
    a) mass (m),
    b) position vector of the centre of mass (CM) in the l.c.s. $(\underline{P}_g)$,
    c) principal axes of inertia defined relative to the l.c.s. through a rotation matrix [B],
    d) moments of inertia about the principal axes passing through the CM (I_x, I_y, I_z).

The above properties thoroughly define the mechanical model. The next step is the determination of the equations that relate all quantities which describe the mechanical behavior of the free-body diagram of the body portion under investigation and, in particular, permit the calculation of the intersegmental force and couple vectors.

Reference is made to the general free-body diagram depicted in Fig. 2a. This free-body diagram consists of n segments. Point R is an arbitrary point at which an external reaction force acting on the s-th segment is applied. Point Q is an arbitrary point to which the intersegmental forces have been reduced. The dynamical equilibrium of the free body requires that the following system of equations be satisfied

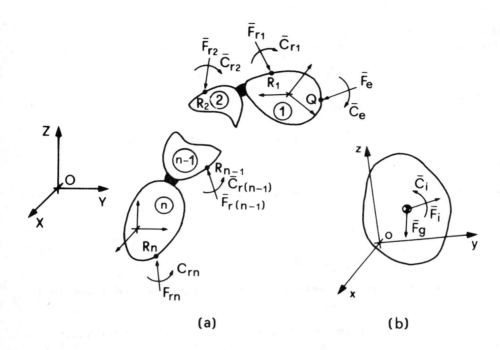

(a)   **(b)**

Fig. 2 (a) Generalized free-body diagram, and (b) a single segment.

$$\underline{F}_g + \underline{F}_i + \underline{F}_r + \underline{F}_e = 0 \tag{2}$$

$$\underline{M}_g + \underline{M}_i + \underline{M}_r + \underline{C}_i + \underline{C}_r + \underline{C}_e = 0 \tag{3}$$

where $\underline{F}_g$, $\underline{F}_i$, $\underline{F}_r$, $\underline{C}_i$, and $\underline{C}_r$ are the resultant vectors of the gravitational, inertial and external reaction forces, and the inertial and external reaction couples acting on the n segments, respectively. $\underline{M}_g$, $\underline{M}_i$, and $\underline{M}_r$ are the resultant moment vectors of the gravitational, inertial, and reaction forces acting on the n segments calculated with respect to point Q, respectively. $\underline{F}_e$ and $\underline{C}_e$ are the intersegmental force and couple vectors.

Taking into consideration an individual segment (Fig. 2b), the gravitational and inertial force vectors referenced to the g.c.s. acting on the segment are given by the following equations (where the subscript designating the segment has been dropped)

$$\underline{F}_g = m \begin{bmatrix} 0 \\ 0 \\ -g \end{bmatrix} \quad , \text{ and } \underline{F}_i = -m \, \underline{\ddot{P}}_g \qquad (4), (5)$$

where $\underline{P}_g = [A] \, \underline{p}_g + \underline{P}_0$

The inertial couple vector, referenced to the g.c.s., is given by

$$\underline{C}_i = -[A][B] \begin{bmatrix} I_x \dot{\omega}_x + (I_z - I_y)\omega_y \omega_z \\ I_y \dot{\omega}_y + (I_x - I_z)\omega_x \omega_z \\ I_z \dot{\omega}_z + (I_y - I_x)\omega_x \omega_y \end{bmatrix} \qquad (6)$$

where

$$\omega_x = \dot{a}_{12} a_{13} + \dot{a}_{22} a_{23} + \dot{a}_{32} a_{33} \quad , \qquad (7)$$

$$\omega_y = \dot{a}_{13} a_{11} + \dot{a}_{23} a_{21} + \dot{a}_{33} a_{31} \quad , \text{ and} \qquad (8)$$

$$\omega_z = \dot{a}_{11} a_{12} + \dot{a}_{21} a_{22} + \dot{a}_{31} a_{32} \quad , \qquad (9)$$

are the segment angular velocity vector components relative to the principal axes of inertia.

The global position vectors of points Q and R_s (s=1,...,n) are also needed for the calculation of $\underline{M}_g$, $\underline{M}_i$, and $\underline{M}_r$. The former position vector is usually given in the l.c.s. and transformed in the g.c.s. using Eqn. 1. The position vectors of points R are usually directly given in the g.c.s.

In summary, if the time functions of the positional variables ($\underline{P}_0$, [A]), the inertial parameters (m, $\underline{p}_g$, [B], I_x, I_y, I_z), and the external reaction vectors $\underline{P}_R$, $\underline{F}_r$, and $\underline{C}_r$ are given for each model segment in addition to the local position vector $\underline{p}_Q$, then the intersegmental force and couple vectors can be calculated using the equations given above. Relative positional information of the adjacent body segments or bones permits the description of the intervening joint kinematics. The screw axis of motion is an effective means for such a description. The six parameters that describe it in each instant of time can be calculated using the time functions of $\underline{P}_0$ and [A] associated with the two segments. Relevant equations are provided by Kinzel et al. and Panjabi et al. (2), among others.

In the following sections, the experimental methods used to determine the above-mentioned segmental positional variables and

inertial parameters are discussed. In particular, as far as the measurement of body segment motion is concerned, the following methods are scrutinized:
    a) stereometry,
    b) exoskeletal linkages,
    c) accelerometry.
Various random measurement errors are introduced while measuring the above-mentioned kinematic variables. Appropriate techniques must therefore be used for the calculus of the first and second derivatives required in Eqns. 5-9. These are discussed in a subsequent section.

3.   STEREOMETRY

This method permits the three-dimensional (3-D) reconstruction of the instantaneous position of a moving point in a laboratory (global) coordinate system. If this is done for at least three noncolinear points fixed in a rigid segment, then the position vector and the rotation matrix of this segment can be derived through simple vector calculations. Based on what was said in the previous section, this represents the fulfillment of a basic experimental need within the solution of the problem with which we are dealing.

Techniques using basic concepts of stereometry include stereophotogrammetry, light scanning, and stereosonic systems. All of these entail that the target points be represented by convenient markers, the physical realization of which depends on the particular technique used. In the present context, the target points are anatomical landmarks, or rigid extensions of them, selected according to practical considerations, which include the following: a) if skin markers are used, relative movement between markers and underlying bone due to soft tissue deformation should be minimal, thus consistent with the assumption of rigidity of the body segment discussed in the previous section, and b) the distances between markers should be sufficiently large for the error propagation from measured marker coordinates to rotation matrix to be minimal.

It is worthwhile emphasizing here that the number of markers needed to describe the kinematics of the free-body diagram under investigation does not necessarily have to be three for each segment. Kinematic constraints imposed on adjacent segments by the intervening joint may be used to lower that number, that is, to lower the mechanical model degrees of freedom.

3.1 Stereophotogrammetry

Close-range photogrammetry permits the achievement of the present experimental objective with an accuracy that is adequate for most gross body movement analyses. It entails the reconstruction of the 3-D coordinates of a target point with respect to a laboratory coordinate system (object space) from the coordinates of the projections of the stated point onto at least two planes (image spaces). The images may be obtained from central projections of the object space onto a light-sensitive image plane through a system of lenses.

3.1.1 Photography. Classical techniques for obtaining photogrammetric measurements use either still cameras or cine cameras. These techniques have been, and still are, extensively used in many scientific fields, and students of live movement appear to have been among the first to appropriate this measuring instrument (3-5). The choice of the actual optical device to be used depends on practical circumstances. Two still cameras with either stationary or continuously moving film (6,7), or two synchronized cine cameras can be used. A single camera can also be used whereby multiple perspective views are provided by mirrors (4,8). Non-metric cameras (i.e., not designed specifically for measurement purposes) are most often used for economic reasons. The markers which designate the anatomical landmark to be tracked may be passive dots or crosses with a color in contrast with the background or active light-emitting diodes (LEDs). The former solution is used with cine cameras, the latter with still cameras. Reflective dots illuminated with a strobe light may also be used instead of LEDs. A projector is used for enlargement of the film negatives and, if necessary, for printing them. Thereafter, the marker image coordinates are digitized.

3.1.2 Opto-electronic devices. In recent years great effort has been devoted to technological improvements connected with stereophotogrammetry in the field of biomechanics. New optoelectronic devices have been developed as alternatives to the conventional photographic cameras, permitting a direct feeding of the point projection information to a digital computer. Their basic characteristics are reported in Table 1. These devices allow the major shortcomings of conventional photogrammetry to be overcome. The operator time required for data reduction from target point projections can be reduced by order of magnitude. The characteristics of the experimental errors can be better assessed and exhibit an enhanced repeatability, therefore allowing for a more effective use of information retrieval procedures.

The first opto-electronic sensors to be used for these automatic motion measurement systems were TV cameras (9-11). In this range, the most updated systems are those developed by Jarrett (11) and Taylor et al. (9). A version of the former system is currently being marketed as VICON (VIdeo CONvertor for biomechanics, trademark of Oxford Medical Computers Ltd., Abingdon Oxon, United Kingdom). TV systems permit the measurement of the 2-D image

	VICON	Taylor et al. (9)	SELSPOT II	CODA-3	CoSTEL
Spatial resolution	hor. 1:1000 vert.1: 300*	1:2000	1:4000	1:16000	1:4000
Sampling frequency (sps)	50	50**	$\dfrac{10000}{\text{N. of markers}}$	600	100
Type of markers	refl.	refl.	IR LED	refl.	IR LED
Max. no. of markers	30	n.s.	128	8+	8

*600 when 25 sps are used
**60 sps with 60 Hz main.
+subject to increase

Table 1 Basic features of motion automatic recording systems (n.s. = not specified)

coordinates of all markers simultaneously on a frame by frame basis. Thereafter, a tracking algorithm must be used to identify individual markers and track their position from frame to frame. This procedure calls for the intervention of an operator in partial interaction with a graphics terminal. TV systems have the disadvantage of a relatively low spatial resolution and sampling frequency (Table 1). In addition, interactive marker tracking inhibits on-line applications.

A different class of sensing devices is used by the SELSPOT and CoSTEL systems. SELSPOT (SElective Light SPOT recognition, trademark of Selective Electronic Co., Mölndal, Sweden) uses camera-mounted lateral effect photodiodes (12). When these detectors are hit by infrared light emitted by an IR LED marker, a photocurrent occurs which is used to obtain two signals linearly related to the image coordinates of the LED. Several markers can be monitored quasi-simultaneously, operating them in time-division multiplex. A drawback of the lateral photo-effect is its sensitivity to spurious light sources, such as reflections. This defect seems to have been partially obviated in the latest version of this system (SELSPOT II). Another problem relates to the power supply to the LED, which, whether realized through a telecontrolled unit or an umbilical cord, causes encumbrance to the subject.

CoSTEL (Coordinate Spaziali mediante Trasduttori Elettronici Lineari, that is spatial coordinates through linear electric transducers) is the name given to an opto-electronic remote sensing device which measures the linear coordinates of projections of an infrared light-emitting marker onto three image space axes (13, 14). These projections are obtained by means of toroidal lenses and the coordinates measured by charge-coupled diode (ccd) linear arrays placed in the focal planes of the objectives. As is the case in the SELSPOT system, the LEDs are time-division multiplexed. The maximal sampling frequency, which is 1000 samples per second, (sps) as far as the electronics is concerned, is, in practice, limited to 100 sps by the amount of marker radiating energy that can reach a ccd photoelement over the working distance for whole-body analyses (5 m). The outputs of the transducers are intrinsically digital and background light noise is automatically compensated for. In order to overcome the above-mentioned inconvenience associated with active markers, a version which uses reflective markers and strobe light is being developed.

3.1.3 X-ray. When accurate quantitative knowledge about the relative motion of two opposing bones is required, Roentgen-stereophotogrammetry may be used. Based on the same principles as conventional photogrammetry, this technique permits the tracking of the motion of radio-opaque markers with respect to a fixed reference frame through two X-ray projections (15). If a dynamic situation is to be analyzed, cineradiography may be used. Markers are usually embedded in the bone in order to avoid spurious soft tissue movements. This technique is intrinsically invasive and represents a health hazard. Its use is thus limited to cadaver specimens. In an experimental set-up established for the study of knee-joint kinematics, de Lange et al. (15) could measure the spatial position of markers with an accuracy of 10 μm.

3.1.4   Analytical photogrammetry. Once the image coordinates of the markers are fed to the computer, either through manual digitization of photographs or automatically using opto-electronic devices, the reconstruction of the relevant object space coordinates must be carried out. This is done through mathematical models (photogrammetric models). Analytical photogrammetry, which deals with this problem, has received renewed attention in recent years among biomechanicians as a consequence of the technological achievements illustrated above (16-21).

The basic concepts which are used for the identification of photogrammetric models are the following (22). Let the position of the target point P be defined with respect to an arbitrary object space coordinate system (X,Y,Z) (o.c.s.); the position of the relevant image point p be defined with respect to an arbitrary image space coordinate system (x,y,z) (i.c.s.) rigid with the light sensitive plane (principal plane) of the camera; the perspective centre, inherent in the system of lenses used, be point 0. Its projection onto the principal plane is the principal point o'. The distance between points 0 and o' is the principal distance, d. These quantities are depicted in Fig. 3. In the i.c.s., the vector defining the position of point p with respect to the perspective centre is given by

$$[p - 0] = \underline{r} = \begin{bmatrix} x_p - x_{o'} \\ y_p - y_{o'} \\ - d \end{bmatrix} \qquad (10)$$

as $z_p = 0$, $z_0 = d$, $x_0 = x_0'$, and $y_0 = y_0'$ by definition. In the o.c.s. and for point P, we have

$$[P - 0] = \underline{R} = \begin{bmatrix} X_p - X_0 \\ Y_p - Y_0 \\ Z_p - Z_0 \end{bmatrix} \qquad (11)$$

If the o.c.s. axes are rotated so as to become parallel to the i.c.s. axes, then the vector $\underline{R}$, in the new frame (X',Y',Z'), is given by

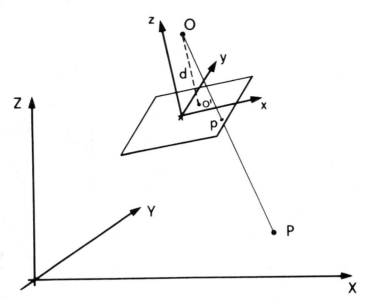

Fig. 3   Object and image coordinate systems; and collinearity
condition.

$$\underline{R}' = \begin{bmatrix} X'_p - X'_0 \\ Y'_p - Y'_0 \\ Z'_p - Z'_0 \end{bmatrix} = [M]\ \underline{R} \tag{12}$$

where $[M]$ is the rotation matrix of the i.c.s. with respect to the
o.c.s. (x,y,z). The optical principles underlying the techniques
through which point P images were obtained entail that the colline-
arity condition hold, that is, the vectors $\underline{r}$ and $\underline{R}'$ be collinear.
Therefore, after the above axis rotation, the vectors $\underline{r}$ and $\underline{R}'$ are
scalar multiples of each other:

$$\underline{R}' = k\ \underline{r} \tag{13}$$

Hence, from Eqns. 12 and 13, a relationship between object space
and image space is obtained:

$$\begin{bmatrix} X_p - X_0 \\ Y_p - Y_0 \\ Z_p - Z_0 \end{bmatrix} = k\ [M]^T \begin{bmatrix} x_p - x_{o'} \\ y_p - y_{o'} \\ -d \end{bmatrix} \tag{14}$$

where k is a variable which depends on the spatial position of P.

In Eqn. 14 a number of parameters appear concerning the characteristics of the photogrammetric set-up used. These parameters are quantitative expressions of the position and orientation of the camera in the o.c.s. (the vector $[X_O, Y_O, Z_O]$ and the matrix [M], respectively), the principal distance of the camera (d), and the image coordinates of the camera principal points $(x_{o'}, y_{o'})$. Parameters defined in the o.c.s. are referred to as external parameters, those defined in the i.c.s., as internal parameters.

If the parameters are assumed to be known and the image coordinates are assumed to be the input variables, Eqn. 14 corresponds to a system of three scalar equations in four unknowns. Therefore, to calculate the object coordinates of P, additional equations, that is, additional camera(s) are needed. With two distinct cameras we would have six equations and -if all four image coordinates were measured- five unknowns. The system of equations would thus be overdetermined. If only three image coordinates were used, then the system would be determined. It should, however, be emphasized that the above-mentioned redundancy lends itself to be exploited for optimizing the solution of the system of equations when the input data is noisy, as in most practical situations. The software packages of the TV and SELSPOT systems mentioned above use data reduction techniques which carry out this optimization. The CoSTEL system uses three cameras each of which measures one image coordinate. Thus, object coordinate reconstruction is based on the solution of a determined system of equations.

Lens distortion and deformation of photographic material, if any is used, may cause a virtual deviation of the light ray from the collinearity situation. In roentgenphotogrammetry other distortitons are introduced by the fact that the virtual perspective centre is not a point but has a finite size and by X-ray refraction. These disturbances must be assessed and refined values of the observed image coordinates must be determined before applying the collinearity condition (Eqn. 14). Different mathematical models are available to carry out the refinement according to the type of distortion with which one is dealing (22).

The solution of the collinearity condition equations poses two problems. Firstly, they are non-linear. Secondly, as mentioned above, more image coordinates are often measured than are necessary for uniquely solving the system of equations. Thus, linearized equations for the collinearity condition have been derived and the method of least squares is used to account for the redundant data. The photogrammetric model developed by Abdel-Aziz and Karara (23) is based on the above considerations. The Direct Linear Transformation (DLT), as it is called, appears to be the most widely-used model in recent biomechanics:

$$x_p = (L_1X_p + L_2Y_p + L_3Z_p + L_4)/(L_gX_p + L_{10}Y_p + L_{11}Z_p + 1)$$

$$y_p = (L_5X_p + L_6Y_p + L_7Z_p + L_8)/(L_9X_p + L_{10}Y_p + L_{11}Z_p + 1) \tag{15}$$

where the coefficients L_1 to L_{11} are functions of the internal and external parameters(6).

3.1.5 Calibration. Another crucial problem is the determination of the values to be given to the photogrammetric model parameters. These parameters are those which appear in Eqn. 14 (or in the system of Eqns. 15), in addition to those that account for the above-mentioned observed image coordinate refinement. The several techniques available for this purpose differ by the parameters that must be measured directly in the field, and those to be estimated through a calibration procedure. The collinearity equations (Eqns. 14 and 15) permit the calculation of the relevant parameters once both the image and object coordinates of an adequate number of target points are known. The information needed for this calculation is provided by a control point distribution, i.e. calibration object, placed within the observation area. The amount of absolute information needed about the geometry of this object differs for different calibration procedures. Marzan and Karara (24) describe a procedure which computes the parameters of the DLT model using the object and image space coordinates of a suitable number of control points. More complex mathematical procedures have been proposed, where limited absolute information is needed about the calibration object (25,26).

3.1.6 Stereometric set-up considerations. The choice of the position and orientation of the two cameras in relation to each other as well as with respect to the measurement field is important. For minimum error propagation to the reconstructed target point position, the best possible solution is achieved when the conjugate rays intersecting in the target point P are orthogonal and when the distances P to camera perspective centres are minimal (22). However, from practical considerations, those conditions cannot always be achieved. The following other factors are to be taken into account:

a) size of the measurement field and overlap area of the fields of view of the two cameras,

b) size of the cone of light emission or reflection of the markers, and

c) shadowing by other body segments.

3.2 Light-Scanning System

The CODA-3 system (Cartesian Optoelectronic Digital Anthropometer, trademark of Movement Techniques Ltd., Barrow-upon-Soar, England) is a light-scanning device in which three fan-shaped beams of white light are swept across the field of view by three rotating multifaceted polygonal mirrors (27). Two of these rotate about parallel axes and one about an axis orthogonal to the others when a beam crosses a marker, in the form of a small pyramidal prism, a brief pulse of light is reflected back along the same path and is ultimately detected by photodiodes in the scanner unit. The time of the returning pulse in relation to the mirror rotation indicates the position of the landmark in the angular field of view. Three of such positions permit the reconstruction of the marker object coordinates. Identification of individual markers is achieved by their distinct colors. As can be seen from the data reported in Table 1, this system exhibits outstanding features, including the use of passive markers. However, no reports of its evaluation in actual biomechanical applications is yet available.

3.3 Stereosonic System

Anatomical landmarks are designated by acoustical transmitters, usually in the ultrasonic range. In the system described by Brumbaugh et al. (28), time-multiplexed pulsed transmittors are used and the detectors are three mutually-orthogonal linear microphones. The time delay between sound impulse emission and detection is measured and used to calculate the distance between emitter and each detector. Three of such distances permit the 3-D reconstruction of the instantaneous marker position. The spatial resolution may be as low as 0.1 mm. The measurement field is, however, small (up to 1 m^3) which represents the basic limitation of the system. Henning and Nicol (29) describe a system which exploits the Doppler-effect. The marker emits a fixed-frequency sound. The sound frequency variations detected by a staionary microphone may be assumed proportional to the rate of variation of the distance between the microphone and the marker. This holds true for relative velocities up to 10 ms^{-1}. Inaccuracy is below 0.5%.

4.   EXOSKELETAL LINKAGES

The gross relative motion between adjacent body segments can be measured using exoskeletal linkage systems. These linkages are attached externally to the body segments, and the relevant angular and linear positions are usually measured using potentiometers. According to the experimental problem to be solved and the accuracy desired, planar, triaxial, or six degree-of-freedom spatial devices are used (30). Several electro-mechanical techniques have been used to construct these devices (2,30-33). The position data provided by electro-mechanical transducers are relative in nature and therefore do not, in general, serve the purpose of determining the intersegmental actions.

If joint kinematics is of interest, the device should be attached directly to the opposing bones. In fact, the soft tissues interposition between linkage attachment and underlying bone would cause relative movement, thereby introducing an error. This restricts this type of experimental approach to in vitro situations (2,34).

5. ACCELEROMETRY

Six properly oriented linear accelerometers permit the description of a 3-D motion of a rigid body (35). Velocity and displacement information can be derived through integration and known initial conditions. Although this is possible in principle, in practice the six differential equations are coupled and can only be solved numerically; but the solution becomes unstable. Use of nine accelerometers allow a stable solution. However, the method also suffers from other limitations. The attachment of a set of accelerometers to the skin may introduce artifacts which can even mask the message signal. The bulkiness of the transducers and related wiring may cause encumbrance to the subject. The determination of the initial conditions may pose technical problems. Data acquisition and reduction is very demanding due to the large number of quantities that have to be measured. Thus, the use of this method for the determination of body segment linkage kinematics does not seem to be competitive with the methods discussed previously. However, there are situations in joint biomechanics where accelerometry plays a fundamental role. This is the case when body segments are subjected to either high frequency vibrations or impulsive external forces (36).

6. BODY SEGMENT INERTIAL PARAMETERS

This section is devoted to the discussion of another important problem in the biomechanics of human movement: the determination of subject-specific segmental inertial parameter values to be assigned to the relevant mechanical model segments. The segmental parameter set is defined in a previous section.

Current methods for the in vivo experimental assessment of these parameters are complex, and some of them may be harmful to the subject's health (e.g. gamma scanning methods). In addition, they do not permit the determination of the necessary parameters independently and often rely on simplifying assumptions such as the uniform density distribution of a segment. Hence the use of these experimental methods for extensive investigations or for routine analyses is debatable.

Prediction techniques, which compute the inertial parameters from anthropometric dimensions, are most often preferable. These techniques can be divided into two major methodological groups of a) estimation through regression equations, and b) geometrical approximation.

The regression equations have been determined through statistical analysis of data obtained from a sample population of subjects. Measurements have been made using cadaver specimens (3,37-41) and living subjects (4,42,43). With the exception of Bernstein (4) and Zatsiorsky and Seluyanov (43), all investigators used relatively small samples (Table 2). Barter (44) derived his regression equations from a statistical combination of the adult male cadaver data of previous authors (3,37,41). The regression equations proposed by some authors use one independent variable only. Body weight is used for segmental mass prediction and either stature or segment length for the calculation of CM loation and radius of gyration (3,4,37,39,41,42). Zatsiorsky and Seluyanov (43) use both body weight and stature simultaneously. Clauser et al. (38) use up to three dimensions chosen among segmental lengths, depths, breadths, and circumferences in addition to body weight. Liu and Wickstrom (40) report regression equations which permit the estimation of the mass, centre of mass, and principal moments of inertia of transverse trunk slices each containing one vertebra from Tl to L5. At present, this is the only data available which permits any given portion of the human trunk to be considered. Statistics were based on seven cadaver specimens. The only study in this category which deals with the determination of the segmental principal axes of inertia is that by Chandler et al. (39). All other authors either explicitly or implicitly make reference to symmetry axes. The magnitude and type of the sample population, the segments taken into consideration and the parameters which may be estimated using the regression equations provided by the different authors are reported in Tables 2 and 3. In Table 3 relevant maximal error ranges are also given either as reported by the authors or as inferred from relevant information.

The geometrical approximation method has been used by several investigators. However, the most thorough studies appear to be those of Hanavan (45), Jensen (46), and Hatze (47). The irregular shapes of the different body segments were represented with standard geometric forms which are capable of simple mathematical description. Hanavan (45) used simple geometric solids (circular ellipsoid, elliptical cylinder, sphere, and frustrum) of uniform density with which he represented 15 body segments. Twenty-five anthropometric measurements are used as inputs to this author's model. Jensen (31) sectioned 16 body segments into elliptical zones. He also assumed uniform density distribution. Dimensions of the elliptical zones were obtained by digitizing photographic records of the side and front view of the subject. Hatze (47)

Author	subjects	age (years)	sex	body mass (kg)	stature (m)
Bernstein	152 live		M		
Dempster	8 cad.	52–83	M	49–72	1.59–1.86
Barter	12 cad.		M		
Drillis and Contini	20 live	20–40	M	76–86	1.67–1.88
Chandler et al.	6 cad.	45–65	M	51–89	1.64–1.81
Clauser et al.	13 cad.	28–74	M	54–88	1.62–1.85
Zatsiorsky and Seluyanov	100 live	19–35	M/F	55–91	1.68–1.80

Table 2 Sample population characteristics (blank space = not specified).

proposes a much more accurate geometrical representation for his 17 segment model. In addition, he accounted for varying densities and made no assumptions about segment symmetries. This permitted him to make a more accurate assessment of the principal axes of inertia and to account for changes in body morphology due to obesity, pregnancy, and other abnormal states. Applicability to children is also an advantage of this method. The price to be paid for such a refinement consists of the 242 anthropometric measurements to be carried out on the subject under investigation.

A brief account of the techniques available for the prediction of body segment parameters has been given above. Which one or ones to use and what accuracy may be expected are the crucial questions that need to be answered in practical circumstances.

Firstly, it must be emphasized that only a very partial validation of the predicted parameter values is possible, in that only a few of these are measurable on living subjects. Hatze (47), for instance, while validating the results of his model, was bound to restrict the comparison between predicted and measured parameters to the segment volumes, CM coordinate along the main axis of the segment and the moments of inertia about the latero-lateral axis of thigh and shank. He reports errors in the range 0.2–5.0%, 0.2–11.0%, and 0.5–5.0%, respectively. As far as the mass moments of inertia are concerned, Hatze (47) estimated that the uniform

density and coronal symmetry assumptions, used in other authors'
geometrical approximation models, introduced errors in the computed
values of these parameters in the range 4-7% and up to 30%, respectively. As far as segment mass prediction is concerned, a possible
overall check is the comparison between the sum of the individual
segment masses and the measured body mass. This, of course,
applies to those techniques for which this comparison does not lead
to an identity by defintion (segmental masses given as percent of
body mass). Miller and Morrison (48) carried out this check using
30 adult male subjects and found that Barter's equations under-
estimate total body mass by about 2%, Clauser et al.'s (38) equations were found to yield overestimations ranging from 2 to 8%.
Zatsiorsky and Seluyanov's were found to overestimate by approximately 2%. It was also inferred that the upper trunk mass
predicted using Liu and Wickstrom's equations was underestimated by
about 20%. This seems to recommend the use of these equations for
within-trunk mass distribution assessment only.

Due to the objective difficulties posed by the segment inertial parameter prediction, the a priori assessment of the relevant
degree of approximation permissible in a given biomechanical analysis is of basic importance. This can be achieved through a sensitivity study of the mathematical model used. Each individual
parameter is perturbed by a quantity equal to the relevant estimated inaccuracy and the consequent variation of the calculated
results observed (49). Of course, when the complexity of the model
equations permits, a sensitivity analysis through proper statistical methods may be carried out instead.

An overall experimental assessment of the parameter prediction
may consist of comparing calculated external reaction forces and
couples, which are highly dependent on many inertial parameters,
with the relevant measured values. Reference to a quasi-static
body movement is advisable, so that the effect on the calculated
force actions of the acceleration estimate inaccuracy is minimized.
This, of course, restricts the error propagation analysis to the
segmental masses and location of the CM. Vaughan et al. (51)
propose a procedure for the optimal selection of segmental parameters which is based on the above comparison. An objective function
is formulated which is given by the difference between calculated
and measured reaction forces. Optimal values of the inertial
parameters are sought which minimize this objective function. If
the number of degrees of freedom of the optimization problem is
kept to a minimum and proper constraint conditions and test movements are used, then this procedure may help in improving the
parameter prediction.

To sum up, when extreme accuracy is required, Hatze's model
seems to represent, at present, the best solution. This author
claims predictions with an overall accuracy better than 3%, and a

Author	segments	mass	location of CM			moments of inertia		
			x	y	z	x	y	z
Bernstein	ua,fa,hn,th,s,f	17-26			9-25			
Dempster	h,t,fa,hn,th,s,f	-						
Barter	h,t,ua,fa,hn,th,s,f	20-48				40-74	40-74	40-94
Drillis and Contini	th,s,f,ua,fa,hn	15-47			-	18-57	18-57	
Chandler et al.	h,t,ua,fa,hn,th,s,f	4-26			-	9-80	8-90	8-150
Clauser et al.	h,t,ua,fa,hn,th,s,f	6-16		6-42	6-16	30-76	30-76	30-84
Zatsiorsky and Seluyanov	h,ut,mt,lt,ua,fa,hn,	12-22			4-10	24-44	24-44	42-78

Table 3 Maximal error ranges associated with parameter prediction (Maximal errors are given in percent). Body segments taken into consideration (h=head, t=trunk, ut=upper trunk, mt=middle trunk, lt=lower trunk, ua=upper arm, fa=forearm, hn=hand, th=thigh, s=shank, f=foot. Blank spaces = parameter not given. Dash = parameter given without relevant accuracy.

maximum error of about 5%, only occasionally reaching 11%. In addition, the large number of body segments taken into consideration allow for a wide range of applications. However, the enormous amount of anthropometric measurements required makes this model unsuitable for field applications such as clinical gait analysis. If regression equations are used, it seems reasonable to recommend that the subject under investigation be of a body configuration and sex consistent with that of the sample population from which the equations were derived (Table 2). Under these circumstances, an approximate idea of the prediction inaccuracy can be obtained by referring to the data reported in Table 3.

7. NUMERICAL DIFFERENTIATION TECHNIQUES

From the previous sections it is understood that a basic interest of the biomechanical analyst is to obtain good estimates of human displacement data, together with their first and second derivatives. The relevant experimental data are affected by relatively large experimental errors, especially when stereometric techniques are used. Numerical differentiation of this data may thus easily lead to unstable solutions. In order to avoid this, appropriate information retrieval procedures must be applied in addition to a wise choice of the motion data sampling frequency.

The experimental errors which affect motion data may be broadly grouped into three types: a) wild points, b) systematic errors, and c) random errors.

Spurious wild points may be introduced into the data by a number of causes, for example, missing data points due to optical occlusion of markers. These points must be corrected prior to any subsequent analysis.

Systematic errors uncorrelated with the movements arise mainly from electro-optical distortions present in the image-processing equipment for which the calibration procedure did not compensate. Certain systematic errors may occur which are correlated with the movements under study; for example, skin marker or exoskeletal linkage movements relative to the underlying skeletal structures. These errors are difficult to eliminate from the acquired data series and may have significant effects on subsequent procedures such as differentiation. These errors may, however, be minimized by the proper design of equipment.

Various random measurement errors are introduced into the data by the methods employed to digitize the marker coordinates. Additional errors of a random nature may also be present due to effects occurring within the image-processing equipment. Due to the inherent high-frequency content, this error, although usually relatively small, can render impossible the direct use of raw experimental data in calculations which entail time differentiation. Classical numerical differentiation procedures would lead to unstable numerical processes. This is a typical problem in experimental biomechanics and its solution is critical.

In the following, reference will be made to an input data series given by

$$v_k = u_k + e_k \quad , \; k = 0, 1, \ldots, N \; ,$$

where u is the underlying function (signal), e_k is the random experimental error (noise), k is the discrete time index.

All numerical differentiation procedures, both for exact and non-exact data, are based on the a priori assumption that little or no detail of the signal gets lost in the sampling process. Thus, a proper choice of the motion data sampling frequency is of crucial importance and worthy of some consideration here.

The choice of the sampling frequency (f_s) is conditioned by two contrasting needs. One aims at the best possible signal and noise description and requires a high f_s. The other is associated with computer memory occupation and running time and, of course, requires that the minimally acceptable number of data points be acquired. In addition, each measurement equipment is characterized by a maximal f_s (see Table 1). A compromising value of f_s is therefore to be sought.

For the above purpose, a possible criterion may be the following. The maximal precision that can be obtained in the calculated n-th derivative is given by (52,53)

$$\sigma_n^2 \geqslant (\sigma_e^2 \, (2 \, \pi f_b)^{2n+1}) / (f_s \, \pi \, (2 \, n + 1)) \qquad ; \tag{16}$$

where σ_n^2 and σ_e^2 are the variances of the estimated n-th derivative error and input data noise, respectively; f_b is the signal band-limit. This formula applies when the measurement random error is white, and when no signal is present above f_b. The lower limit of σ_n^2 applies when a perfect differentiation operator is used below f_b and the signal above f_b is zero.

In order to calculate the theoretical minimal value of f_s, σ_e^2, σ_n^2, and f_b must be given. The variance of the input data series may be assessed through ad hoc experiments (54) and is usually typical of the given experimental set-up. The variance of the n-th derivative is given a value according to the desired accuracy of the end results. The signal bandlimit may be inferred using knowledge relative to the basic characteristics of the phenomenon under investigation or through the spectral analysis of some related quantity which is accurately measurable. A typical example of such a quantity is an external reaction force given by a linear combination of body segment accelerations. The determination of the factor by which the minimal value of f_s should be multiplied in order to obtain the actual value to be used is a mere matter of experience. The author found a factor of approximately 1.3 satisfactory in most circumstances.

The methods commonly used to carry out the estimation of the signal u_k and/or its first and second derivatives can be grouped under the two headings below.

7.1 Time Domain Techniques

These techniques require that the structure of the underlying function be known and a homogeneous set of analytical functions be associated with it. In other words, reference is made to a model of the phenomenon under investigation. The analytical function which, within the given set, best fits the input data is typically found through a least squares procedure. This requires that the noise samples e_k be uncorrelated and the relevant variance be a priori known. If this latter variance is not available, then interactive decision-making procedures must be used. Single approximating functions can be used for the totality of the input data points (global approach), or for a small number of data points, and applied sequentially (local approach). Derivatives are thereafter generated through analytical differentiation. It should be emphasized that equidistant time points are not necessarily required by these techniques and that estimated functions can be re-sampled at any given rate, thus permitting interpolation between data points.

Techniques within the above methodological group which are described in biomechanical literature are the following. Plagenhoef (55) used global Chebyshev polynomial functions. Lanshammar (53) illustrates the application of local second-order polynomial functions fitted over five data points and of fourth-order polynomial functions fitted over nine data points. Both cubic and quintic spline functions have been proposed for use in the present context (56,57). Techniques using the Fourier series have also been reported (50,58). As discussed below, due to the particular approximating function used, these latter techniques may also be placed within the frequency domain group.

7.2 Frequency Domain Techniques

These techniques are often referred to as filters, either differentiating or not, and may be divided into two subgroups according to whether or not they require the explicit calculation of the Fourier transform of the data. This latter group entails

the numerical calculation of the convolution integral of the data
series and the filter impulse response. The other techniques
require that the calculated data periodogram be multiplied by a
suitably-designed window. Thereafter, the inverse Fourier transform is calculated.

The central assumption on which all of these techniques are
based is the statistical stationary of the noise which was not
required by the time domain techniques. In addition, detrended and
equally-spaced in time data points are required. The convolution
integral approach does not permit interpolation between data
points, while the spectral approach allows it.

The techniques belonging to this group which have been described in biomechanical literature are the following. A phase-
cancelled second-order Butterworth low pass filter is used by
Winter et al. (59). This is a recursive infinite-response filter
(IIR). Other IIR filters have been described by Woltring (17) and
Gustafsson and Lanshammar (60). Lesh et al. (61) reported on the
use of non-recursive finite-impulse response filters (FIR) designed
employing the algorithm provided by McClellan et al. (62). The use
of another FIR filter designed using the Kaiser window method is
reported by Andrews et al. (63). For general information concerning these filters see, for instance, Hamming (64). These techniques use filters, the transfer function of which approximates a
single step function eventually followed by derivative factors.
The design of these filters requires the a priori knowledge of the
signal bandlimit which is assumed as the filter cut-off frequency.
Alternatively, the filter low-pass characteristics can be determined for each data sequence by seeking a cut-off frequency for
which the variance of the filter residuals equals that of the
noise. For this procedure, an estimate of the noise variance is
required. The cut-off frequency selection can also be carried out
through mathematical algorithms and using the relevant statistical
information contained in the data spectrum (64).

The harmonic regression technique referred to above may be
considered as adopting a spectral approach, in that the signal
periodogram is calculated. This technique uses a step function
window in the strict sense. It should be emphasized that the use
of a step function window is based on the assumption that the
spectrum of the data shows a clear division between signal and
noise. If this is not the case and a "transition" frequency range
exists where signal and noise have comparable spectral power, then
better results are obtained using a window tapered in this frequency range (65). This type of window is used in an algorithm
implemented by Andrews et al. (63), which may be outlined in the
following way. A ramp-shaped function is chosen having a value of
unity at low frequencies, a linear transition trend and zero value
for the upper frequency range. This function is fitted to a

smoothed periodogram of the data sequence. Hatze (66) uses a similar but more advanced procedure whereby the window is chosen so as to optimize the signal derivative estimation.

Some of the aforementioned techniques have been the object of comparative evaluation which are, however, incomplete and most of them suffer from a qualitative approach. At the present therefore, it is impossible to say which of the above techniques is "the best" for a given sequence.

REFERENCES

1. Kinzel, G.L., Hall, A.S., Jr. and B.M. Hillberry. Measurement of the Total Motion between Two Body Segments-I. Analytical Development. J. Biomechanics 5 (1972) 93-105.

2. Panjabi, M.M., Krag, M.M., and V.K. Goel. A Technique for Measurement and Description of Three-Dimensional Six Degrees-of-Freedom Motion of a Body Joint with an Application to the Human Spine. J. Biomechanics 14 (1981) 447-460.

3. Braune, C.W. and O. Fisher. Der Gang des Menshen I. Abb. Math. Phys. Cl. Kon. Sachs. Ges. Wissensch. 21 (1895) 151-324.

4. Bernstein, N.A. The Coordination and Regulation of Movements (Pergamon Press Ltd., 1967).

5. Marey, E.J. La Methode Graphique dans les Sciences Experimentales, 2nd edition with supplement: le Development de la Methode Graphique par la Photographie (Paris: G. Masson, 1885).

6. Cappozzo, A. Stereophotogrammetric System for Kinesiological Studies. Med. and Biol. Eng. and Comput. 21 (1983) 217-223.

7. Wyss, U.P., and V.A. Pollak. Kinematic Data Acquisition System for Two-or Three-Dimensional Motion Analysis. Med. and Biol. Eng. and Comput. 19 (1981) 287-290.

8. Morasso, P. and V. Tagliasco. Analysis of Human Movements: Spatial Localization with Multiple Perspective Views. Med. and Biol. Engng. and Comput. 21 (1983) 74-82.

9. Taylor, K.D., Mottier, F.M., Simmons, D.W., Cohen, W., Pavlack Jr., R., Cornell, P., and Haukins, G.B. An Automated Motion Measurement System for Clinical Gait Analysis. J. Biomechanics 15 (1982) 505-516.

10. Winter, D.A., Greenlaw, R.K., and D.A. Hobson. Television-Computer Analysis of Kinematics of Human Gait. Comp. Biomed. Res. 5 (1972) 498-504.

11. Jarret, M.O., Andrews, B.J., and J.P. Paul. Quantitative Analysis of Locomotion Using Television. ISPO World Congress, Montreaux, Switzerland, 1974.

12. Lindholm, L.E.   An Optoelectronic Instrument for Remote On-Line Movement Monitoring.   In R.C. Nelson and C.A. Morehouse ed.s (Baltimore: University Park Press, 1974), pp. 510-512.

13. Leo, T. and V. Macellari.   On Line Microcomputer System for Gait Analysis Data Acquisition Based on Commercially Available Optoelectronic Devices.   In A. Morecki, K. Fidelus, K. Kedzior, and A. Wit ed.s, Biomechanics VII-B (Baltimore, University Park Press, 1981) pp. 163-169.

14. Macellari, V. CoSTEL: a Computer Peripheral Remote Sensing Device for 3-Dimensional Monitoring of Human Motion. Med. and Biol. Engng. and Comp. 21 (1983) 311-318.

15. de Lange, A., van Dijk, R., Huiskes, R., Selvik, G., and Th. J.G. van Rens.   The Application of Roentgenstereophotogrammetry for Evaluation of Knee-Joint Kinematics in Vitro. In R. Huiskes, D. Van Campen and J. De Wijn ed.s, Biomechanics: Principles and Applications (The Hague: Martinus Nijhoff Publishers, 1982), pp. 177-184.

16. Ayoub, M.A., Ayoub, M.M. and J.D. Ramsey. A Stereometric System for Measuring Human Motion. Human Factors 12 (1970) 523-535.

17. Woltring, H.J. Calibration and Measurement in 3-D Monitoring of Human Motion.   II: Experimental Results and Discussion. Biotelemetry 3 (1976) 65-97.

18. Shapiro, R.   The Direct Linear Transformation Method for Three-Dimensional Cinematography. Res.Q. 49 (1978) 197-205.

19. Andriacchi, T.P., Hampton, S.J., Shultz, A.B. and J.O. Galante.   Three Dimensional Coordinate Data Processing in Human Motion Analysis.   J. Biomech. Engng.   101 (1979) 279-283.

20. Dapena, J., Harman, E.A., and J.A. Miller.   Three Dimensional Cinematography with Control Object of Unknown Shape.   J. Biomechanics 15 (1982) 11-19.

21. Miller, N.R., Shapiro, R., and T.M. McLaughlin. A Technique for Obtaining Spatial Kinematic Parameters of Segments of Biomechanical Systems from Cinematographic Data.   J. Biomechanics 13 (1980) 535-547.

22. Gosh, S.K. Analytical Photogrammetry. (New York, Pergamon Press Ltd., 1979).

23. Abdel-Aziz, Y.I. and H.M. Karara.   Direct Linear Transformation from Comparator Coordinates into Object Space Coordinates in Close Range Photogrammetry. Proceedings of the ASP/UI Symposium on Close Range Photogrammetry, Urbana, Illinois, 1971.

24. Marzan, T. and H.M. Karara.   A Computer Program for Direct Linear Transformation of the Colinearity Condition and some Applications of it. Symposium on Close Range Photogrammetric Systems.   American Society of Photogrammetry, Falls Church (1975) 420-476.

25. Kenefick, J.F., Gyer, M.S., and B.F. Harp. Analytical Self-calibration. Photogramm. Engng. 38 (1972) 1117-1126.
26. Woltring, H.J. Planar Control in Multi-Camera Calibration for 3-D Gait Studies. J. Biomechanics 13 (1980) 39-48.
27. Mitchelson, D. Recording of Movement Without Photography. In D.W. Grieve, D. Miller, D. Mitchelson, J.P. Paul and A.J. Smith, Techniques for the Analysis of Human Movement (London: Lepus Books, 1975).
28. Brumbaugh, R.B., Crowninshield, R.D., Blair, W.F. and J.G. Andrews. An In-vivo Study of Normal Wrist Kinematics. J. Biomech. Engng. 104 (1982) 176-181.
29. Hennig, E.M. and K. Nicol. Velocity Measurement without Contact on Body Surface Points by Means of the Acoustical Doppler Effect. In P. V. Komi ed., Biomechanics V-B (Baltimore: University Park Press, 1976), pp. 449-455.
30. Chao, E.Y. Justification of Triaxial Goniometer for the Measurement of Joint Rotation. J. Biomechanics 13 (1980) 989-1006.
31. Johnston, R.C. and G.L. Smidt. Measurement of Hip Joint Motion during Walking. Evaluation of an Electrogoniometric Method. J. Bone Jnt. Surg. 51A (1969) 1083-1094.
32. Lamoreux, L.W. Kinematic Measurements in the Study of Human Walking. Bulletin of Prosthetic Research. BPR-10-15 (1971) 3-84.
33. Townsend, M.A., Izak, M. and R.W. Jackson. Total Motion Knee Goniometry. J. Biomechanics 10 (1977) 183-193.
34. Kinzel, G.L., Hillberry, B.M., Hall, A.S., Jr., Van Sickle, D.C., and W.M. Harvey. Measurement of the Total Motion between Two Body Segments--II. Description of Application. J. Biomechanics 5 (1972) 283-293.
35. Morris, J.R.W. Accelerometry - A Technique for the Measurement of Human Body Movements. J. Biomechanics 6 (1973) 729-736.
36. Light, L.H., McLellan, G. and L. Klenerman. Skeletal Transients on Heel Strike in Normal Walking with Different Footwear. J. Biomechanics 13 (1980) 477-480.
37. Dempster, W.T. Space Requirements of the Seated Operator. WADC Technical Report 55-159, Wright-Patterson AFB, Ohio (1955).
38. Clauser, C.E., McConville, J.T. and J.W. Young. Weight, Volume and Centre of Mass of Segments of the Human Body. Report No. AMRL-TR-69-70, Wright-Patterson AFB, Ohio (1969).
39. Chandler, R.F., Clauser, C.E., McConville, J.T., Reynolds, H.M. and J.W. Young. Investigation of Inertial Properties of the Human Body. Report No. AMRL-TR-74-137, Wright-Patterson AFB, Ohio (1975).
40. Liu, Y.K. and J.K. Wickstrom. Estimation of the Inertial Property Distribution of the Human Torso from Segmented Cadaveric Data. In R.M. Kenedi ed., Perspectives in Biomedical Engineering (London: MacMillan Press, 1973), pp. 203-213.

41. Fisher, O. Der Gang des Menschen, Abh. Math. Phys. Cl. Kon.
     Sachs. Ges. Wissensch. II-25 (1900) 1-130. III-26 (1901)
     85-170. IV-26 (1901) 469-556. V-28 (1904) 319-418. VI-28
     (1904) 531-617.
42. Drillis, R.J. and Contini, R.   Body Segment Parameters.
     Technical Report No. 1166.03. School of Engineering and
     Science, New York Univ. (1966).
43. Zatsiorsky, V. and V. Seluyanov. The Gamma Mass Scanning
     Technique for Inertial Anthropometric Measurement.   J.
     Biomechanics (in press).
44. Barter, J.T. Estimation of the Mass of Body Segments. WADC
     Technical Report 57-260, Wright-Patterson Air Force Base,
     Ohio, (1957).
45. Hanavan, E.P. A Mathematical Model of the Human Body. Report
     No. AMRL-TR-102, Wright-Patterson AFB, Ohio (1964).
46. Jensen, R.K. Estimation of the Biomechanical Properties of
     Three Body Types Using a Photogrammetric Method.   J.
     Biomechanics 11 (1978) 349-358.
47. Hatze, H. A Mathematical Model for the Computational
     Determination of Parameter Values of Anthropomorphic Segments.
     J. Biomechanics 13 (1980) 833-843.
48. Miller, D.J. and W.E. Morrison. Prediction of Segmental
     Parameters Using the Hanavan Human Body Model. Med. Sci.
     Sports 7 (1975) 207-212.
49. Cappozzo, A. The Forces and Couples in the Human Trunk during
     Level Walking. J. Biomechanics 16 (1983) 265-277.
50. Cappozzo, A., Leo, T. and A. Pedotti. A General Computing
     Method for the Analysis of Human Locomotion. J. Biomechanics
     8 (1975) 307-320.
51. Vaughan, C.L., Andrews, J.G. and J.G. Hay. Selection of Body
     Segment Parameters by Optimization Methods. J. Biomech.
     Engng. 104 (1982) 38-44.
52. Andrews, B. and D. Jones. A Note on the Differentiation of
     Human Kinematic Data. Dig. 11-th Internat. Conf. on Medical
     and Biological Engng. (Ottawa, 1976), pp. 88-89.
53. Lanshammar, H. On Practical Evaluation of Differentiation
     Techniques for Human Gait Analysis. J. Biomechanics 15 (1982)
     99-105.
54. Cappozzo, A., Leo, T. and V. Macellari. The CoSTEL Kinematics
     Monitoring System: Performance and Use in Human Movement
     Measurements.   In   H.   Matsui   and   K.   Kobayashi   ed.s,
     Biomechanics VIII-A (Champaign: Human Kinetics Pub, 1982).
55. Plagenhoef, S.C. Computer Programs for Obtaining Kinetic Data
     on Human Movements. J. Biomechanics 1 (1968) 221-234.
56. Dierckx, P. An Algorithm for Smoothing, Differentiation and
     Integration of Experimental Data Using Spline Functions.   J.
     Comp. appl. Nat. 1 (1975) 165-184.
57. Wood, G.A. and L.S. Jennings. On the Use of Spline Functions
     for Data Smoothing. J. Biomechanics 12 (1979) 477-479.

58. Jackson, M.K. Fitting of Mathematical Functions to Biomechanical Data. IEEE Trans. Biomed. Eng. BME-26 2 (1979) 122-124.

59. Winter, D.A., Sidwall, H.G. and D.A. Hobson. Measurements and Reduction of Noise in Kinematics of Locomotion. J. Biomechanics 7 (1974) 157-159.

60. Gustafsson, L. and H. Lanshammar. ENOCH An Integrated System for Measurement and Analysis of Human Gait. Institute of Technology, Uppsala University, S-751-21, Uppsala, Sweden (1977).

61. Lesh, M.D., Mansour, J.M. and S.R. Simon. A Gait Analysis Subsystem for Smoothing and Differentiation of Human Motion Data. Trans. ASME J. Biomech. Eng. 101 (1979) 205-212.

62. McClellan, J.H., Parks, T.W., and L.R. Rabiner. A Computer Program for Designing Optimum FIR Linear Phase Filters. IEEE Tran. Audio Electroac. AU-21 (1973) 506-526.

63. Andrews, B., Cappozzo, A. and F. Gazzani. A Quantitative Method for Assessment of Differentiation Techniques Used for Locomotion Analysis. In J. P. Paul, M. W. Ferguson-Pell, M. M. Jordan and B.J. Andrews ed.s, Computing in Medicine (London: The MacMillan Press, 1982), pp. 146-154.

64. Hamming, R.W. Digital Filters. (Englewood Cliffs, Prentice Hall, 1977).

65. Anderssen, R.S. and P. Bloomfield. Numerical Differentiation Procedures for Non-Exact Data. Numer. Math. 22 (1974) 157-182.

66. Hatze, H. The Use of Optimally Regularized Fourier Series for Estimating Higher-Order Derivatives of Noisy Biomechanical Data. J. Biomechanics 14 (1981) 13-18.

GAIT ANALYSIS AS A TOOL TO ASSESS JOINT KINETICS

T. P. Andriacchi and A. B. Strickland

Rush-Presbyterian-St. Luke's Medical Center
Department of Orthopedic Surgery
1753 West Congress Parkway
Chicago, Illinois 60612

1. INTRODUCTION

There has been an increasing interest in the use of gait analysis as a clinical and research tool in recent years. The development of computerized systems for acquisition and processing of gait measurements has made large scale use of gait analysis feasible. Analysis and interpretation of the vast quantity of measurements that come from the gait laboratories have become the major problem associated with their use. There is clearly a need for careful planning in the preparation of a gait analysis study. Such a study should be sufficiently focused to achieve an understanding of either the normal or pathological processes that could not be obtained subjectively from general observations (1,2).

Some guidelines to consider in the planning of a study of normal or pathological gait are the following: a) the need to address a specific question. This involves forming a hypothesis and methods to test the hypothesis. b) Careful control of interdependent gait variables should be maintained. For example, the speed of walking greatly influences quantitative measures of most gait variables. c) Careful selection criteria among patient groups should be defined. This is quite crucial to provide valid statistical comparison among experimental groupings. d) A knowledge of the sensitivity of the measurement system is required. Also, one should have an understanding of the variation of particular measurements in a normal population. e) Variables with physical meaning should be selected. This is important when attempting to look at the theoretical basis for understanding the causes and effects of gait abnormalities in patient groups.

The above points will be illustrated by examples of two studies of patients treated with total hip and total knee replacement.

The approach to these total joint replacement studies was to use an analysis of limb kinetics (relating force to motion). This served as the theoretical basis for addressing several specific questions related to the design and usage of these total joint implants. This is a reasonable basis for a study because level walking is achieved by angular movement of limb segments. Angular segmental motion is related to the moments generated by the muscles. Furthermore, externally measured moments can be related to internal forces acting on the joints and in particular on the implants and in the muscles. The approach we have taken is a classical approach that has been understood and described in the literature. The following is a brief background of some of the relevant literature.

1.1 Background

Quantitative description of human locomotion in kinetic terms has been in the literature for over 100 years (3-5). In more recent times the approach to this problem has been to record limb motion and foot-ground reaction force simultaneously (6-11), in order to carry out a mechanical analysis of the forces, moments and limb motion of the thigh, shank and foot segments during walking. Other investigators, (12) have attempted to reconstruct the kinetics of walking by relying only on the measurement of motion and the approximation of the limb segment inertia property of each of the segments of the lower extremities and torso. The forces necessary to produce the observed motions must then be calculated using the equations of dynamics.

In general, kinetic studies of gait have combined the gait observations with mathematical models (13-18) to compute forces and moments at the joints. Several studies have focused on a single joint and have used either reduction methods or optimization techniques to estimate internal muscle and joint forces. There has also been some analysis of the relationship between generalized force magnitudes acting at the joints and speed of walking (10,15).

A common difficulty in applying these studies to the interpretation of normal gait is the small number of observations. This limitation was due in part to the amount of time required for data acquisition and reduction. Computerization of data acquisition and reduction has made it practical to use kinetic measurements in gait analysis studies.

Kinematic and kinetic measurements have been applied to several studies of patients with total joint replacements. Rydell

(19) studied and compared the gait of two patients with instrumented Austin-Moore type prostheses. This study provided quantitative information on the in vivo forces occurring at the joints during activities of daily living. Because of the obvious difficulties of doing a larger study of this nature and the fact that these two patients were not walking normally, it was difficult to extrapolate the results of this study to normal locomotion or even patients with other types of total hip replacement.

Murray, et al. (20) reported two dimensional kinematic measurements during walking in 30 patients before and following the McKee-Farrar total hip reconstruction. The results showed improvement in patients following hip reconstruction, but still subnormal function in some time-distance and sagittal plane motion measurements at 6 months post-operation. McGrouther (18) examined the pre and post-operative gait of three patients who had undergone Charnley-type hip reconstruction. Results indicated grossly abnormal joint moments prior to surgery with improvement following reconstruction. However, the post-operative moments were still abnormal. This study was conducted in only three patients. In a more recent study Johnson, et al. (21) mathematically predicted the forces acting about the reconstructed hip joint based on the three dimensional kinematic and kinetic measurements of one normal subject. The assumption was made that gait patterns would not be altered by slight displacement of the location of the hip joint center. Their results showed that the hip joint loading can be greatly altered by displacement of the center of the joint.

Several studies have evaluated gait patterns in patients with knee disease. These investigations included kinematic measurements (22-27) and force plate measurements. There have also been several kinetic and force analysis studies of function in normal subjects and in patients after treatment for knee disability (16-18). The common finding among these studies was that patients who appeared to be clinically asymptomatic after joint replacement have abnormal gait patterns. There is still much to investigate concerning the nature of the gait abnormalities in patients following total joint replacement, its relationship to the design of the total joint replacements or its effect on the mechanical life of the joint replacement. Questions of this kind can be addressed through appropriate kinetic analysis of normal and abnormal gait following total joint replacement.

2. METHODOLOGY FOR KINETIC MEASUREMENT OF GAIT

2.1 Theoretical Basis and Simplifying Assumptions

The analysis of the motion of the limb segments requires the definition of a set of governing equations and assumptions. If each limb segment is idealized as a rigid body moving in three dimensional space, there are six scalar equations defining the general three dimensional forces and motion of each segment (6).

These six equations can be solved for the extrinsic forces and moments acting at the joints by measuring the ground reaction force and limb motion. The joint reactions are sequentially obtained starting with the foot ground reaction force moving up to the ankle, the knee, and the hip during support phase.

To implement this approach the leg was conceptualized as shown in Fig. 1 with lump mass approximations for the thigh segment and shank and foot segment. Several investigators have done an analysis of the influence of the inertial approximation (29,30) on the calculation of joint reaction forces and moments. During stance phase these factors play a much less significant role than the influence of the foot ground reaction force since the accelerations are relatively low. However, during swing phase appropriate inertial modeling may be more critical.

2.2   Estimate of Joint Center Error

Another factor limiting the accuracy of the calculation of joint reaction moment is the location of the actual joint center from external markers. Shown in Fig. 2 are the placements of six external markers located with light emitting diodes at the anterior-superior iliac spine, greater trochanter, center of the lateral joint line of the knee, lateral malleolus, lateral aspect of the calcaneus and base of the fifth metatarsal. The positions of the joint centers at the hip, knee and ankle were located in the sagittal plane by the position of the light emitting diodes at the greater trochanter, lateral joint line of the knee, and lateral malleolus, respectively. The frontal plane position of the center of the knee joint was located by identifying the mid-point of the line between the peripheral margins of the medial and lateral plateau at the level of the joint surface. Similarly, the ankle joint center was estimated at the mid-point of a line from the tip of the lateral malleolus to the tip of the medial malleolus. The center of the hip joint was located at 1.5 cm distal to the mid-point of a line from the anterior-superior iliac spine to the pubic symphysis. Since it is not always possible to take X-rays of the joints of patients who will be candidates for gait analysis, it is important to have an estimate of the error and the approximation of the joint center position.

A study was conducted to predict the error associated with the joint center placements as described above. The hip was selected as the joint where maximum error would occur. Twenty patients free of hip pathology were studied. Antero-posterior pelvic X-rays were taken with markers located on the greater trochanter to represent

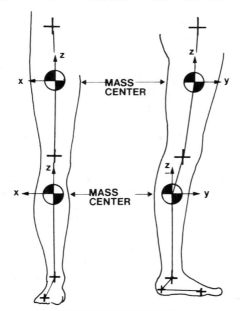

LIMB DYNAMIC MODEL

Fig. 1 A lumped mass model of the lower extremities for approximating inertial properties.

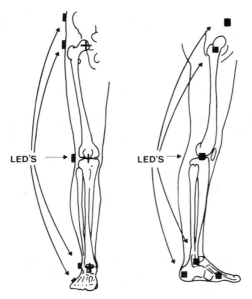

LED PLACEMENT

Fig. 2 The position of the external markers used for positional measurements indicated by the LED. Also shown are the corrected location of the joint centers.

the location of the LED marker used in gait analysis. A scale was also located in each X-ray to adjust for magnification. The hip joint center was approximated on each patient using the method described above on the marker location. In addition, the true location of the hip joint relative to the marker was measured in each X-ray. The average of error between the surface measurements and the actual measurements from the X-rays was 0.79 cm.

A study was conducted to determine the influence of this error on the calculation of the joint reaction moment, since this quantity would be most greatly influenced by this error. Shown in Fig. 3 is the effect of an LED location error on the normal pattern of hip flexion extension moment when the joint center was moved 1.6 cm anterior and 1.6 cm posterior to the nominal joint center position. These errors are superimposed on the intrinsic errors associated with the instrumentation, photogrametric techniques (31), and filtering schemes. The perturbation approach shown in Fig. 3 was conducted for each joint in each component direction to give an estimate of sensitivity of the joint moments to net system errors. This information allowed us to define the sensitivity window of our measurements.

The instrumentation (31,32) used for the studies described in this chapter included an opto-electronic system for motion analysis, a piezo-electric force plate and a mini-computer system for data acquisition and processing. The two cameras of the opto-electronic system were placed symmetrically with respect to the walkway.

3.   NORMAL VARIATION IN JOINT MOMENTS DURING LEVEL WALKING

The methodology previously described was used to record and analyze more than 300 gait cycles over a range of walking speeds in 29 normal subjects. It was hypothesized that we would be able to identify patterns of moments that would fall within a range of normal variation that would account for individual differences, retest variability, sexual differences, and walking speed. The three dimensional moments acting at the hip, knee and ankle joints during level walking were studied.

Twenty-nine normal adults (15 females and 14 males) were studied. The average age of the entire group was 39.4 years, (female group was 40.5 and the male group was 38.9). No musculo-skeletal or neurological abnormalities existed, and on visual gait observation, all subjects walked without a limp.

Each subject was observed bilaterally, wearing shoes, over 12 stride cycles, 6 on the left side and 6 on the right side. A stride cycle was defined as the interval between successive heel-

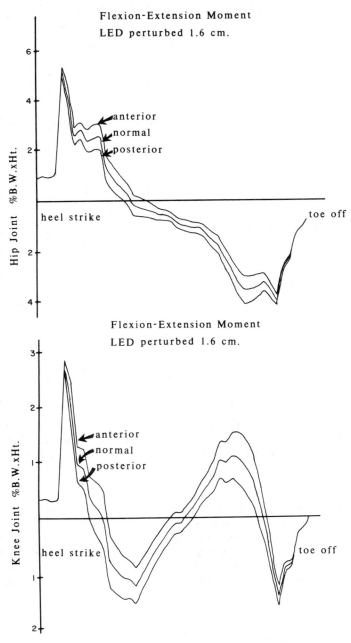

Fig. 3 The influence of an anterior and posterior positional error of the joint centers on the flexion—extension moment of the hip and knee.

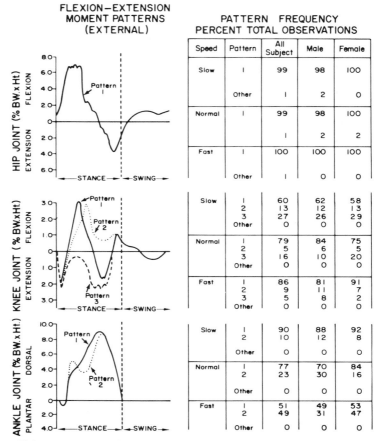

FLEXION–EXTENSION
MOMENT PATTERNS
(EXTERNAL)

PATTERN FREQUENCY
PERCENT TOTAL OBSERVATIONS

Speed	Pattern	All Subject	Male	Female
Slow	I	99	98	100
	Other	I	2	0
Normal	I	99	98	100
		I	2	2
Fast	I	100	100	100
	Other	I	0	0
Slow	I	60	62	58
	2	13	12	13
	3	27	26	29
	Other	0	0	0
Normal	I	79	84	75
	2	5	6	5
	3	16	10	20
	Other	0	0	0
Fast	I	86	81	91
	2	9	11	7
	3	5	8	2
	Other	0	0	0
Slow	I	90	88	92
	2	10	12	8
	Other	0	0	0
Normal	I	77	70	84
	2	23	30	16
	Other	0	0	0
Fast	I	51	49	53
	2	49	31	47
	Other	0	0	0

Fig. 4 An illustration of the most frequently occurring patterns of
flexion-extension moments at the hip, knee, and ankle joint. The
table gives the percentages out of 316 stride cycles that each
pattern occurs.

strikes on the same foot including the support and swing phase. A
total of 348 stride cycles were measured in this study. One stride
cycle was observed for traverse of a 10 meter walkway. However,
for various reasons 316 of the 348 observations were analyzed. The
primary reason for not including all stride cycles was marker
blockage during the stride cycle, usually due to arm movement.

3.1 Results

At the hip joint, the flexion-extension moment in 99
percent of all stride cycles had the same pattern (Fig. 4). The
same pattern was used by both males and females. There was also no
change in this pattern with walking speed. However, as will be

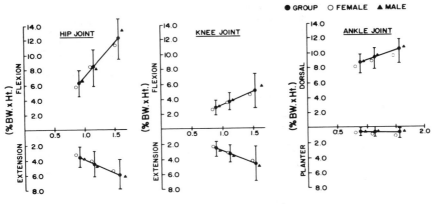

Fig. 5 The variation of the maximum amplitude of the flexion-extension moment with walking speed at the hip, knee and ankle joint.

described later, the maximum magnitudes of the moments increased with walking speed.

At the knee joint three patterns of normal moments were identified in the flexion-extension direction (Fig. 4). The most frequently occurring pattern (Pattern 1) was present in 79 percent of all stride cycles at a normal walking speed. The predominance of Pattern 1 seems to be dependent on walking speed. At a slow walking speed there was an increase in both Pattern 2 and Pattern 3, similarly at a fast walking speed Pattern 1 moments tended to increase.

At the ankle joint two patterns of flexion-extension moment were identified. Pattern 1 occurred in 77 percent of total observations at a normal walking speed. In this pattern the external moment tended to plantar flex the ankle throughout the major portion of stance phase.

The maximum amplitudes of the flexion-extension moments at the hip, knee and ankle joints were influenced by the speed of walking (Fig. 5). It should be noted that all magnitudes reported here were normalized to percent body weight times height. Using this normalization we found no difference between the magnitudes of the moments in males and females. However, before normalization there was a statistically significant ($p < 0.05$) difference between males and females when compared as showed in Fig. 5.

The pattern of abduction-adduction moment at the hip joint was the same for all subjects (Fig. 6). A similar pattern of

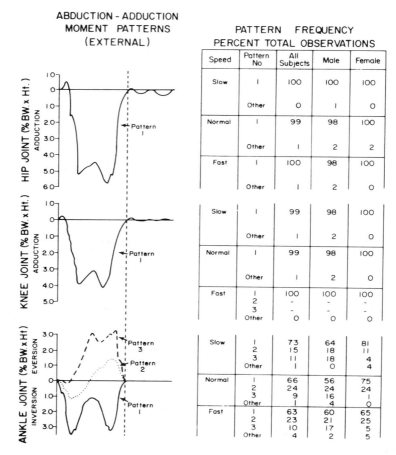

Fig. 6 An illustration of the most frequently occurring pattern of abduction-adduction moment at the hip, knee and ankle joints. The table gives the percentages out of 316 stride cycles that each pattern occurs.

abduction-adduction moment was observed at the knee joint. This pattern was also predominant among all subjects male and female and at all walking speeds. At the ankle joint there were three common patterns of inversion-eversion moments. The predominant pattern occurring in 66 percent of the observations tended to invert the ankle throughout stance phase. The moments at the ankle joint tended to show the greatest individual variation from subject to subject.

No significant relationship between the magnitudes of the abduction-adduction moment and walking speed could be identified.

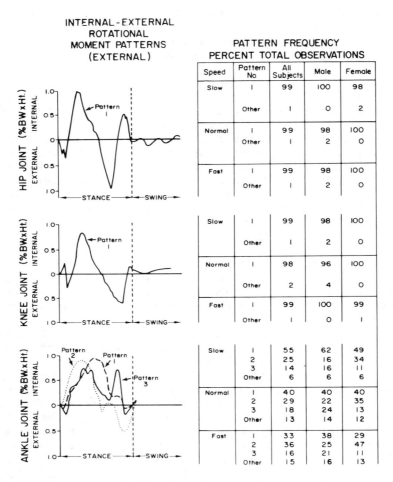

Fig. 7 An illustration of the most frequently occurring patterns of internal-external rotation moments at the hip, knee and ankle joints. The table gives the percentages out of 316 stride cycles that each pattern occurs.

The magnitudes for the normal walking speed were statistically the same for the slow and fast speeds.

The internal-external rotation moment at the hip joint (Fig. 7) was also quite consistent. One pattern was observed in more than 99 percent of all observations in both male and female subjects at all walking speeds. A similar pattern was found at the knee with same frequency of occurrence. Again, the ankle joint showed the largest variation among subjects. Three patterns were observed to occur at the ankle joint. Pattern 1 occurring in

40 percent of the total observations at a normal walking speed was
the most frequent. There were no significant trends in the
magnitudes of the internal-external rotation moments at the hip,
knee or ankle joints with walking speed.

3.2 Discussion

     The moments determined in this study were acting externally on
the hip, knee and ankle joints. However, basic mechanical princi-
pals require that these external moments be balanced, in a dynamic
sense by equal and opposite internal moments. The muscles are the
primary internal structures capable of generating internal moments
sufficient to balance these externally generated moments. In some
cases, the moments were probably balanced by a combination of
muscle forces, ligamentous tension and joint contact forces.
Therefore, the joint contact forces are also proportional to the
moments acting on the joints.

     The appropriate application of these parameters to the study
of normal and abnormal function requires an understanding of the
variability that can be expected in a population of normal
subjects. The study demonstrates that many of the components of
the moments are reprducible among normal subjects. The moments
acting at the hip joint were the most reproducible. The knee joint
moment patterns had somewhat more variability than the hip. More
variability was found at slower speeds at the knee. In testing
patients with knee disabilities one should be aware of the possible
variations in these patterns at the slower speeds. If possible,
knee patients should be tested at walking speeds of at least 1
meter per second or faster to reduce interobservation variability.
The ankle joint has the most variation in patterns of moments of
the three joints. It should be noted that these variations
exceeded the type that result from system errors, discussed
earlier, and thus could be attributed to actual variations among
normal walking patterns.

     It is important to account for influences of walking speed
when evaluating the magnitudes of the moments. The maximum
amplitude of the moments in the flexion and extension directions
increase with walking speed. The largest changes with speed occur
in the magnitude of the moment tending to flex the hip joint.
These changes are probably related to increase in stride length
with walking speed.

     The magnitudes of the moment tending to abduct and adduct the
joints should not be ignored when calculating forces exerted on the
joints. Large moments tend to adduct the joints throughout the
stance phase. At the knee joint, the magnitude of the adduction
moment is larger than the flexion or extension moments. The moment

in this direction would tend to compress the medial compartment of the knee and stretch the lateral soft tissue.

The magnitude of the internal-external rotation moments during level walking are relatively small and probably do not produce significant stresses on the joints or soft tissue during normal level walking. However, other activities in daily living may produce significantly higher stresses in these directions.

The size of the subject is also an important consideration when attempting to compare moment magnitudes among normal subjects. The size-normalization factors selected for this study was the product of body weight and height. This measurement is easily obtained, reproducible and easily identified. It non-dimensionalizes the moment magnitude, and seems to account for subject size variation. For example, if the average size difference between the male and female subjects in this study were not accounted for, the magnitudes of the moments would differ by as much as 40 percent between male and female subjects. After normalization the moment magnitudes were statistically the same.

The application of joint reaction moments to the study of normal and abnormal function during gait has received increased interest in recent years. These parameters are useful indicators of function during gait and may have useful clinical applications. They provide the most direct non-invasive method for observing kinetic function and inferring muscle action without requiring sophisticated mathematical models. Other gait measurements such as time-distance and kinematic parameters are useful indicators of the presence of a gait abnormality, but the joint moments have the potential of providing a way to find the cause and source of these abnormalities.

4.   THE INFLUENCE OF HIP RECONSTRUCTION ON GAIT

The hypothesis addressed in this study (33) was that the placement of the femoral head at a reconstructed hip would influence the abduction-adduction and flexion-extension moments as well as motion at the hip joint. Specifically, we hypothesized that mechanically shortening the moment arm of the hip abductor would be reflected in modified abduction-adduction moments at the joint.

Thirty subjects were studied. Twenty of these were taken from a population of patients who had undergone unilateral hip reconstruction performed by a single primary surgeon. The remaining 10 subjects were an age-matched group of normal subjects without previous musculoskeletal trauma or disease. The selection criteria for the 20 patients included the following: a) unilateral primary

degenerative joint disease or traumatic arthritis, b) a hip reconstruction using the Charnley—Mueller prosthesis without trochan-
teric osteotomy, c) a minimum post-operative follow-up of 12
months, d) an age between 50 and 80 years, e) an excellent clinical
result on the basis of a Harris hip score of 95 or greater, and f)
less than 1 cm of leg length discrepancy.

The patients were separated into two groups based on the
radiographically determined length of the hip abductor moment arm.
The hip abductor arm was measured relative to the non-operated
side. The patients were placed in one group (Group 1) if the
abductor of the moment arm was shortened by at least 8 mm. The
other patients (Group 2) was selected to have a hip abductor moment
arm that was shortened by not more than 1 mm when compared to the
contralateral side.

4.1 Results

Surprisingly, there was no statistically significant difference in the magnitude of the abduction-adduction moment that could
be correlated to the difference in the abductor moment arms of the
two groups. There was however a statistically different magnitude
of flexion-extension moment in the patient group with unshortened
(Group 2) abductor moment arm. Further the group of patients with
the unshortened abductor moment arm had a lower than normal range
of flexion-extension motion at the hip joint. The average flexion-
extension motion for this group was 27 degrees compared to 40
degrees in normals. This range of motion also was significantly
different than the 38 degrees of motion found in the reconstructed
hip of the group with the shortened abductor moment arm. The
difference in the range of flexion-extension motion was coupled to
a difference in the magnitude of the maximum flexion moment at the
hip joint in the patient group (Group 2) with the unshortened
abductor moment arm. The magnitude of this moment was significantly higher than normal, whereas in the group with the shortened
moment arm the peak flexion moment was statistically normal. The
group of patients with the shortened abductor moment arm had a gait
that was indistinguishable from normal.

4.2 Discussion

The results of the study did not support our initial hypothesis. However, the results have some important implications on
total hip reconstruction. The valgus position of the femoral
component associated with the shortening of the abductor moment arm
as in the Group 1 patient appears to be favorable from both the
clinical viewpoint and from a functional viewpoint during gait.
Results of this study provide additional explanation for the
apparent improved clinical result in patients with femoral components placed in a valgus position. For example, the higher
moment tending to flex the hip joint would require a higher than

normal extensor force at heel strike in the patients with the abnormal gait (Group 2). This could have adverse long term effects. These patients are placing increased demands on the hip extensors and this increased force would also increase the magnitude of the resultant force on the femoral head.

The search for an explanation in the Group 2 patients must go beyond the antero-posterior dimensional changes in the center of the hip joint. The gait abnormality seems to indicate that changes in the sagittal plane orientation of the joint center and femoral neck angle should be investigated. This would include the degree of antiversion of the prosthetic femoral neck. This feature has not been studied in these patients and may well provide an explanation of the observed gait patterns. Clearly, these studies indicate that the orthopedic surgeon and the biomechanical engineer responsible for design should realize that changes in joint center location can affect gait patterns as well as load transmission at the hip joint which will affect the long term results of hip replacement.

5.   THE INFLUENCE OF TOTAL KNEE REPLACEMENT ON GAIT

The hypothesis of this study (32) was that one can identify a relationship between gait and total knee replacement design. Five prosthetic knees were selected for this study that were considered to be representative of cruciate ligament sacrificing and sparing designs with varying amounts of constraint.

Twenty-six patients, in five experimental groups were studied during level walking and stair climbing. The five implants selected for this study were the Geomedic, Gunston, total condylar, duopatellar, and Cloutier designs. The patients selected for this study were rated according to post-operative pain, function, passive range of motion, and joint stability. A point system based on the Hospital for Special Surgery knee rating system was used to quantitate post-operative status. All patients were evaluated at least one year post-operatively, and to qualify for this study a score of 85 or more on the basis of this system was required. Therefore, all patients had an excellent clinical result, were able to walk without aids, had little or no pain, were able to climb stairs in reciprocal manner. The resultant population for the experimental study consisted of 36 knees in 26 patients. No attempt was made to match the patients in terms of diagnosis, involvement of other joints, sex distribution, age or presence of bilateral total knee replacements. However, patients with moderate or severe involvement of other joints that was associated with pain were not included in the study.

An aged-matched control population of 14 healthy adults (7 men and 7 women) with an average age of 62.4 were also studied. The

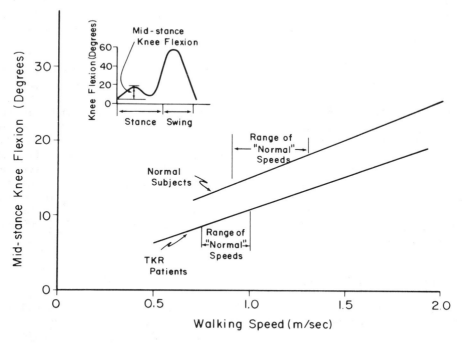

Fig. 8 An illustration of difference in the change of the relationship between knee flexion during stance and walking speed in control subjects and in patients (reproduced from Ref. 32).

gait of both the normal subjects and patients were measured during
12 stride cycles, each of which occurred mid-way during a separate
walking trial on a 10 meter walkway. Each subject was instructed
to walk at three nominal speeds: slow, normal and fast. Each
subject was also observed while ascending and descending a three
step staircase (32).

The range of self selected speeds tended to overlap those of
the three nominal speed categories. Nevertheless, for approximately 80 percent of the time patients' chosen speeds were within
their nominal range. Each of the other measurements (moments and
motion) of gait were considered with walking speed as an independent variable in order to separate differences in gait that were
due to factors other than changes in speed.

5.1   Results

The stride length of the patients with total knee replacement
was shorter than normal over the range of walking speeds. Simi-

Range of Knee Motion Climbing Up Stairs

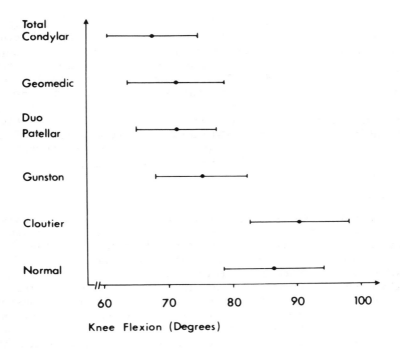

Fig. 9 The differences in the total range of motion of the knee while climbing up stairs among the five groups of patients and the control subjects. The patients with the Cloutier prostheses were the only group whose range of motion did not differ from that of the control group (reproduced from Ref. 32).

larly, the change in angle of knee flexion during stance phase (Fig. 8) was also significantly less in patients. In both parameters (stride length and stance knee flexion) there were no differences between the patients in terms of the different designs of prosthesis.

The third characteristic of the abnormal gait in the patients with total knee replacement was a pattern of external flexion-extension moment at the knee joint. The moments were compared by selecting the test conducted at a walking speed that was closest to 1 meter per second for each subject. Two abnormal moment patterns were found in the total knee replacement group. The two abnormal patterns, observed in the majority of patients were external moments predominantly tending to either flex or extend the joint throughout stance phase. Normally, the external moment oscillates between flexion and extension. The abnormalities in both the flexional and extensional moment patterns occurred during the middle portion of stance phase.

In contrast to level walking, patient function during stair climbing was clearly dependent on the design of the prosthesis. The Cloutier group (cruciate retaining unconstrained design) has statistically normal range of knee motion while climbing up and down the stairs (Fig. 9). The reduced range of motion during ascending the stairs was associated with the pattern of knee flexion-extension moments. The patients with the Cloutier prosthesis had a normal pattern of flexion-extension moment which tends to predominantly flex the knee. Patients with reduced range of motion had a moment pattern that was characterized by a sign reversal from flexion to extension at 44 percent of stance phase.

5.2 Discussion

This study presents evidence which reports the hypothesis that total knee replacement has a substantial influence on function. An analysis of the characteristics of the gait abnormalities and stair climbing abnormalities indicates that the abnormal function was associated with abnormal patterns of flexion-extension moments about the knee. These findings point to a potential explanation indicating that total knee replacement design has a substantial influence on the action of the knee musculature. Since all patient groups in this study had the same passive range of motion, the possibility exists that the interaction of the kinematics of the knee joint with the surrounding ligaments and muscles produce functional differences between designs. Normally, as the knee flexes between 0 and 90 degrees, the contact areas between the femur and tibia were moved posteriorly, increasing the mechanical advantage of the quadriceps significantly by increasing their moment arm about the condylar contact point. The mechanical advantage of this posterior movement may not be possible to the same degree in more constrained designs and thus gait during stair-climbing is potentially compromised. This explanation is consistent with the biomechanical findings of this study.

REFERENCES

1. Brand, R.A. and Crownshield, R.D. Comment on Criteria Patient
    Evaluation. J. Biomechanics, 14 (1980), 655.
2. Cappozzo, A. Consideration on Clinical Gait Evaluation. J.
    Biomechanics, 16 (1983), 302.
3. Braune, C.W., Fischer, O. Der Gan des Menschen. (Abhand
    lunger der Saechs. Gessellschaft der Wissenschaften, 1898),
    21-28.

4. Muybridge, E. The Human Figure in Motion. (Chapman and Hall, 1901).

5. Marey, E.J. LaMethode Graphique dans les Sciences Experimentales, (Masson, 1885).

6. Bresler, B. Frankel, J.P. The Forces and Moments in the Leg During Walking. Transactions of the American Society of Mechanical Engineering, 72 (1950), 27-36.

7. Cappozzo, A., Figura, F., Marchetti, M., Pedotti, A. The Interplay of Muscular and External Forces in Human Ambulation. Journal of Biomechanics, 6 (1976), 35-43.

8. Andriacchi, T.P., Andersson, G.B.J., Fermier, R.W., Stern, D., Galante, J.O. A Study of Lower Limb Mechanics During Stair-Climbing. Journal of Bone and Joint Surgery, 62-A (1980), 749-757.

9. Boccardi, S., Pedotti, A., Rodano, R., Santambrogio, G. Evaluation of Muscular Moments at the Lower Limb Joints by an On-Line Processing of Kinematics Data and Ground Reaction. Journal of Biomechanics, 14 (1981), 35-45.

10. Cavanagh, P.R., Gregor, R.J. Knee Joint Torque During the Swing Phase of Normal Treadmill Walking. Journal of Bio-mechanics, 8 (1975), 337-344.

11. Winter, D.A. Overall Principle of Lower Limb Support During Stance Phase of Gait. Journal of Biomechanics, 13 (1980), 923-927.

12. Zarrugh, M.Y. Kinematic Prediction of Intersegmental Loads and Power at the Joints of the Leg in Walking. Journal of Biomechanics, 14 (1981), 713-725.

13. Morrison, J.B. The Mechanics of the Knee Joint in Relation to Normal Walking. Journal of Biomechanics, 3 (1970), 51-61.

14. Paul, J.J. Force Actions Transmitted in the Knee of Normal Subjects and by Prosthetic Joint Replacements. Total Knee Replacement (The Institution of Mechanical Engineers, 1974).

15. Crowninshield, R.D., Johnston, R.C., Andrews, J.C., Brand, R.A. A Biomechanical Investigation of the Human Hip. Journal of Biomechanics, 11 (1978), 75-85.

16. Harrington, I.J. A Bioengineering Analysis of Force Actions At the Knee in Normal and Pathological Gait. Biomedical Engineering, May (1976), 167-172.

17. Johnson, F., Waugh, W. Method for Routine Clinical Assessment of Knee Joint Forces. Med. Biology Eng., 17 (1979), 145-154.

18. McGrouther, D.A. Evaluation of a Total Hip Replacement. Journal of Biomed. Mater. Res. Symp., No. 5 (Part 2) (1974), 271-283.

19. Rydell, N.W. Forces Acting on the Femoral Head-Prosthesis. Acta Orthopaedica Scandinavica, Supplement 88, 37 (1966).

20. Murray, M.P., Brewer, B.J., and Zuege, R.C. Kinesiologic Measurements of Functional Performance Before and After McKee-Farrar Total Hip Replacement. J. Bone and Joint Surg., 54-A (1972), 237-255.

21. Johnson, R.C., Brand, R.A., and Crowninshield, R.D. Reconstruction of the Hip. J. Bone and Joint Surg., 61-A (1979), 639-652.

22. Andriacchi, T.P., Ogle, J.A., and Galante, J.O. Walking Speed as a Basis for Normal and Abnormal Gait Measurements. Journal of Biomechanics, 10 (1977), 261-268.

23. Chao, E.Y. Functional Evaluation of Total Knee Replacement Patients Through Gait Analysis. (American Society of Mechanical Engineers, Publication 75-APMB-5, 1975).

24. Chao, E.Y., Laughman, R.K., and Stauffer, R.N. Biomechanical Gait Evaluation of Pre and Postoperative Total Knee Replacement Patients. Arch. Orthop. Traumat. Surg., 97 (1980), 309-317.

25. Goldflies, M.L., Andriacchi, T.P., and Galante, J.O. The Relationship between Varus Deformity and Moments at the Knee During Gait and the Changes at the Knee after High Tibial Osteotomy. Trans. Orthop. Res. Soc., 6 (1981), 54.

26. Kettelkamp, D.B., and Leaverton, P.E. Gait Characteristics of the Rheumatoid Knee. Arch. Surg., 104 (1972), 30-34.

27. Rittmen, Nancy, Kettlekamp, D.B., Prior, Philip, Schwartzkopf, G.L., and Hillberry, Ben. Analysis of Patterns of Knee Motion Walking for Four Types of Total Knee Implants. Clin. Orthop., 155 (1981), 111-117.

28. Dempster, W.T., Gaughran, R.L. Properties of Body Segments Based on Size and Weight. American Journal of Anatomy, 120 (1967), 33-54.

29. Mikosz, R.P., Andriacchi, T.P., Hampton, S.J., Galante, J.O. The Importance of Limb Segment Inertia on Joint Loads During Gait. (Transactions of the 99th Winter Annual Meeting of the A.S.M.E., San Francisco, 1978).

30. Wells, R.P. The Projection of the Ground Reaction Force as a Predictor of Internal Joint Moments. Bull. of Prosth. Res. 18:1 (1981), 15-19.

31. Andriacchi, T.P., Hampton, S.S., Schultz, A.B., and Galante, J.O. Three Dimensional Coordinate Data Processing In Human Motion Analysis. J. of Biomechanical Engineering, 101 (1978) 279-288.

32. Andriacchi, T.P., Galante, J.O. and Fermer, R.W. The Influence of Total Knee Replacement On Function During Walking and Stair Climbing. 64A:9 (1982), 1328-1335.

33. Hodge, W.A., Andriacchi, T.P., and Galante, J.O. Influence of Hip Reconstruction on Gait. (Am. College of Surgeons, Surgical Forum, Vol. XXXI), 517-519.

BIOMECHANICS OF THE JOINTS IN THE LEG

J. P. Paul

Bioengineering Unit, University of Strathclyde
Glasgow, Scotland, U.K.

Biomechanical analysis is frequently used with reference to Wolff's Law (1) to explain the disposition of material in anatomical structures particularly with regard to the orientation of the trabeculae in the bone of the upper femoral shaft, neck and head. Most workers except Wolff's Law as an article of faith since it seems eminently reasonable; although to the knowledge of the present author there has been no scientific validation of its relevance nor indeed an exploration of its modus operandi. For instance, it is not known whether the structure of the bone corresponds to the integral over a long period of the average value of loading experienced by the bone or whether it corresponds to the load actions developing higher than average stresses on a restricted number of occasions. Similarly, it is easy to conceive that there will be minimum and maximum thresholds corresponding to no laying down of bone or resorption of bone respectively. It is interesting to note that the lines of the trabeculae in the proximal femur are frequently associated with the lines of principal stress obtained by various means related to the loading of the head of femur and the greater trochanter. Rarely is the loading due to muscular forces included and few such studies assess the sensitivity of the position of the stress lines to the assumed direction of loading on the femoral head.

Ideally in the assessment of the function and loading of joint replacement one should consider the full three dimensional loading system, although frequently the two dimensional situation of one legged standing is used for this purpose. This situation is not the same as the transient situation during the stance phase of walking since in one legged standing the displacement of the center of mass over the supporting foot corresponds to greater angles of

adduction of the femur that occur in the walking cycle. This view
is useful however in the assessment of the effect of placing of the
acetabular cup on the loading to be expected in the muscles and the
joints. Fig. 1 shows the ground force acting on the supporting leg
during single support passing medial to the hip joint and balance
being maintained by tension in some of the abductor muscles. In
Fig. 1(a) the effect is shown of placement of the acetabular cup in
superior position to the natural anatomical situation as frequently
occurs during surgery. The lever arm of the external force is
unchanged and there is very little change in the lever arm of the
abductor muscles, as can be seen by comparison of the dotted
perpendicular line to the full perpendicular line. Where there is
a significant change is in the effective length of the muscles and
it may be expected that following this procedure the behavior of
the muscle will be altered corresponding to a movement along the
length/tension diagram towards the origin. This may account for
delayed strengthening of the abductor muscles in the period of
rehabilitation following surgery.

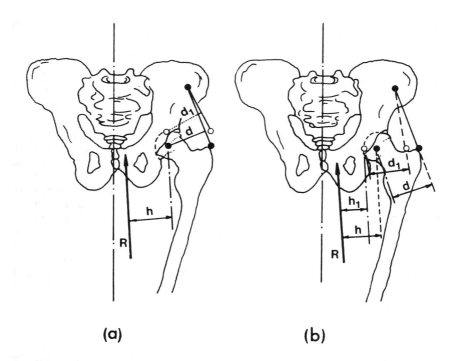

(a)   (b)

Fig. 1 The effect of acetabular cup placement on abductor muscle
and external load lever arms: (a) cup placed superior to the
natural anatomical joint, and (b) cup placed medial to the natural
anatomical joint. (Dots indicate the natural joint, and circles
indicate joint geometry after anthroplasty).

   In Fig. 1(b) the effect of more medial placement of the
acetabular cup is shown and this does not greatly affect the lever
arm of the abductor muscles; but by reduction of the lever arm of
the external force the required tension in the abductors is reduced
and the joint force will therefore be reduced. It is worth noting
however that, because of the movement medially, the line of action
of the abductor muscles will move closer to the vertical and thus
the line of action of the resultant joint force will be even closer
to the vertical. In these circumstances there is a danger that
most of the load on the acetabular cup will be transmitted at its
surface rim leading possibly to enhanced wear or plastic deformation or to the possibility of subluxation, if there is any defi-
ciency in the effective function of the inward rotator group of
muscles. This effect will be increased also if, as frequently
happens, the effective length of the femoral neck is reduced by the
surgical procedure on the femur.

ACTIVITY		JOINT FORCE MAXIMA*		
		Hip	Knee	Ankle
Level Walking	1.1 m/s	4.9	2.7	---
	1.5 m/s	4.9	2.8	3.85
	2.0 m/s	7.6	4.3	---
Stairs	Ascent	7.2	4.4	---
	Descent	7.1	4.9	---
Ramp	Ascent	5.9	3.7	---
	Descent	5.1	4.4	___

Table 1 Maximum values of forces at leg joints in various
activities.

*Forces are expressed in multiples of body weight.

If data from locomotion tests on normal individuals are analysed and the hip joint force is obtained by consideration of muscles in anatomically and functionally selected groups as mentioned in the chapter on mathematical modeling, then the values of load calculated for the hip joint are shown in Table 1, for walking in a straight line on a level surface at uniform speeds and also for walking on stairs and ramps. The high values of force seen at the hip joint correspond not to changes in the values of ground/foot force relative to those experienced while standing stationary but rather to the structural effect due to the line of action of the ground force being offset from the axes through the hip joint and therefore causing moments resisted by muscular tension. The lever arms of the muscles are generally less than the lever arms of the external load and therefore the joint forces are considerably higher due to this structural effect. The magnitude and direction of the joint force can be obtained in approximate terms by considering only the ground to foot force, resisted by muscle and ligament, but the values mentioned in the table have had the total dynamic situation considered in respect of gravitational and inertial load actions corresponding to the masses of the proximal body segments using the segmental mass properties quoted by Contini and Drillis (2).

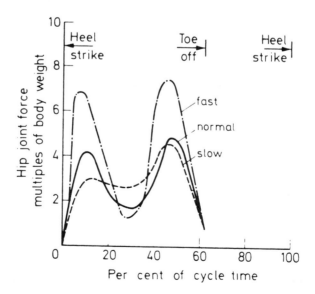

Fig. 2 Hip joint force at different walking speeds.

The variation with time for the hip joint force at walking speeds is shown in Fig. 2, maximum joint forces are obviously occurring in stance phase and show a double peaked variation with time.

In engineering analysis the direction of a force is frequently more important than its actual value and Fig. 3 shows the directions of hip joint force seen with respect to the proximal femur in the frontal and lateral views. The two arrows in each case refer respectively to the first and second maxima in the curve of variations of load with time. It is of interest to note the forward and backward component of load on the femoral head which must inevitably give rise to a twisting load action being transferred between any surgical implant and the shaft of femur.

Since Wolff's Law (1) is not specific on the question of whether a few isolated load cycles of higher magnitude will give rise to remodeling of bone it appears reasonable to bear in mind the analysis of joint replacement loading that normal individuals undertake occasionally activities which may be more stressful than level surface walking. Table 1 shows also th effect on the hip joint of stair and ramp negotiation. Elsewhere in this book results for runners in side stepping as far as the moments

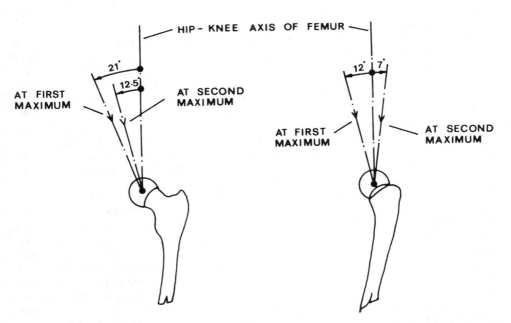

Fig. 3 Direction of hip joint force relative to the proximal femur in the frontal and lateral views.

transmitted at the hip are concerned are also reported. However, there has been no analysis known to this author of such side stepping, at normal walking pace, as required to negotiate obstacle or in busy streets or on cornering or access to motor vehicles. These may be expected to yield quite high results for torsional loading.

The natural knee is a complex structure, involving a patello-femoral joint and a two compartment bibiofemoral joint and the analysis of this by Morrison (3) has been altered only in detail by subsequent authors. The analysis is realistic in respect of flexion/extension loading and adduction/abduction loading, although were it to be applied to situations of severe torsion as in sports injuries leading to torn ligaments then some refinement might be necessary. In this analysis loading intended to flex the knee is considered to be resisted by tension in the patellar ligament and the reference axis system is taken to be centered in the joint space at the position of closest approach of the bony structures as of the femur and tibia as shown in lateral X-ray. In the lateral view this position is consistently just within the interior posterior border of the cortical shaft of the tibia even for quite large flexion angles. Lever arms are then determined for the muscle structures relative to this axis system. In the frontal view of the leg longitudial force will be distributed between the medial and lateral compartments of the knee joint depending on the bending moment which accompany the longitudial load. As the bending moment increases in the adducting direction which is the direction generally found through the stance phase of gait, the load taken by the medial compartment will progressively increase relative to that of the lateral. The situation frequently arises that the line of action of the resultant ground force lies outside of the joint capsule and in these circumstances the joint space tends to open on the lateral side if not prevented by external structures in tension, such as the lateral collateral ligaments or iliotibial tract. The same effect could be produced if there were different levels of force transmitted by the medial and lateral heads of hamstrings or by the corresponding heads of gastrocnemius. If the tension occurs in the passive structures it will obviously be one of the loads summing up to the total joint force. The tendency for anterior posterior movement of the tibia relative to the femur is resisted principally by the cruciate ligaments. In most analyses these, being passive structures, are taken to have no load in them except where this is nevessary to balance the components of the muscular and other ligamentous forces. The lines of action of forces corresponding to the situation described are shown in Fig. 4. If the external loading system is tending to extend the knee the muscles resisting this will be generally either the hamstrings or the gastrocnemius since studies show that these two groups are rarely active simultaneously. In this situation a decision is made corresponding to the EMG known to be developed at the phase of the gait cycle under consideration. In either situation the flexing/extending, abducting/adducting muscle forces are calculated and their longitudinal and anterior-posterior force components allow the calculation of the values of the forces in the internal structures and consequently the joint itself. Values of joint force for level walking activities are shown in Table 1, for a series of test subjects in the category of young, healthy individuals with no known disability.

It is of interest to look at some data relating to the performance of patients following joint replacement surgery. Data from a series of tests conducted at the University of Strathclyde, Glasgow, are shown in Fig. 5. Figure 5(b) shows a bar diagram indicating the magnitude of the force at the hip joint, expressed in multiples of body weight. Comparison is made between a normal population corresponding to the patients tested and the double

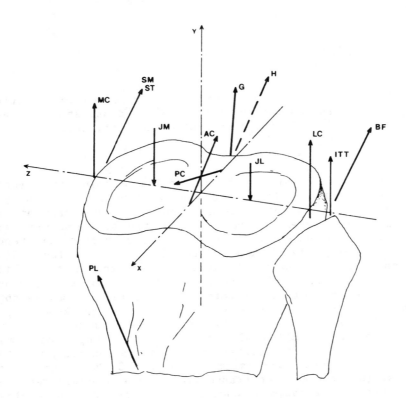

Fig 4. Lines of action of forces acting on the proximal tibia (see text).

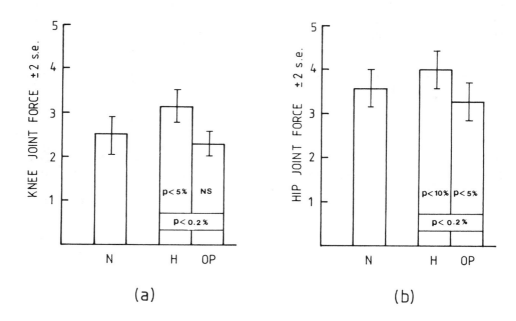

Fig 5. (a) Knee, and (b) hip joint forces expressed in multiples of body weight for the normal population (N), and operated (OP) and non-operated (H) sides of hip joint replacement patients.

block corresponds to the hip which has received a joint replacement and the contralateral side: bars indicate mean value and $\pm$ 2 standard errors. It is interesting to note how the force on the non-operated side is greater than that on the operated side and also is greater than the normal population although this difference is not statistically significant at the 95% level. Figure 5(a) shows corresponding values of the force transmitted at the tibio-femoral joint for patients who have received hip joint replacement. As before, the ordinate is joint force in multiples of body weight. Of interest there is the enhanced value of force at the knee on the side which did not receive the hip joint replacement and it is understood that it is clinical experience that this joint may frequently present with difficulties in the situation following the replacement of the contra-lateral hip. Figure 3 shows ,the direction and position of the force transmitted to the proximal femur at the three instances of maximum load, shown in Fig. 2. It is clear that the interface between the joint replacement and the bone will be loaded in a way which will give uneven pressure on the under-lying bone and may lead to eventual tilting of the prosthesis if there is a breakdown of the cement or of the underlying bony structure.

In the analysis of the biomechanics of the ankle joint it is unreasonable to define an orthogonal axis system since the directions of the axes of the talocrural and talocruralnavicular joints are inclined relative to the sagittal and frontal planes in the general anatomical situation. Loads transmitted by ground to foot can be resolved to give the resultant forces together with the moments about these two axes at the ankle. It may be noted however that in general one would modify the external load actions by the effects of gravity and acceleration on the masses of the segments intervening between the ground and the axes of interest. Even at the hip joint the inclusion of such terms affect the resultant load actions by at worst, approximately 10%, and thus their exclusion in particular analyses does not affect the end results greatly. The data in this chapter has however included the effect of gravitational and inertial effects where appropriate. The analysis presented here relates to the situation in level walking where inversion/eversion and plantar/dorsi flexion are not limited by ligamentous restraints since the test subject will be walking within the middle range of these angles (4, 5). Gastrocnemius and soleus are plantar flexors and invertors and they are treated as one muscle group for the analysis. The posterior tibial muscle tibialis posterior, flexors, hallucis longus and flexor digitorum longus are also plantar flexors and invertors and are treated as a second group. The third group is the peroneal group, peroneus brevis and peroneus longus, their basic action is plantar flexion together with eversion. The only muscle which produces dorsi flexion and inversion is tibialis anterior; this is treated on its own. Finally, the extensors of the great and small toe tend to dorsi flex and evert and are treated as one group. To obtain a solution in the first instance, those muscles are taken to be active whose principal action resists the rotating tendency of the external load system at that particular instant in time. If the equilibrium of the connection of the foot to the shank is defined by the appropriate equations, with selection of appropriate muscle groups, one can obtain data such as in Fig. 6(a) indicating the variation with time of the forces in the calf group and the anterior tibial group of muscles during one walking cycle for seven test subjects walking at a uniform speed in a straight line on a level surface. Fig 6(b) shows the corresponding joint force resultant which has two peaks corresponding, firstly to the action of the anterior tibial muscles and secondly to the calf muscles. It will be noted that the value of joint force at between 3.5 and 4 times body weight is intermediate between those of the hip and the knee.

For the leg, there are obviously data relating to some of the regularly occurring activities, and it is probably realistic that

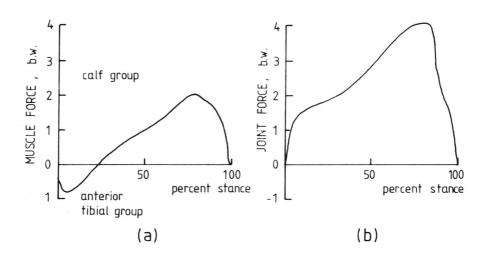

Fig. 6 (a) Force developed by the calf group and anterior tibial group of muscles during locomotion, and (b) the corresponding talocrural joint force, in multiples of body weight.

the design process for joint replacement should be undertaken relative to walking as an action corresponding to high loads on the joints which is repeated between one and two million times per annum possibly. Further attention should be paid to extending the range of data even in the fields which have been described here, but also in such maneuver as cornering and side stepping and in situations such as walking on busy pavements or walking on rough surfaces. Ideally one would have a measurement system with which the test subject could be freely ambulant.

REFERENCES

1.   Wolff, J.   Das Gesetz der Transformation der Knochen.   A Hirschwald, Berlin (1892).
2.   Contini, R. and Drillis, R.S.   Body Segment Mass Properties, Tech. Report 1166.03, New York University (1966).
3.   Morrison, J.B.   Bioengineering Analysis of Force Actions Transmitted by the Knee Joint.   Biomedical Engineering 3, (1968), 164.

4.   Procter, P. Berme, N. and Paul, J.P.   Ankle Joint Biome-
     chanics.   Biomechanics VII-A (Ed: Morecki et al.)   PWN,
     Warszawa and University Park Press, Baltimore (1981), 52.
5.   Procter, P. and Paul, J.P.   Ankle Joint Biomechanics.   J.
     Biomechanics 15(9), (1982), 627.

BIOMECHANICS OF THE JOINTS IN THE UPPER LIMB

N. Berme, G. Heydinger and A.E. Engin*

Department of Mechanical Engineering, *Department of
Engineering Mechanics, The Ohio State University,
Columbus, Ohio 43210, U.S.A.

1. INTRODUCTION

The upper limb, with its mobile shoulder, its extensible and
folding member, the arm and forearm, and its terminal working tool
the hand, is versatile and has a large range of movement allowing
the manipulation of objects. Loss of function in any one of the
upper limb joints translates into reduced function of the hand,
which could hamper such daily activities as eating, dressing, and
personal hygiene. Furthermore, in patients who's lower limb joints
are affected by disease, or who suffer from a neuromuscular
disorder, the upper limb also assumes a weight bearing function. A
significant portion of the body weight can be carried by the upper
limbs in assisting to rise from the seated position, turning in bed
or in using a walking aid. These two conflicting requirements of
mobility and stability as well as its overall versatility makes the
assessment of the function, and loading of joint replacements for
the upper limb significantly more complicated than those for the
lower limb. Although a significant amount of research has been
carried out on upper limb biomechanics, particularly in the
kinematics and myoelectric activities of its muscles, our knowledge
of upper limb joints is by no means complete. This chapter gives a
review of the state-of-the-art knowledge in this field.

2. THE SHOULDER COMPLEX

The shoulder complex can be defined as the group of structures
which connect the arm to the thorax. The interaction of these
structures make the shoulder the most mobile and complex joint in
the human body. The wide range of motion that the shoulder complex

provides for the arm conflicts with the need for a stable base of operation for the upper limb. Static and dynamic stability, regardless of the position of the arm, are obtained by the muscles and ligaments associated with the shoulder.

The shoulder complex consists of the scapula, clavicle, and humerus, and four articulations; the sternoclavicular, the acromioclavicular, the scapulathoracic, and the glenohumeral (Fig. 1). A brief examination of these articulations individually will aid in the understanding of their interactive relationships and shoulder mechanics as a whole.

The sternoclavicular joint, the only bony connection of the upper limb to the trunk is a plane synovial joint that connects the proximal end of the clavical to the sternum. The clavicle holds the shoulder at its proper distance from the midline of body and part of the force on the shoulder is transmitted to the thorax through the clavicle. Superior-inferior, anterio-posterior, and rotatory movements are all allowed at the sternoclavicular joint.

The acromioclavicular joint is also a plane synovial joint which connects the proximal acromion of the scapula to the distal end of the clavicle. This joint permits the scapula to rotate, relative to the clavicle, about a horizontal axis in the frontal plane, and about a vertical axis in the sagittal plane. Forces are transmitted from the scapula to the clavicle via the strong coracoclavicular ligament which unites the lower lateral third of the clavicle to the coracoid process of the scapula. The coracoclavicular ligament, because of its length, allows for some relative motion between the clavicle and scapula, but ensures that during movement of considerable extent the two bones move together.

The scapulothoracic articulation has none of the usual joint characteristics, therefore it is not a true anatomic joint. The scapula does not have bony or ligamentous connection to the thorax, except for its attachment through the acromioclavicular and sternoclavicular joints. The broad anterior surface of the scapula is separated from the rib cage by two muscles which slide across one another as the scapula moves.

The glenohumeral joint is a ball-and-socket synovial joint connecting the head of the humerus with the distal portion of the scapula, the glenoid fossa. The nearly hemispherical head of the humerus has a surface area considerably larger than the area of the glenoid, thus allowing much freedom of movement of the humeral head on the glenoid. Much of the stability of the glenohumeral joint comes from the muscles, which originate from the scapula and have tendinous insertions in the glenohumeral joint capsule, that compose the musculotendinous cuff. The musculotendinous cuff stabilizes the joint by compressing the humeral head into the

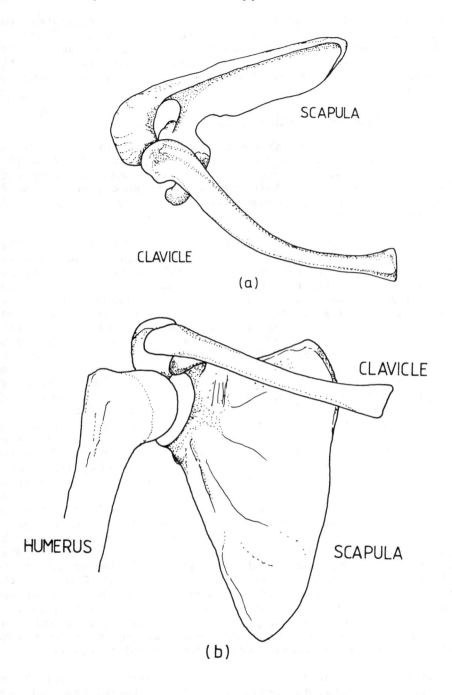

Fig.1   a) Right shoulder girdle from above, and b) anterior view.

glenoid fossa. The coracohumeral ligament, which originates from the coracoid process and blends with the superior joint capsule, passively supports the upper limb against the force of gravity. The anatomical structure of the glenohumeral joint varies greatly among individuals, and dislocations in the anterior, posterior, or inferior directions are not uncommon.

2.1 Kinematics of the Shoulder Complex

Shoulder movement is obtained by a combination of motions at the four articulations of the shoulder complex. The clavicle, scapula, and humerus all move during shoulder motion. Ranges of motion of the arm and shoulder are easily measured, but an understanding of individual component motions of the shoulder complex is a more difficult task.

In elevation of the arm four phases can be identified (1). The first phase extends from zero to 30 degrees in abduction and zero to 60 degrees in flexion. During this phase the scapula and clavicle positions vary relative to the frame of the body until the end of the phase, when the conoid ligament becomes taut and the two links act practically as one (the claviscapular link). Phase two, which lasts to about 100 degrees abduction or flexion, is characterized by claviscapular link rotation about an imaginary anterioposterior axis extending from the sternoclavicular joint to the root of the spine of the scapula. The scapula and clavicle acting together as a single link provides stability to the shoulder yet mobility is retained via phase two rotation. For each ten degrees of glenohumeral rotation the scapula rotates five degrees, (this 2:1 ratio continues throughout elevation). Phase two is completed when further rotation about the anterioposterior axis is rendered impossible due to ligament structures. During phase three the clavicle rotates about its long axis and the scapula rotates inferolaterally with the acromioclavicular joint as the center of rotation. The clavicle and scapula no longer move as a single link but resume their mechanism qualities until the beginning of phase four when the relative motion in the acromioclavicular joint ceases. During phase four, which lasts to maximum elevation, the scapula and clavicle, moving again as a link, rotate about an axis determined by the sternoclavicular and acromioclavicular joints and the humerus finishes its rotation in the glenoid. Sometimes the last two phases of this motion is combined and described as one phase (2). Most authors, however, agree that the initial portion of elevation is strongly dependent on the scapulothoracic and sternoclavicular joints, while the remaining motion becomes more dependent on the glenohumeral and acromioclavicular joints.

Three types of motion occur at the glenohumeral joint. These are rotation, rolling, and translation of the humeral head relative to the scapula. Flexion-extension, abduction-adduction, and medial-lateral rotation about the long axis of the humerus can all occur with a combination of these three types of motion.

A fairly detailed description of shoulder ranges of motion and movements of the joints and links during these motions are given by Kapandji (3). He gives ranges of motion for flexion-extension, abduction-adduction, and rotation about the humeral axis, and discusses forward displacement (antepulsion) and backward displacement (retropulsion), as well as inferior and superior displacements of the shoulder. He also indicates that the true plane of abduction of the shoulder is not in the frontal plane but in a plane forming an angle of about 30 degrees in front of the frontal plane, which in the body corresponds to the angle of the shoulder blade.

2.2 Electromyography of the Shoulder

Electromyographic (EMG) studies are useful in determining the actions of individual and groups of muscles during contraction. Although they do not give rise to direct qualitative muscle force calculations, they can help in the formulation of muscle prediction models, or can be used as a check to determine the accuracy of a model. Various researchers have investigated, using EMG's, different shoulder movements and positions to determine which muscles are active. Due to the infinite number of movements possible at the shoulder and to the individual variations of muscle activity during the same movement, it is difficult to say which muscles will be active during any particular activity. Should stability is partially maintained by antagonistic muscle action, therefore at any given position of the shoulder many muscles, other than the prime movers, may be active.

The three abductors and flexors of the humerus, the deltoid, pectoralis major, and supraspinatus, and the three depressors of the humerus; the subscopularis, infraspinatus, and teres minor are continuously active throughout both abduction and flexion, thus indicating antagonistic stabilizing muscle actions (4). EMG's have also shown that the teres major is not stabilizing the joint in a static position. The muscles that rotate the scapula during elevation, specifically the trapezius, rhomboids, anterior serratus, and levator scapulae, bring about the rotary motion of the scapula necessary for elevation (4).

EMG studies of the anterior, middle, and posterior portions of the deltoid muscle and sternal portion of the pectoralis major were performed by Sullivan and Portney (5). They investigated four different upper extremity diagonal movement patterns (combinations of flexion or extension, adduction or abduction, and external or internal rotation) and reported the primary role of the muscles considered, as well as the effect of flexing or extending the elbow during the activity. The muscles were least active when the arm was moved in the opposite direction to what caused maximum activity. Similar results were reported by Ekholm et al. (6), who investigated EMG signals of various muscles during diagonal shoulder movements resisted by weight-and-pulley circuit.

An EMG study of the biceps brachii in movements at the gleno-humeral joint during extension, abduction, adduction, and medial and lateral rotation of the arm with the elbow flexed and extended, and with and without a resistive load, indicate that both the long and short heads of the biceps are active during flexion of the arm regardless of elbow position (7). The biceps is inactive in all the extension activities and inactive in most of the abduction and rotation cases. The long head is not active during adduction but the short head of the biceps is active in nearly half of the cases indicating that individual variations do arise in the activities of various muscles.

Electromyography can be used to determine when a muscle becomes fatigued. While the arm is held at 90 degrees of forward flexion and at 90 degrees abduction electromyographic signs of fatigue in the upper part of the trapezius and the supraspinatus muscle can be noticed within a few minutes (8). Fatigue of the biceps, deltoid, and infrospiratus also occur after longer periods of time.

2.3 Forces at the Shoulder Complex

Due to the complexity of the shoulder joint complex, predicting the forces in the joints and muscles associated with the shoulder is a difficult task. Quantitative analyses of the forces transmitted through the scapula and clavicle and their associated muscles and ligaments are virtually nonexistent. Forces at the glenohumeral joint have been predicted, and intersegmental forces and moments at the shoulder joint, as well as torques around the humeral axis, determined for various activities.

Glenohumeral joint force during isometric abduction in the plane of the scapula was calculated by Poppen and Walker (9). They measured the EMG activity in the supraspinatus, subscapularis, infraspinatus, latissimus dorsi, and the anterior, middle, and posterior deltoid muscles. Muscle lines of action and the center of rotation of the humeral head were determined from cadaver x-rays. The resultant force between the humeral head and the glenoid was resolved into a shearing component and a compressive component. To obtain a solution they assumed that the force in a particular muscle was proportional to the muscle cross-sectional area times the integrated EMG signal. They found the resultant force to reach a maximum of 0.89 times body weight at 90 degrees of abduction and a maximum shearing force up the face of the scapula to peak at 0.42 times body weight at 60 degrees of abduction. The maximum compressive force is also at 90 degrees abduction and is found to exceed 0.8 times body weight. The forces obtained by Poppen and Walker were nearly twice as large as those obtained in Inman et al. (4), but this is attributed to the fact that different lines of action for some of the muscles were used. They also investigated the effect that external and internal rotations would have on the force vector. Based on the criterion that the joint is more stable when the force vector acts closer to the center of the glenoid, they concluded that external rotation provides greater stability than internal rotation.

A technique for calculating the force generated by individual muscles that contribute to isometric abduction of the upper limb in the coronal plane with the humerus medially rotated was developed by DeDuca and Forrest (10). Their two dimensional model included the supraspinatus muscle and the anterior, middle, and posterior portions of the deltoid muscle. They assumed that the ratio of the force developed in each muscle group remained constant and the force generated was a function of the muscle cross-sectional area. Although no muscle force or glenohumeral joint force information is provided, a means of calculating these forces is presented via a simplifying model with the shortcoming that other muscles surrounding the shoulder joint are also involved in abduction to some degree.

To procure data that could be used for the development of a more realistic shoulder model for use within a total-human-body model, Engin determined the passive resistive forces and moments as well as active muscle moments at the shoulder complex (11, 12). Details of this study are presented elsewhere in this book.

3. THE ELBOW COMPLEX

The elbow complex is a compound synovial joint which contains three articulations within a common fibrous capsule (Fig. 2). The trochlea of the humerus with the semilunar notch of the ulna form the humeroulnar joint, the capitulum of the humerus and the head of the radius for the humeroradial joint, and the head of the radius in the radial notch of the ulna form the superior radioulna joint. (The ulna and radius also articulate near the wrist forming the inferior radioulna joint.) The humeroulnar and humeroradial joints are hinge type joints which allow for flexion and extension of the forearm. The head of the radius is also free to rotate on the capitulum of the humerus and does so during pronation and supination. The radioulnar articulation is a pivot type joint in which the head of the radius spins in the radial notch when the forearm is rotated.

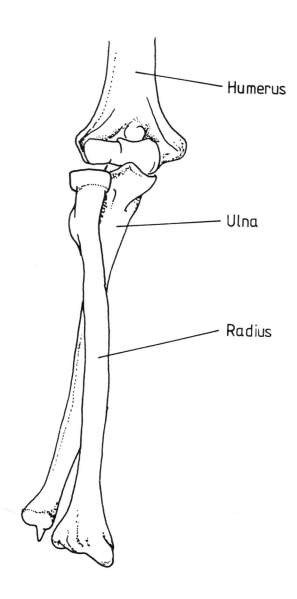

Fig. 2 Anterior view of right arm bones (hand pronated).

The bony interlocking of the ulna with the humerus provides much stability to the elbow joint. Three ligaments are also major contributors to this joints stability. The medial and lateral ligaments of the elbow help prevent undesired valgus and varus motion. The annular ligament wraps around the head of the radius and holds it in its place in the radial notch, thus forming an articulating surface with the radius and providing stability to the radioulnar joint. The muscles that cross the elbow also help provide stability during contractions in that they compress the joint surfaces together.

3.1 Kinematics of the Elbow

The flexion-extension axis of the elbow joint passes through the center of the trochlea of the humerus and changes only slightly during complete flexion-extension. As viewed from the sagittal plane, locus of the instantaneous centers of rotation of the elbow in flexion-extension is located in the center of the throchlea and varies within a range of only 2-3 mm. The instantaneous center of rotation also varies slightly translationally because of the variations in the geometry of the articulating surfaces (13).

Elbow extension is limited by the bony interference of the olecranon process of the ulna in the olecranon fossa of the humerus. Normal full extension is considered zero degrees although individual variations can be a few degrees positive or negative (hyperextension). Active flexion of the elbow ranges from 135 to 145 degrees and passive flexion is from 150 to 160 degrees. The rotatary position of the forearm and the position of the shoulder affect the range of flexion of the elbow.

The axis of rotation of the forearm for supination or pronation is through the head of the radius and distal ulnar head. The radium rotates around the relatively fixed ulna during pronation-supination. The proximal end of the ulna does not move during pronation-supination, and the distal end translates slightly while the radius moves circularly around it (14). The average normal ranges of forearm pronation and supination are approximately 70 degress and 85 degrees respectively. Differing ranges can be found in the literature with fairly large standard deviations due to individual variations.

The upper arm and the forearm form an angle in the valgus-varus direction known as the carrying angle. In a full extension this angle is generally 10 to 15 degrees valgus for males and 20 to 25 degrees valgus for females. The carrying angle changes, due to the fact that the trochlea is not symmetrical, to about 6 to 10 degrees varus when the elbow is fully flexed. (This feature allows for the hand to be easily brought to the face during activities such as eating and drinking.) Changes in the carrying angle are not greatly influenced by the pronation or supination of the forearm. Chao and Morrey (13) reported that the angle varies linearly with the flexion angle to full flexion, but Youm et al. (14) reported that deviations from a linearly varying carrying angle up to 90 degrees flexion occur and that the carrying angle does not change beyond 90 degrees elbow flexion.

3.2 Electromyography of the Elbow

Electromyographic analyses of the muscles crossing the elbow joint show that the primary elbow flexors are the brachialis, the long and short heads of the biceps, and the brachioradialis, whereas the major extensors of the elbow are the three heads of the triceps and the anconeus. The major pronating muscles include the pronator teres and the pronator quadratus while the supinator and biceps muscles act as primary supinators. Since the biceps inserts in the radius it can act as a supinator and its action as a flexor can change, with respect to the other flexors, depending on the position of the forearm.

A detailed electromyographic study of both heads of the biceps, the brachialis, and the brachioradialis was performed by Basmajian and Latiff (15). They found a wide range in the degrees of activity of some of the muscles and in the sequence of appearance and disappearance of activity during various movements. General trends were however noted. The short and long heads of biceps have similar actions except that the long head is generally more active. The biceps is a flexor, both isometric and isotonic, when the forearm is pronated. The biceps EMG amplitude is over two times larger during supination than in pronation for isometric tension (16). The brachialis is active during forearm flexion regardless of the position of the forearm, while the brachio-radialis is active during quick flexion of the forearm and during flexion in the prone and semiprone forearm positions. Antagonistic activities of the flexors during extension show variable patterns, depending on forearm position, with the brachialis generally being active.

EMG patterns of the biceps, brachioradialis, and triceps during isometric flexion of the elbow show that tricep's EMG is of low level compared to the biceps and brachioradials. Integrated rectified EMG's of the biceps and brachioradialis have been used to make relation correlations between the forces in these two muscles and the externally applied torques (17). Other EMG studies indicate that the pronator quadratus is always the prime pronator muscle and that the pronator teres acts as an auxiliary muscle which reinforces the quadratus during fast pronation or pronation against resistance (18).

With the shoulder flexed 90 degrees, the elbow fully extended, and with a force applied at the wrist, increasing to 22 Newtons, the biceps shows no significant increase in EMG activity. The brachialis and brachioradialis EMG activity increases significantly only after a load of +8N is applied, indicating that these muscles are secondary to ligaments in elbow joint support for this particular dislocating force (19).

3.3 Forces at the Elbow

Since the elbow joint is not nearly as complicated as the shoulder complex, more realistic estimates of the joint, muscle, and ligament forces are available (21-25). By measuring the external loading on the limb, noting the limb's position, and making simplifying assumptions a model can be developed to predict structural forces. Some simplifying assumptions commonly used which make the system statically determinate are grouping certain muscles together, assuming no antagonistic muscle action, assuming negligible joint friction, and assuming that joint surfaces have geometrically specified contours, as well as other constrait conditions on the muscles, ligaments, and lines of force. Many of these assumptions and possibly others were made during the following analyses so they will not be repeated.

After an extensive examination of the musculature of the upper limb Amis et al. (20) predicted maximum forces up to 3 kN during flexion on both the humero-radial and humero-ulnar articulations. These values are higher than those found by previous analyses, but it is suggested that this is caused by a more realistic assessment of the muscle forces applied to the bones of the forearm.

A biomechanical analysis of elbow joint function by Berme et al. (21) was carried out investigating eating, dressing, pulling a heavy object (table) and assisted standing from the sitting position. They found compressive loads of 300 N acting on both sides of the trochlear notch during the dressing and eating activities, and that the total joint load reaches peaks up to 2500 N in the seat rise and table pull activities. These forces represent typical values that are encountered in daily activities.

Strenuous isometric action can produce a maximum humero-ulnar force of 3.2 kN at 120 degrees flexion, which corresponds to a triceps tendon force of 2.9 kN. Amis et al. (22, 23) calculated that the humero-radial and humero-ulnar articulations can both have compressive loads of several kilo-Newtons and the medial, but not lateral, collateral ligament is heavily loaded during some strenuous activities. Based on this analysis they suggest that the radial head component should be considered by the designer of a total elbow replacement. After predicting torques of 66 Nm at the elbow caused by humeral rotation, they also conclude that the poor

history of elbow prosthesis loosening is caused by torsional forces
at the prosthetic stem.

Elbow joint forces in patients with rheumatoid arthritis were
also studied by Amis et al. (24). Forces up to 2.4 kN were
predicted to act on the distal humerus, with similar forces acting
on both the radius and ulna showing that even though the subjects,
who were mostly joint replacement candidates, experienced pain,
they could still perform activities that caused joint forces over
2 kN.

4.   THE WRIST AND HAND COMPLEX

The human wrist and hand complex has contributed significantly
to the development of man. The wrist provides fine placement of
the hand in space and adds additional degrees of freedom to the
upper limb. The wrist also controls the length-tension relationships of the hand muscles which cross the wrist, thus allowing for
fine adjustment of grip. This control of the extrinsic hand
muscles, combined with the intrinsic musculature of the digits
(fingers and thumb), makes the hand a very versatile and powerful
tool which, because of the mobility of the thumb, is unique to man.

The skeleton of the wrist and hand is subdivided into three
groups; the carpals or wrist-bones, the metacarpals or bones of the
palm, and the phalanges or bones of the digits. (Fig. 3)

The eight bones of the wrist form two rows. The bones of the
proximal row, from the radial to the ulnar side, are the scaphoid,
lunate, triquetrum, and pisiform, while those of the distal row,
also from the radial to the ulnar side, are the trapezium,
trapezoid, capitate, and hamate. Movements of the wrist complex
are rendered by two compound joints; the radiocarpal and the midcarpal joints. The ellipsoidal radiocarpal joint if formed by the
scaphoid, lumate, and triquetrum distally and by the radius and
radioulnar disc proximally. Because the radioulnar disc is interposed between the carpals and the ulna, the ulna is not part of the
articulation.

The midcarpal joint is formed by the two rows of carpals.
(The pisiform does not participate in this articulation, but
functions entirely as a sesamoid bone.) Unlike the radiocarpal
joint, the midcarpal joint does not have its own capsule or form a
single uninterrupted articular surface. There is, however, an
intercarpal joint capsule that is continuous between the intercarpal articulations. This intercarpal joint capsule allows for
only a little gliding movement between the bones in one row, but
allows for the relative free movement between the proximal and
distal rows.

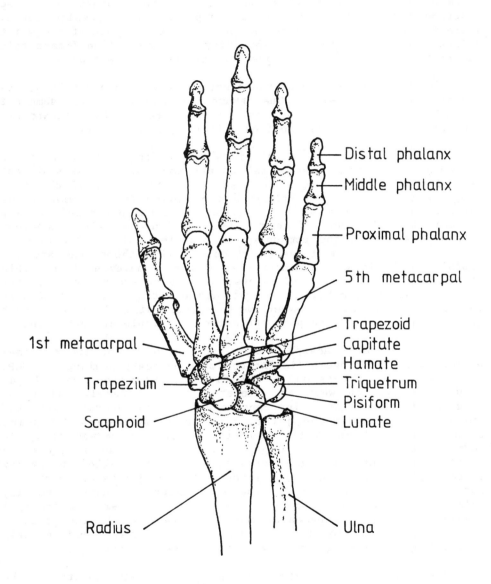

Fig. 3 Dorsal aspect of the bones of right hand and wrist.

Numerous ligaments give support to the wrist complex. There are ligaments, on both the dorsal and volar surfaces of the wrist, which cross both the radiocarpal and the midcarpal joints. These ligaments not only provide support for the joints but also contribute to wrist motion by the application of passive force. There are also smaller ligaments, which cross only one of the wrist joints, which maintain joint integrity and play a significant role in wrist motion by checking movement between joint surfaces.

The hand is made up of the nineteen bones and nineteen joints distal to the wrist. The thumb, although it is somewhat structurally similar to the fingers, will be examined separately from fingers because its function differs significantly.

The carpometacarpal (CMC) joints of the fingers consist of the articulations between the distal carpal row and the bases of the second through fifth metacarpals. The CMC joints of the four fingers are plane synovial joints enclosed in a common joint capsule and allow one degree of freedom: flexion-extension. The metacarpals of the fingers also articulate with adjacent metacarpals within the common joint capsule. The metacarpals of the index and middle fingers articulate with themselves and the distal carpals in such a manner that almost no movement is possible at the second and third CMC joints, but the metacarpal of the ring finger is slightly mobile, and that of the little finger still more mobile. Strong transverse and weaker longitudinal ligaments, both volarly and dorsally, support the motion available at each joint.

Between the metacarpal heads and the bases of the proximal phalanges of the fingers lie the condylar metacarpophalangeal (MCP) joints. These joints allow for flexion-extension, as well as abduction-adduction when the fingers are not flexed. When the fingers are flexed the joint capsule and two collateral ligaments, one on each side of the joint, associated with each MCP joint become taut and check the abduction-adduction movements. In addition to the collateral ligaments, each MCP joint is protected on its flexor surface by a fibrocartilaginous pad called the palmar ligament, which restricts hyperextension. The joints are protected dorsally by an expansion of the long extensor tendons, usually called the extensor hoods. The deep transverse metacarpal ligaments connect the heads of the metacarpals of the four fingers together and attach to the palmar ligaments, thus greatly restricting transverse mobility of the finger metacarpals.

The proximal and distal interphalangeal (IP) joints of the fingers and the interphalangeal joint of the thumb are all composed of the head of a phalanx and the base of the phalanx proximal to it. The IP joints are synovial hinge joints which allow for flexion and extension and are enclosed in a joint capsule. Similar to the MCP joints of the fingers, each IP joint has two collateral ligaments and one palmar ligament. The collateral ligaments of the IP joints always remain taut and provide stability while the palmar ligament prevents excessive hyperextension. The distal IP joints of the fingers and the IP joint of the thumb allow for some hyperextension, but the .proximal finger IP joints allow practically none.

The carpometacarpal joint of the thumb is a saddle joint enclosed in its own capsule. If the articular surfaces, the trapezium and the base of the first metacarpal, are kept in opposition by muscle forces then their profile would dictate that the joint has two degrees of freedom, flexion-extension and abduction-adduction. The joint also permits some axial rotation which occurs concurrently with the other motions. There are varying opinions as to what causes the axial rotation of the first metacarpal (29).

The metacarpophalangeal joint of the thumb is a condyloid joint which allows for flexion-extension and abduction-adduction, and has a joint capsule and collateral ligaments similar to the other MCP joints. Unlike the MCP joints of the fingers, this joint is reinforced volarly by two sesamoid bones. These bones are held in place by an intersesamoid ligament and by fibers from the collaterals.

4.1 Kinematics of the Wrist and Hand

The wrist complex is biaxial, with motions of flexion-extension and abduction-adduction. The wrist behaves like a simple hinge joint during each motion and functions essentially like a universal joint having slightly offset orthogonal axes that pass through the capitate (25).

Motion during flexion and extension of the wrist takes place at the radiocarpal and midcarpal joints. Significant disagreement about the relative contributions of these two joints to flexion-extension, and about the overall ranges of motion provided by the wrist exists. Sarafian et al. (26) express the average range of wrist flexion-extension (the range between the radius and capitate) as 66 degrees of flexion (ranges from 38 to 102 degrees) and 55 degrees of extension (ranges from 31 to 79 degrees). These large ranges of motion are attributed to individual differences in the bony structure of wrist as well as the static and dynamic interplay of the carpals. Most of the flexion motion of the wrist occurs at the midcarpal joint while the radiocarpal joint contributes a greater range of motion during wrist extension. The scaphoid, which is anatomically considered part of the first row of carpals, is functionally part of the first carpal row during flexion but belongs to the second row during extension due to the tightening of ligamentous structures (26).

The maximum ranges of radial-ulnar deviation of the wrist, which occur when the wrist is in neutral flexion-extension, are approximately 20-25 degrees radial deviation and 30-35 degrees ulnar deviation. When the wrist is fully extended or flexed very little, radial or ulnar deviation is possible due to the positions of the carpals and ligaments. Radial deviation from a neutral position consists initially and predominately of the distal carpal row moving radially on the proximal row, until ligamentous and bony structures lock the two rows together, and the carpals, as a single unit, slide slightly ulnary on the radius until full radial deviation is obtained. Ulnar deviation occurs initially at the midcarpal joint until motion is checked by the ligaments, and continues at the radiocarpal joint until maximum deviation occurs. The relative sliding of the carpals within each row also add to radial-ulnar wrist deviations (27).

The range of motion of the carpometacarpal joints of the fingers increases from the radial to the ulnar side of the hand. While the second CMC joint is essentially immobile, the fifth CMC joint allows for flexion to a maximum range of 20 degrees and for slight adduction. The movements at the CMC joints of the fingers allow for the cupping of the palm, thus allowing the hand to conform to the shape of an object placed in the palm.

Flexion-extension of the thumb at the CMC joint occur in a plane nearly parallel to the palm, while abduction-adduction occur almost perpendicular to the palm. The CMC joint of the thumb allows for a much wider range of motion than those of the fingers. It is this large range of motion, plus the direction of the motion, which allow for opposition of the thumb, or movement of the thumb toward the little finger. Opposition of the thumb allows for precision handling as well as various power grips.

The range of motion for flexion-extension provided by the metacarpophalangeal joints of the fingers also increases radially to ulnarly. The index finger can flex approximately 98 degrees while the little finger can go to 100 degrees flexion. The index and little fingers have greater mobility at the MCP joint in the abduction-adduction plane than do the other two fingers. The MCP joint of the thumb is more restricted in flexion than the MCP joints of the fingers. Hyperextension and abduction-adduction are extremely limited at the MCP joint of the thumb.

The interphalangeal joints of the fingers also provide more flexion-extension ulnarly than radially. Greater flexion-extension is provided at the proximal IP joints than at the distal ones.

The essential activities of the hand, although the possible number of activities is infinite, are generally divided into power grasp and precision handling or pinch. Power grasp is the forceful act, using all three joints of the fingers, of holding an object between the fingers and palm. The thumb is often active in power grip as a stabilizing element. Precision handling is the manipulation of small objects between the fingers or between the fingers and thumb. These two functions are extremely important to the performance of daily activities (28).

4.2 Electromyography of the Wrist and Hand

Extensive electromyographic studies pertaining to the wrist and hand have been performed during many different activities (e.g. See Refs. 29-31). These studies include both extrinsic and intrinsic hand musculature during such activities as pinching, strong grasp, writing, and game playing, as well as unresisted movements of the wrist and digits. The findings of EMG studies of the hand are valid only for the particular activity under study, as changes in the configurations of the wrist or digits could influence muscle activity.

Electromyography has been useful in indicating the actions of the many muscles associated with the wrist and hand. The major actions of these muscles can be found in many anatomy texts. The hand has many intrinsic muscles which act to move the digits, as well as various extrinsic muscles, some of which act on the digits and wrist and others which only act on the wrist complex. While the musculature of the four fingers is similar, that of the thumb differs significantly due to its anatomical and functional differences.

4.3 Forces at the Wrist and Hand

Complete three dimensional analyses, which include joint, tendon, and ligament forces, are rare for the hand and nonexistent for the wrist. The complexity of these structures make generating a useful model for predicting accurate loads difficult, and oversimplification of the structures results in errors. Considerably more work has been done pertaining to grip and pinch strengths provided by the hand and digits. The complete force analyses that have been done are limited in that only a few hand positions have been studied. Slight changes in the hand or wrist position can significantly change the results, and individual variations, even for similar activities, makes generalizations inappropriate.

Studies of normal grip strength indicate that grip strength decreases with age, is greater for males, and is greater in the dominant hand. The ratio of dominant to nondominant hand grip strength is slightly greater than unity for normal individuals, and can thus be used as a stable parameter in the evaluation of pathological conditions (32).

A three dimensional normal model of the anatomical structures of the human hand is presented by Chao et al. (33). Joint and tendon orientations are given as well as the force and moment potentials of the tendons. A detailed description, however, of the ligamentous structures is not provided in this model.

The metacarpophalangeal joint of the index finger was bio-mechanically analyzed in three dimensions by Berme et al. (34). They measured the external forces on the index finger during an isometric tap turning test and a pinching test. The flexor and extensor tendons, the collateral ligaments, and the interosseus muscles were included in the model. Joint, muscle, and ligament forces were predicted to be considerably higher than the external loading. Resultant compressive forces up to 190 N were calculated to be acting on the MCP joint surface. The joint forces they present are considered to be the lowest possible for this situation, because of some of the simplifications of the muscle system and tendon lines of action that were made.

A similar analysis was performed by Chao et al. (28) during four isometric hand functions; tip, lateral and ulnar pinch, and grasp. Tendon and joint forces for all the finger joints are presented, but ligamentous forces were not considered. Measure-ments of the external force on the fingers is not reported but instead the forces are given in units of applied loads. A general trend was noted in that the compressive joint force is least in the DIP joint and becomes progressively larger from the PIP joint to the MCP joint.

The MCP resultant joint forces predicted by Chao et al. (28) were about two-thirds those predicted by Berme et al. (34) for a similar pinching activity. Berme et al. attributed this to the fact that the ligaments contributed to the joint loading, that the external loading conditions differed, and the finger configurations may have been different.

Studies similar to those just described for the fingers have been done for the thumb during various isometric activities. Toft and Berme (35) predicted joint reactions that were about twice the external load for the interphalangeal joint and three times for the metacarpophalangeal joint during pinch activities. They suggested that the inclusion of antagonist muscle activity could double these figures.

Higher thumb joint forces have been reported, for slightly different pinch activities, by Cooney and Chao (36). They also predicted forces at the carpometacarpal joint of the thumb and found them to be approximately twice the forces at the metacarpophalangeal joint. During a strong grasp activity they estimated joint force to externally applied load ratios to be of similar magnitudes as during the pinch activities. They stated, however, that the thumb joint forces during grasp are considerably higher since the external loading on the thumb during grasp can be about ten times the loading during pinch.

REFERENCES

1. Driv, Z. and Berme, N., The Shoulder Complex in Elevation of the Arm: A Mechanism Approach. J. Biomech., 11(5), (1978) 219-225.
2. Saha, A.K., The Classic Mechanism of Shoulder Movements and a Plea for the Recognition of Zero Position of Glenohumeral Joint. Clin. Orthop., 173, (1983) 3-10.
3. Kapandji, I.A., The Shoulder. Clin. Rheum. Dis., 8(3), (1982) 595-616.
4. Inman, V.T., Abbott, L., and Saunders, J.B., Observations on the Function of the Shoulder Joint. J. Bone Joint Surg., 26(1), (1944) 1-30.
5. Sullivan, P.E. and Protney, L.G., Electromyographic Activity of Shoulder Muscles During Unilateral Upper Extremity Proprioceptive Neuromuscular Facilitation Patterns. Phys. Ther., 60(3), (1980) 283-288.
6. Ekholm, J., Arborelius, U.P., Hillered, L., and Ortquist, A., Shoulder Muscle EMG and Resisting Moment During Diagonal Exercise Movements Resisted by Weight-and-Pully-Circuit. Scand. J. Rehabil. Med., Vol. 10(4), (1978) 179-185.
7. Furlani, J., Electromyographic Study of the M. Biceps Brachii in Movements at the Glenohumeral Joint. Acta. Anat., 96(2), (1976) 270-284.
8. Hagberg, M., Electromyographic Signs of Shoulder Muscular Fatigue in Two Elevated Arm Positions. Am. J. Phys. Med., 60(3), (1981) 111-121.
9. Poppen, N.K. and Walker, P.S., Forces at the Glenohumeral Joint in Abduction. Clin. Orthop., 135, (1978) 165-170.
10. DeDuca, C.J. and Forrest, W.J., Force Analysis of Individual Muscles Acting Simultaneously on the Shoulder Joint During Isometric Abduction. J. Biomech. 6, (1973) 385-391.
11. Engin, A.E., On the Biomechanics of the Shoulder Complex. J. Biomech., 13(7), (1980) 575-90.
12. Engin, A.E. and Kazarian, L., Active Muscle Force and Moment Response to the Human Arm and Shoulder. Aviat. Space Environ Med., 52(9), (1981) 523-530.

13. Chao, E.Y. and Morrey, B.F., Three-Dimensional Rotation of the Elbows. J. Biomech., 11, (1978) 57-73.

14. Youm, Y., Dryer, R.F., Thambyrajah, K., Flatt, A.E., and Sprague, B.L., Biomechanical Analyses of Forearm Pronation-Supination and Elbow Flexion-Extension. J. Biomech., 12 (1979) 245-255.

15. Basmajian, J.V. and Latif, A., Integrated Actions and Functions of Chief Flexors of the Elbow. J. Bone Jt. Surg., 39A, (1957).

16. Simons, D.G. and Zuniga, E.N., Effect of Wrist Rotation on the XY Ploy of Averaged Biceps EMG and Isometric Tension. Amer. Jour. Phys. Med. 49, (4), (1970) 253-256.

17. Cnockaert, J.C., Lensel, G., and Pertuzon, E., Relative Contribution of Individual Muscles to the Isometric Contraction of a Muscular Group. J. Biomech, 8, (1975) 191-197.

18. Basmajian, J.V. and Travill, A., Electromyography of the Pronator Muscles in the Forearm. Ant. Rec., 139, (1961) 45-49.

19. Hanson, C.T., Joslow, B., Danoff, J.V. and Alon, G., Electromyographic Response of the Elbow Flexors to a Changing Dislocating Force. Arch. Phys. Med. Rehabil., 62, (1981) 631-634.

20. Amis, A.A., Dowson, D. and Wright, V., Muscle Strengths and Musclo-Skeletal Geometry of the Upper Limb. Engr. in Med., 8, (1979) 41-48.

21. Berme, N., Nicol, A.C., and Paul, J.P., A Biomechanical Analysis of Elbow Joint Function. I. Mech., E., (1977) 46-51.

22. Amis, A.A., Dowson, D., and Wright, V., Elbow Joint Force Predictions for Some Strenuous Isometric Actions. J. Biomech., 13, (1980) 765-775.

23. Amis, A.A., Dowson, D., and Wright V., Analysis of Elbow Forces Due to High-Speed Forearm Movements. J. Biomech., 13, (1980) 825-831.

24. Amis, A.A., Hughes, S., Meller, J.H., Wright, V. and Dowson, D., Elbow Joint Forces in Patients with Rheumatoid Arthritis. Rheum. Rehab., 18, (1979) 230-234.

25. Andrews, J. and Youm, Y. A Biomechanical Investigation of Wrist Kinematics. J. Biomech., 12, (1979) 83-93.

26. Sarrafian, S., Melamed, J., and Goshgarin, G., Study of Wrist Motion in Flexion and Extension. Clin. Orthop., 126, (1977) 153-159.

27. Youm, Y., McMurtry, R., Flatt, A., and Gillespie, T., Kinematics of the Wrist. J. Bone Jt. Surg., 60A(4), (1978) 423-431.

28. Chao, E., Opgrande, J., and Axmear, F., Three-Dimension Force Analysis of Finger Joints in Selected Isometric Hand Functions. J. Biomech., Vol. 9, (1976) 387-96.

29. Long, C., Intrinsic-Extrinsic Muscle Control of the Fingers. J. Bone Jt. Surg., 50A(5), (1968) 973-984.

30. Trombly, C. and Cole, J., Electromyographic Study of Four Hand Muscles During Selected Activities. Amer. J. Occup. Ther., 33(7), (1979) 440-449.
31. Delagi, E. and Perotto, A., Clinical Electromyography of the Hand. Arch. Phys. Med. Rehabil., 57, (1976) 66-69.
32. Thorngren, K. and Werner, C., Normal Grip Strength. Acta. Orthop. Scand., 50, (1979) 255-559.
33. Chao, E., Cooney, W. and Linscheid, R. Normative Model of Human Hand for Biomechanical Analysis. J. Biomech., 12, (1979) 775-788.
34. Berme, N., Paul, J., and Purves, W., A Biomechanical Analysis of the Metacarpophalangeal Joint. J. Biomech., 10, (1977) 405-412.
35. Toft, R. and Berme, N., A Biomechanical Analysis of the Joints of the Thumb. J. Biomech. 13, (1980) 353-360.
36. Cooney, W. and Chao, E., Biomechanical Analysis of Static Forces in the Thumb during Hand Function. J. Bone Jt. Surg., 59A(1), (1977) 27-36.

BIBLIOGRAPHY

1. Armstrong, T. and Chaffin, D., An Investigation of the Relationship Between Displacements of the Finger and Wrist Joints and the Extrinsic Finger Flexor Tendons. J. Biomech., 11, (1978).
2. Brand, P., Beach, R., and Thompson, D. Relative Tension and Potential Excursion of Muscles in the Forearm and Hand. J. Hand Surg., 6, (3), (1981) 210-219.
3. Ejeskar, A. and Ortengren, R. Isolated Finger Flexion Force--A Methodological Study. The Hand, 13, (3) (1981) 223-229.
4. Mayfield, J., Johnson, R., and Kilcoyne, R. The Ligaments of the Human Wrist and Their Functional Significance. Anat. Rec., 186, (1976) 417-428.
5. Storace, A. and Wolf, B. Kinematic Analysis of the Role of the Finger Tendons. J. Biomech., 15, (1982) 391-393.
6. Youm, Y., Gillespie, T., Flatt, A., and Sprague, B. Kinematic Investigation of Normal MCP Joint. J. Biomech., 11, (1978) 109-118.
7. Youm, Y. and Yoon, Y. Analytical Development in Investigation of Wrist Kinematics. J. Biomech., 12, (1979) 613-621.
8. Volz, R., Lieb, M., and Benjamin, J. Biomechanics of the Wrist. Clin. Ortho., 149, (1980) 112-117.

PASSIVE AND ACTIVE RESISTIVE FORCE CHARACTERISTICS IN MAJOR HUMAN JOINTS

A. E. Engin

Department of Engineering Mechanics, The Ohio State University, Columbus, Ohio 43210 U.S.A.

1. INTRODUCTION

Effectiveness of the multi-segmented total-human-body models to predict realistically live human response depends heavily on the proper biomechanical description and simulation of the major articulating joints of the body. Short time transient response of the multi-segmented models requires proper characterization of the passive resistive force and moment data in articulating joints. Simulation of biodynamic events lasting more than a fraction of a second will also require the incorporation of active muscles into the multi-segmented models and constitute long-time response of the model.

The most sophisticated versions of these total-human-body models, in particular vehicle-occupant models, are articulated and multi-segmented to simulate all the major articulating joints and segments of the human body. During the last two decades there have been as many as ten distinct vehicle-occupant models developed in the U.S.A. alone. Formulation of the equations of motion in these models has been done by utilization of Lagrange's equations, Euler's rigid body equations, and Lagrange's form of d'Alembert's principle. Naturally, the first models developed have been two-dimensional and they take their impetus from the original work of McHenry (1). Since this work, refinements and other two-dimensional models appeared in the crash victim simulation literature (2-6). The development of the three-dimensional models followed the two-dimensional ones in various research centers (7-12). A comprehensive review of both two- and three-dimensional mathematical models simulating biodynamic response of the human body was provided by King and Chou (13).

In this chapter, first a brief background information on major human joints and their models according to the order of increasing complexity is presented. This background information is followed by a section dealing with theoretical aspects of relative motion between two body segments. In the subsequent section a description of a research program specially designed to supply the data on passive and active resistive force and moment vectors in major human articulating joints is provided. The chapter is concluded by presentation of some representative results on the shoulder, elbow, hip, knee and ankle joints. These results include information on the range of motion, values for the resistive force and moments in the joints, and resistive torques about the long-bone axes of the body segments.

2.   BRIEF REVIEW OF HUMAN ARTICULATING JOINTS AND THEIR MODELS

Joints in the human skeletal structure can be roughly classified into three categories according to the amount of movement
which is available at the joint. These categories are named
Synarthroses (immovable), Amphiarthroses (slightly movable) and
Diarthroses (freely movable). The skull sutures is an example of a
synarthordial joint. Examples of an amphiarthrodial joint are
junctions between the vertebral bodies and the distal tibiofibular
joint. Our main interest here is the biomechanics of the major
articulating joints of the upper and lower extremities which belong
to the last category' i.e. the diarthroses. In general, the diarthrodial joint has a joint cavity which is bounded by articular
cartilage of the bone ends and the joint capsule.

The "bearing surface" of the articular cartilage is almost
free of collogen fibres and is thus true hyaline cartilage. From a
biomechanics point of view, articular cartilage may be described as
a poroelastic material composed of solid and fluid constituents.
When the cartilage is compressed, liquid is squeezed out, and, when
the load is removed, the cartilage returns gradually to its original state by absorbing liquid in the process. The time dependent
behavior of cartilage suggests that the articular cartilage might
also be modeled as a viscoelastic material, in particular, as a
Kelvin solid.

The joint capsule encircles the joint and its shape is
dependent on the joint geometry. The capsule wall is externally
covered by the ligamentous or fibrous structure (fibrous capsule)
and internally by synovial membrane which also covers intra-
articular ligaments. Synovial membrane secretes the synovial fluid
which is believed to perform two major functions: it serves as a
lubricant between cartilage surfaces and also carries out metabolic
functions by providing nutrients to the articular cartilage. The
synovial fluid is non-Newtonian in behavior, i.e. its viscosity

depends on the velocity gradient. Cartilage and synovial fluid interact to provide remarkable bearing qualities for the articulating joints. More information on properties of articular cartilage and synovial fluid can be found in reference (14) and in another chapter of this book.

Structural integrity of the articulating joints is maintained by capsular ligaments and both extra- and intra-articular ligaments. Capsular ligaments are formed by thickening of the capsule walls where functional demands are greatest. As the names imply, extra- and intra-articular ligaments at the joints reside external to and internal to the joint capsule, respectively. Extra-articular ligaments have several shapes, e.g. cord-like or flat depending on their locations and functions. These types of ligaments appear abundantly at the articulating joints. However, only the shoulder, hip and knee joints contain intra-articular ligaments. For example, the cruciate ligaments at the knee joint are probably the most well known intra-articular ligaments. Further information about the structure and mechanics of the human joints can be found in reference (15).

Returning to the modeling aspects of the articulating joints, in particular, kinematic behavior of the joints it can be stated that in each articulating human joint, a total of six degrees of freedom exist to some extent. One must emphasize the point that the "degrees of freedom" used here should be understood in the sense it is defined in mechanics, because the majority of the anatomists and the medical people have different understanding of this concept; e.g. both Steindler (16) and MacConaill (17) imply that three degrees of freedom is the maximum number required for anatomical motion.

Major articulating joints of the human have been studied and modeled by means of various joint models possessing single and multiple degrees of freedom. Among the various joint models the hinge or revolute joint is probably the most widely used articulating joint model because of its simplicity and its single degree of freedom character. When the articulation between two body segments is assumed to be a hinge type, the motion between these two segments is characterized by only one independent coordinate which describes the amount of rotation about a single axis fixed in one of the segments. Although the most frequent application of the hinge joint model has been the knee, the other major joints have been treated as hinge joints in the literature, sometimes with the assumption of the motion to take place only in a particular plane, especially when the shoulder and the hip joints are considered.

When the degrees of freedom allowed in a joint model are increased from one to two, one obtains a special case of the three-degrees-of-freedom spherical or ball and socket joint. There are

two versions of this spherical joint which have received some
attention in the literature. In the first version no axial rotation of the body segment is allowed and the motion is determined by
the two independent spherical coordinates ϕ and θ. In the second
version, the axial rotation is allowed but the motion is restricted
to a particular plane passing through the center of the sphere.
Again, most of the major joints have been modeled by the two-
degree-freedom spherical joint models by various investigators.

If we increase the degrees of freedom to three, we get the two
obvious joint models, namely, the ball and socket joint model and
the planar joint model. For the ball and socket joint model in
addition to ϕ and θ, a third independent coordinate, ψ, which
represents the axial rotation of one of the body segments, is
introduced. The planar joint model, as the title suggests, permits
the motion on a single plane and is characterized by two cartesian
coordinates of the instantaneous center of rotation and one coordinate, θ, defining the amount of rotation about an axis perpendicular to the plane of motion. Dempster (18) appears to be the first
one who applied the instant centers technique to the planar motion
study of the knee joint.

The six-degrees-of-freedom joint (general joint) allows all
possible motions between two body segments. A good example of a
general joint is the shoulder complex, which exhibits four independent articulations among the humerus, scapula, clavicle, and
thorax. Of course at the shoulder complex, the six degrees of
freedom refers to the motion of the humerus relative to the torso.
If one considers the total number of degrees of freedom for the
motions executed by the various bones of the shoulder complex one
can easily get a number much higher than six even with the proper
consideration of various constraints present in the joint complex.

The basic concept for the study of the general joint is quite
fundamental and its origin probably goes back to the classical work
by Chasles (19). The relative motion between two body segments A
and B can be characterized by a unique axis called the screw axis
as shown in Fig. 1. The relative displacement of segment B, from
one position to another one, can be defined in terms of a rotation
$\Delta\alpha$ about and translation Δs along the screw axis. For each incremental displacement of segment B with respect to segment A, a new
screw axis is defined. In fact, if the increments taken by segment
B are made infinitesimal in size, the collection of the screw axes
will form a ruled surface called an axode. There are two unique
axodes, one associated with the motion of segment B with respect to
segment A, and another one is associated with the motion of A with
respect to B. During the relative motion the two axodes roll and
slide relative to each other along a generator which is momentarily
common to both axode surfaces, (20). Incidentally, the screw axes
and axodes are the generalization for spatial motion of the instant

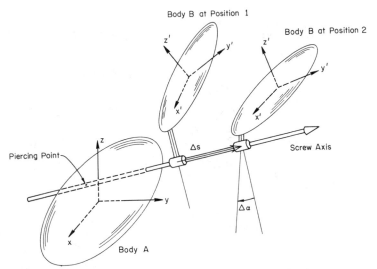

Fig. 1   General motion of two body segments and the screw axis used in characterization of the relative motion.

centers and centrodes associated with the general planar motion. For a planar motion, the axodes become two rolling cylinders, and for the spherical joint they become two rolling cones with common apexes at the center of the sphere.   For the revolute joint they simply degenerate to a single axis.   Of course, in each of the specialized cases the translation, Δs, along the screw axis becomes zero.

3.   THEORETICAL ASPECTS OF RELATIVE MOTION BETWEEN TWO BODY
     SEGMENTS

The quantitative determination of the nature of the relative motion between two body segments which are connected with a complex anatomical joint is of prime importance to biomechanicians as well as to those in medicine.   In the previous section we briefly reviewed various joint models applied in examining the relative motion between two body segments.   These joint models range from a simple hinge joint with one degree of freedom to the most general joint model possessing six degrees of freedom.   In this section some theoretical aspects of the kinematics of the relative motion in three dimensional space will be presented by considering the motion of the upper arm with respect to the torso.

Let us consider the relative motion of arm designated as body segment B in Fig. 2 with respect to the torso which is designated as body segment A.   For the intention of studying the relative

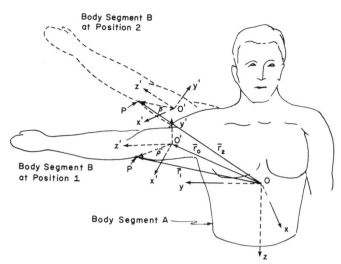

Fig. 2 Motion of body segment B with respect to body segment A in
three dimensional space. Displacement of body segment B from
position 1 to position 2 is illustrated.

motion between these two body segments, let us assume that one of
them e.g., body segment A, be fixed and the other one, body segment
B, is moving relative to body segment A. Note that the range of
motion between body segments A and B is controlled by the joint
anatomy and ligamentous as well as muscle forces present during
motion. It is very essential to point out before we proceed
further that no human body segment is a rigid body in the sense
defined in mechanics. However, for the purposes of studying the
nature of motion in a given anatomical joint the adjacent body
segments to this joint can be assumed to be rigid bodies if certain
precautions are observed. Let the unprimed xyz and the primed
x'y'z' cartesian coordinate systems be attached to the body segments A and B, respectively. These coordinate systems can be also
referred to as fixed and moving coordinate systems since body
segment A is assumed to be fixed and body segment B is considered
to be moving.

Let P be an arbitrary point in body segment B whose position
is designated by vectors $\underline{\rho}$ and $\underline{r}_1$ ($\underline{r}_1$ @ position 1; $\underline{r}_2$ @ position
2) in references x'y'z' and xyz, respectively. Since point P is
fixed in a moving body segment, the components of vector $\underline{\rho}$ in
reference x'y'z' will remain constant, whereas the components of
vector $\underline{r}_1$ will change as the body segment B moves relative to body
segment A. In fact, the relative position of the moving segment is
considered completely determined with respect to the fixed segment
if for every point in the moving segment and its associated local

position vector ρ, the corresponding $\underline{r}_1$ can be found. From Fig. 2 the relationship between vectors $\underline{r}_1$, $\underline{r}_o$ and $\underline{\rho}$ can be written in a compact matrix form

$$[r_1] = [r_o] + [T][\rho] \tag{1}$$

where the elements of matrix T, t_{ij} are the direction cosines of the $O'x'$, $O'y'$ and $O'z'$ axes relative to the axes of the xyz reference. Thus, matrix T represents rotational orientation of $x'y'z'$, whereas matrix $[r_o]$ represents separation of $x'y'z'$ with respect to the fixed xyz reference. It is more convenient to express Eq. 1 in terms of augmented vectors r_{1a}, ρ_a whose first component is 1, and a single 4 x 4 matrix T_a by adding the equation $1 = 1$ to the system of equations contained in Eq. 1. Thus, Eq. 1 takes the following expanded and compact forms:

$$\begin{bmatrix} 1 \\ x_1 \\ y_1 \\ z_1 \end{bmatrix} = \begin{bmatrix} 1 & 0 & 0 & 0 \\ x_o & t_{11} & t_{12} & t_{13} \\ y_o & t_{21} & t_{22} & t_{23} \\ z_o & t_{31} & t_{32} & t_{33} \end{bmatrix} \begin{bmatrix} 1 \\ x_1' \\ y_1' \\ z_1' \end{bmatrix} \quad \text{or} \quad [r_{1a}] = [T_a][\rho_a] \tag{2}$$

Note that there is a new matrix T_a for each position of body segment B, however, at a given position the matrix T_a is the same for all points of body segment B. Hence, determination of the matrix T_a is sufficient to know the position of the moving body segment relative to the fixed one.

For the total description of the relative motion between two body segments, besides the knowledge of the instantaneous positions of the one body segment relative to another, we must have a description of the nature of the displacement during the motion of the moving segment from position 1 to position 2. Needless to say, instantaneous positions and displacements are very closely related. Displacement analysis results in determination of the set of screw axes; thus, it is essential for the accurate determination of the locations of the joint centers. As was stated in the previous section, displacement of body segment B from position 1 to position 2 can be defined in terms of a rotation   about and translation s along the screw axis, Fig. 3. If the two positions considered are close enough, then the displacements are incremental and refer to a new screw axis each time.

Let us consider a point P fixed in body segment B. As the body segment B moves from position 1 to position 2, we can define

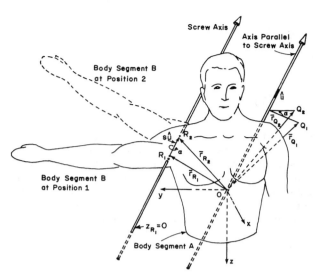

Fig. 3 Representation of the motion of body segment B from position 1 to position 2 in terms of a rotation α about and translation
s along the screw axis.

the position vectors $\underline{r}_1$ and $\underline{r}_2$ which are expressed in terms of
components in xyz references:

$$\underline{r}_1 = x_1\hat{i} + y_1\hat{j} + z_1\hat{k} \quad \text{and} \quad \underline{r}_2 = x_2\hat{i} + y_2\hat{j} + z_2\hat{k} \tag{3}$$

The components of $\underline{r}_2$ will be related to the components of $\underline{r}_1$ by the
following special case of an affine transformation (21):

$$\begin{bmatrix} x_2 \\ y_2 \\ z_2 \end{bmatrix} = \begin{bmatrix} m_{11} & m_{12} & m_{13} \\ m_{21} & m_{22} & m_{23} \\ m_{31} & m_{32} & m_{33} \end{bmatrix} \begin{bmatrix} x_1 \\ y_1 \\ z_1 \end{bmatrix} + \begin{bmatrix} a_x \\ a_y \\ a_z \end{bmatrix} \tag{4}$$

Eq. 4 can be written in augmented form as

$$\begin{bmatrix} 1 \\ x_2 \\ y_2 \\ z_2 \end{bmatrix} = \begin{bmatrix} 1 & 0 & 0 & 0 \\ a_x & m_{11} & m_{12} & m_{13} \\ a_y & m_{21} & m_{22} & m_{23} \\ a_z & m_{31} & m_{32} & m_{33} \end{bmatrix} \begin{bmatrix} 1 \\ x_1 \\ y_1 \\ z_1 \end{bmatrix} \tag{5}$$

Eqs. 4 and 5 can be expressed in a more compact form as

$$[r_2] = [M][r_1] + [a] \quad \text{and} \quad [r_{2a}] = [M_a][r_{1a}] \quad , \tag{6a,b}$$

respectively. From a mathematical point of view, the augmented form describes the motion of a three-dimensional set of points contained within body segment B relative to a hyperplane, (22). In Eq. 6a matrix M represents a pure rotation about the screw axis and also contains direction cosines information for the screw axis. The augmented matrix M_a in Eqs. 5 and 6b has the total information for determination of the displacement of the moving body. It can be shown that (23,24) the matrix M_a can be computed from the following equation

$$[M_a] = [T_{2a}][T_{1a}]^{-1} \tag{7}$$

where T_{1a} and T_{2a} are the coordinate transformation matrices between xyz and x'y'z' references for positions 1 and 2. An exoskeletal device (ESD) which is attached to both body segments A and B can monitor the necessary parameters for the evaluation of T_a matrices.

4. EXPERIMENTAL DETERMINATION OF THE RESISTIVE FORCE & MOMENT VECTORS IN MAJOR HUMAN ARTICULATING JOINTS

In general, we can identify two basic types of resistive force and moments at the articulating joints. The first type is associated with a rotational motion on a plane whose normal, for all practical purposes, is also normal to the long-bone axis of the moving body segment. Flexion-extension and abduction-adduction, which take place in the traditional anatomical planes, and the associated resistive force and moments are examples of the first type. The second type of resistive moment designated as resistive torque in this chapter is associated with the rotational motion of a body segment about its long-bone axis. External and internal rotations of the body segments are examples of the second type. Of course, one can also attach the words <u>passive</u> and <u>active</u> to these two basic types of resistive force and moments depending upon absence or presence of the active muscle forces. The major components of the experimental phase of the research program which was developed to collect the resistive force and moment data are a subject restraint system, a global force applicator (GFA), and the exoskeletal device (ESD). A brief description of these experimental apparatus will be presented next.

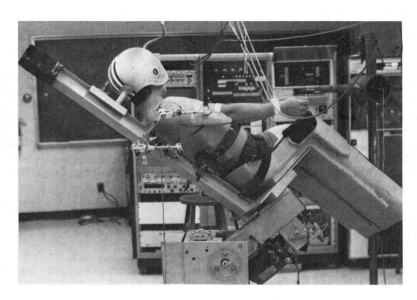

Fig. 4 Overall view of the subject restraint system.

        The subject restraint system as shown in Fig. 4 is used to
orient the torso of the subject in various spatial positions during
the resistive force tests associated with shoulder and hip joints.
This is an important feature of the subject restraint system which
assists in the mobilization of subject's appropriate body segment
at a constant elevation while the experimentor moves the body
segment by means of the GFA throughout its entire range of motion.
To eliminate the gravitational component of the moment values at
the joint centers, the force application to the moving body segment
is made in a horizontal plane while the elevation of the moving
body segment is maintained by a support line in such a way that in
the direction of the force application a relaxed floating type of
motion of the moving body segment is achieved.

        Forces are applied to the moving body segments by means of the
GFA (Fig. 5) which consists of one stationary link and a series of
four moving links attached together with eight revolute joints
containing high precision potentiometers. The outputs of the
potentiometers and the length dimensions of the links are utilized
to obtain the direction as well as the point of application of the
force vector.   The GFA is terminated by a force transducer and a
force cuff which is free to rotate about its axis.   The force
transducer was designed and built to measure all three components
of the force and moment vectors. Of course, the predominant force
component is the one along the direction of the last link of the
GFA and all the other force as well as the moment components are

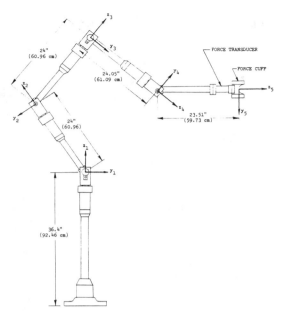

Fig. 5   Schematic drawing of the global force applicator (GFA).

relatively small in magnitude if one maintains approximately perpendicular force application on the moving body segment.

The third major component of the experimental apparatus is the
ESD as shown in Fig. 6.   The ESD was designed with a capability
suitable to study the most complicated joint, i.e. the shoulder
complex; it also consists of eight revolute joints whose rotations
are monitored by means of high precision potentiometers.   Although
there are major design differences between the ESD and the GFA,
from the kinematics point of view the ESD can be considered as a
miniaturized version of the GFA.   Fundamental design requirements
of the ESD were (a) capability of providing complete freedom of
motion between two adjacent body segments and (b) capability of
providing   sufficient   data   to   determine   the   values   of   the
T_a matrices defined by Eq. 2 for all possible motions at the
joints.   Incidentally, any endeavor to measure directly the so-
called rigid-body characteristics of two body segments must include
an understanding of certain factors such as: (a) the human body
segments have no definite physical demarcation points; (b) no human
body segment is a rigid body; (c) the physical structure of these
body segments varies from one individual to another.   The treatment
of these factors varies with respect to the particular joint under
study.   However, common to the study of all joints is utilization
of the principles of orthopedic bracing in attaching the ends of
the ESD to the moving and the fixed body segments.   Thus, heat

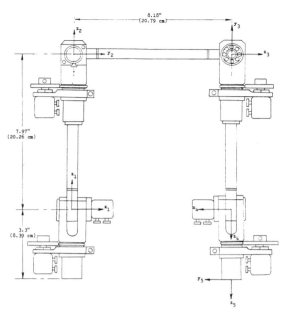

Fig. 6 Schematic drawing of the exoskeletal device (ESD).

formable plastic material was used in forming individually fitted
shells for the body segments. Special care was given to locate the
bony landmarks of the body segments to minimize relative soft
tissue motion. This was also achieved by the light weight and very
low friction construction of the ESD. In fact, the ESD is balanced
by means of pulleys and small weights in such a way that the subject does not feel its presence or, stated differently, the ESD
creates only very negligible resistance to the motion of the moving
body segment. More details on the GFA and the ESD can be found in
reference (25). Fig. 7 shows both the ESD and the GFA during data
collection on the shoulder complex.

5.   NUMERICAL RESULTS

      The developments of the ESD, the GFA, the subject restraint
system, and the associated theoretical concepts which have been
presented in the previous sections were made to achieve following
major tasks. The first one is determination of the joint stop
envelopes which define the range of motion in various directions;
the second one is quantitative determination of resistive force and
moments in major articulating joints; the third task is quantitative determination of both passive and active torques about the
long-bone axes of the body segments connected to the major articulating joints. Accomplishment of these tasks and the knowledge

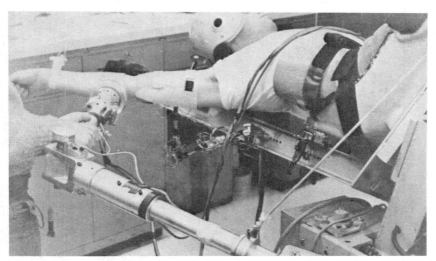

Fig. 7 Force application by means of the GFA on a subject's arm.

gained from them is extremely important in increasing the validity
of the multi-segmented biodynamic models of the human body.   We
will next present some numerical results in regard to these three
tasks.

In this research program three male subjects were tested and
for each joint the tests were repeated three times.   Thus, the
results presented here are either for one subject or for all subjects for a typical test.   Fig. 8 shows the cartesian coordinate
systems of the fixed-body segments and the ESD attachment point
locations.   Fig. 9 shows θ and ϕ angles which define the orientation of the upper arm with respect to the torso.   Thus,
$\phi=90°$ corresponds to the motion in the frontal plane.   Fig. 9 also
shows a centrode path for the shoulder complex when the arm is
elevated in the frontal plane.   The points of this particular
centrode path are obtained by the intersection of the screw axes
with the frontal plane.   Similar centrode paths can be obtained for
various values of constant ϕ, each defining a plane passing through
a point such as S in Fig. 9.   The significance of the shape of the
centrode path can be examined in the light of the anatomical structure of the shoulder joint complex.   The most striking feature of
the shoulder complex is the presence of four independent articulations.   These are: 1. The glenohumeral joint which is a ball and
socket joint where the humerus mates with the glenoid cavity of the
scapula.   2. The acromioclavicular joint where the clavicle meets
the acromion process of the scapula.   3. The sternoclavicular joint
where the clavicle meets the manubrium of sternum.   4. The scapulothoracic joint where the scapula rotates on the thorax.   In the
true sense, the scapulothoracic articulation is not a joint, but

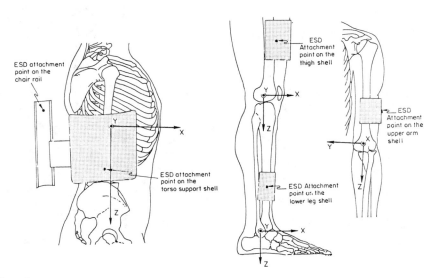

Fig. 8   Coordinate systems of the fixed-body segments and the ESD
attachment point locations.

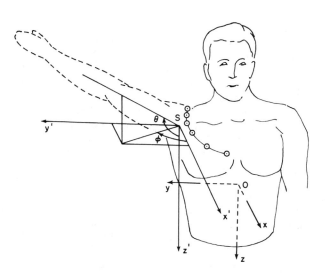

Fig. 9   Centrode curve for the shoulder joint for a motion corresponding to the elevation of the arm in the frontal plane.

this definition is of value when describing the movements of the scapula over the thorax. There are numerous ligaments connecting various components of the shoulder complex. In Fig. 9 the point closest to the origin of the xyz coordinate system corresponds to the initial phase of the arm elevation ($\theta \simeq 25°$). As the angle of elevation increases, the centrode path curves upward, indicating dependence of the joint motion on the glenohumeral and acromio-clavicular joints, whereas the initial phases of the arm extension utilizes primarily sternoclavicular and scapulothoracic articulations.

In Figs. 10-12 various aspects of passive resistive forces and moments at the shoulder complex of a test subject are presented. In particular, Fig. 10 contains plots of the magnitudes of the passive resistive force and moment vectors during forced sweep of the subject's arm by means of the GFA for shoulder ab/ad duction (abduction/adduction). Components of the passive resistive moment vector calculated at a point S with coordinates x=0, y=0.186m, z=-0.156m with respect to the thorax coordinate system, are displayed in Fig. 10b. The choice of point S is arbitrary; since for any other point in the shoulder joint complex the corresponding moment vector is addition of the moment vector given at point S and the vector obtained by the cross product of the position vector, which extends from that point to point S, and the force vector itself. Note that in these figures, θ and ϕ angles define the orientation of the moving body segment with respect to the fixed one. For the shoulder and the upper arm, the θ angle refers to the angle between the z-axis of the torso and the long-bone axis of the upper arm (this angle also defines the shoulder flexion-extension in the sagittal plane). The ϕ angle refers to the angle between

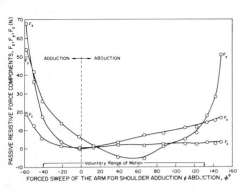

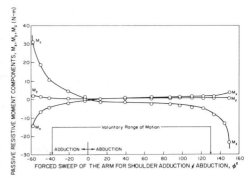

(a)   (b)

Fig. 10 Components of the passive resistive force (a) and moment vectors (b) at the shoulder complex during forced sweep of the arm for shoulder ab/ad duction.

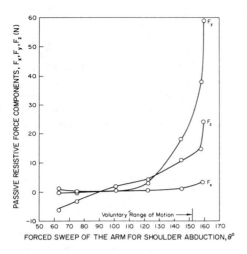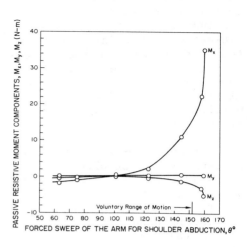

(a)   (b)

Fig. 11 Components of the passive resistive force (a) and moment vectors (b) at the shoulder complex during forced sweep of the arm for shoulder abduction in the frontal plane.

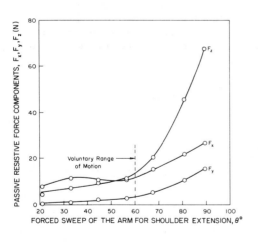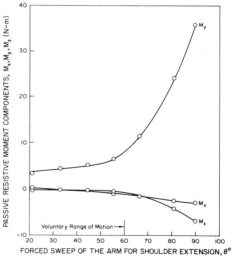

(a)   (b)

Fig. 12 Components of the passive resistive force (a) and moment vectors (b) at the shoulder complex during forced sweep of the arm for shoulder extension.

the projection of the long-bone axis of the upper arm on the xy-plane and the x-axis (the positive and negative values of this angle also define the shoulder abduction and adduction, respectively). In Figs. 10-12 and the subsequent figures the voluntary range of motion information is also included on the abscissa of the

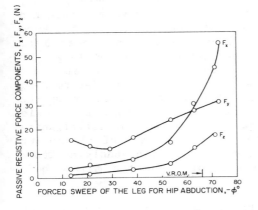
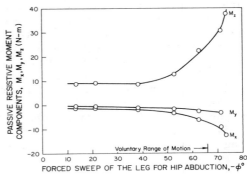

(a)   (b)

Fig. 13 Components of the passive resistive force (a) and moment vectors (b) at the hip joint during forced sweep of the leg for hip abduction.

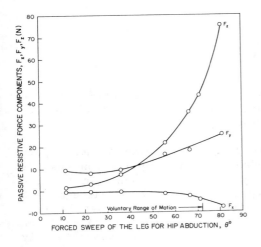
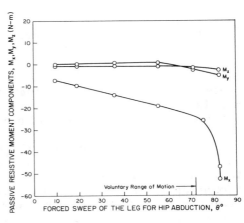

(a)   (b)

Fig. 14 Components of the passive resistive force (a) and moment vectors (b) at the hip joint during forced sweep of the leg for hip abduction in the frontal plane.

graphs. Passive resistive force and moment results for the hip, elbow, knee and ankle joints are displayed in Figs. 13-17, respectively.

Next set of figures are related to the passive resistive torques about the long-bone axes of the body segments attached to the major articulating joints. The joints and associated body segments about which the passive resistive torques were determined are: the shoulder and upper arm, the hip and upper leg, the knee and lower leg, elbow and lower arm, and ankle and lower leg. Determination of the passive resistive torques about the long bone axes of the body segments requires proper execution of at least three major tasks. These tasks are: a) capability of determining the kinematics of the moving body segment, e.g. monitoring the rotational motion of the upper arm about its long bone axis (humeral rotation) during the torque application, b) establishing means of applying torques about the long bone axes of the moving body segments under in vivo conditions, c) simultaneously monitoring torque as well as the constraint forces on the moving body segment.

The first task was accomplished by means of the ESD and the rotations, , about the long bone axis of a body segment was considered equivalent to the rotations about the respective screw axes; thus, the magnitudes of the rotations about the long bone axis are determined by adding the incremental screw axis rotations, $\Delta\alpha_i$, previously obtained (23,24) and given below:

$$\psi = \sum_{i=1}^{k} \Delta\alpha_i = \sum_{i=1}^{k} \cos^{-1}\left(\frac{m_{11} - u_x^2}{1 - u_x^2}\right)_i \tag{8}$$

where u_x is one of the direction cosines of the screw axis and m_{11} is the first term of the rotation matrix, M, which can be obtained from the information provided by ESD.

Collecting the torque data from the live human subjects puts much heavier demands on the methods of torque application than if it were done on human cadavers. With cadavers, one can fix the torque application device directly to the long bone whereas with live human subjects a completely different approach must be followed. The method devised for the torque application utilized the adjacent body segment, which was maintained at an approximately 90° orientation to the axis of the bone whose torque values were to be determined. By applying forces on the adjacent body segment, one could indirectly apply torques about the axis of the long bone of interest.

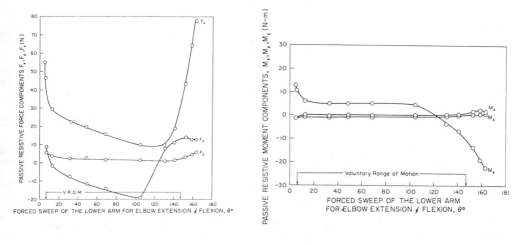

(a)   (b)

Fig. 15 Components of the passive resistive force (a) and moment vectors (b) at the elbow joint during forced sweep of the lower arm.

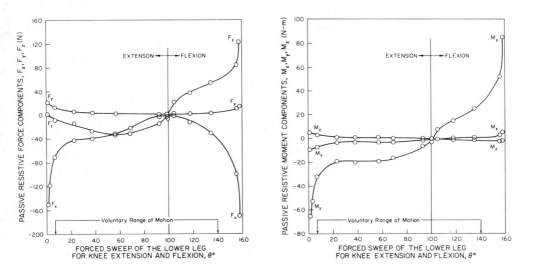

(a)   (b)

Fig. 16 Components of the passive resistive force (a) and moment vectors (b) at the knee joint during forced sweep of the lower leg.

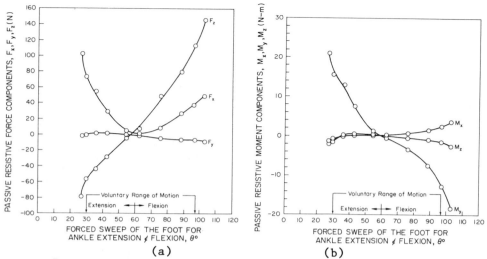

Fig. 17   Components of the passive resistive force (a) and moment
vectors (b) at the ankle joint during forced sweep of the foot.

To achieve the task of torque application about the long
bones, body segment shells were designed and built. For the
shoulder, hip, and knee joints, the design of the shells was similar, i.e. they involved an "L" shape construction. For the
shoulder joint, the L was fitted to the upper arm and the lower arm
by keeping the elbow joint at a 90° flexion as shown in Fig. 18.
The same was done for the hip joint shell, where the L was fitted
to the upper and the lower leg. For knee joint, the foot was
fitted with an L-shaped half boot covering the sides of the ankle
and terminating above the malleoli. For the elbow and ankle torque
measurements, design of the shells was quite different from the
ones mentioned above. The shell designed for the elbow torque
measurements was fist fitted; it covered most of the fist and had a
sufficient opening to put the hand in it. The shell for the ankle
was almost like a shoe with an opening at the toes region and some
opening on the top. All the shells were made by heat-formable
plastic material and their strength was reinforced by fiberglass
compound. To each shell, a steel inverted T-shape rail was also
attached rigidly so that the top part of the T was buried in fiberglass at the shell, leaving only the lower part exposed. This
exposed part was parallel to the lower arm in the shoulder shell
and thus perpendicular to the upper arm. When the torque transducer was attached to the exposed portion of the rail and aligned
properly, its axis coincided closely with the humeral axis. Similar statements apply to the other shells.

A typical test procedure consisted of a) preparation of the
appropriate shell segments to which the ends of the ESD were

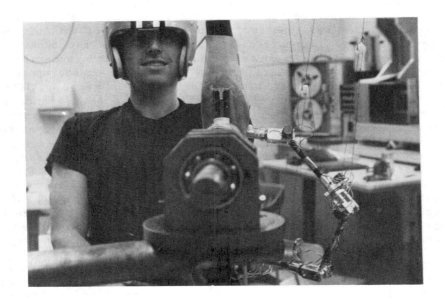

Fig. 18   Torque application on the upper arm along the long bone axis.

attached, b) fitting of the shell segments to the body segments, c) alignment of the torque transducer with the long bone axis, and d) application of the torques via torque transducer. For the shoulder and hip joints, the stationary end of the ESD was attached to the torso shell, which was snugly fitted around the posterior half of the torso. Because of the three-dimensional force and moment vector measuring capability of the force transducer, in addition to the torque values about the axis of the transducer, the other components of the moment vector as well as all three components of the constraint force vector were also measured. Since our interest in this investigation was quantitative determination of the passive resistive torques about the long bone axes, the subjects were asked to relax as much as possible before the experimentor rotated their body segments. The body segment was rotated manually by rotating the shaft to which the torque transducer and the body segment shell was attached. The rotation motion was started from an initial configuration and continued till the experimentor was verbally commanded by the subject to stop.

The plots of the passive resistive torques about the long bone axes for all three subjects are given in Figs. 19-21. Subjects were first asked to rotate their moving body segments voluntarily and data were collected for this voluntary motion. Later, the same rotational motion was repeated by the application of the torques by the experimentor. In particular, Fig. 19a shows the behavior of the passive resistive torques about the upper arm (humeral) axis during the medial and lateral torque application on the upper arm. For this test, the upper arm was oriented along the positive x direction and the zero value of the angle ψ corresponds to a 45° medially rotated lower arm position. Here, the positive x direction refers to the anterior direction, positive y direction to the right lateral and, naturally, positive z direction refers to the inferior direction if the origin of the right-handed cartesian coordinate system is fixed in the mid-torso location. Note that the data presented in Fig. 19a correspond to only one specific orientation of the upper arm, by changing the orientation of the upper arm and repeating the torque tests, one can get a more complete picture of the passive resistive torque behavior about the humeral axis of the shoulder complex.

The passive resistive torques about the femoral axis are shown in Fig. 20a. The orientation of the upper leg was along the positive x direction and the zero value of ψ corresponds to the lower leg orientation along the positive z axis. The comments made above for the orientation of the upper arm and the associated torque values also apply here for the orientation of the upper leg. During most of these torque tests, and especially for the hip torques for which the values are relatively high, 1-2° (not more than 2% of the total range of the forced motion) of shell rotation with respect to the body segments were observed at the higher torqued limits of the motion. Of course, this was a direct consequence of applying the torque on the shell. In Fig. 20b, passive resistive torques about the tibial axis for 90° of knee flexion are plotted. The same is done for 90° of elbow flexion for the torques about the lower arm (Fig. 19b). Fig. 21 shows the torques for the ankle rotation. For the knee and the elbow torques, the boundaries of the forced movement for both plots may contain motion—some ankle motion for the knee torques and some wrist motion for the elbow torques. This extraneous motion was carefully monitored, and minimized when observed. One very apparent conclusion that can be drawn from the results presented in Figs. 19-21 is that the maximum tolerable passive resistive torques associated with the long bones of the lower extremities are more than twice the ones associated with the long bones of the upper extremities. In fact, the magnitudes of the tolerable passive resistive torques about the long bones increase at the joints in the order of elbow, shoulder, ankle, knee and hip.

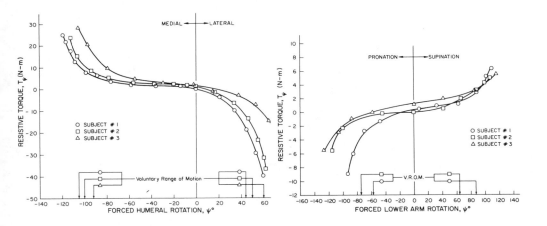

(a)   (b)

Fig. 19 Passive resistive torques (a) about the humeral axis of
the shoulder complex (b) about the radius–ulna axis of the elbow
joint of the three subjects during torque applications on the upper
and the lower arm, respectively.

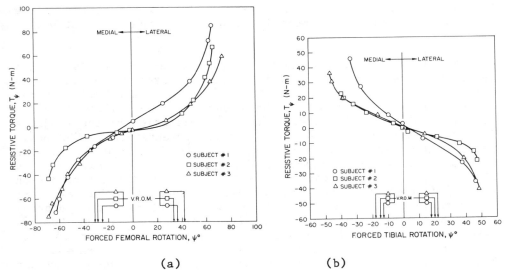

(a)   (b)

Fig. 20 Passive resistive torques (a) about the femoral axis of
the hip joint (b) about the tibial axis of the knee joint of the
three subjects during torque applications on the upper and the
lower leg, respectively.

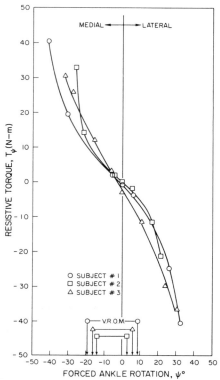

Fig. 21   Passive resistive torques for the ankle rotation of the
three subjects during the medial and lateral torque application.

Finally, some representative results on active muscle torques
about the upper arm and upper leg long-bone axes are displayed in
Figs. 22a & b.   In particular, Fig. 22a shows the behavior of the
active muscle torques about the upper arm axis during internal
(medial) and external (lateral) torque application by the subjects
for various internally rotated upper arm orientations.   The positions indicated on the abscissa of this figure describe the
internal angular orientation of the upper arm whose axis remains
fixed parallel to the positive x direction.   The initial condition
(i.e. $\psi = 0^{o}$) of the upper arm was defined such that the lower arm
was parallel to the z axis.   With the exception of the internal
rotation limits, the subjects applied torques about the humeral
axis in both internal and external directions, as shown in Fig.
22a.   The active muscle torques about the femoral axis are shown in
Fig. 22b.   For these tests the orientation of the upper leg was
along the positive x direction and the zero value of ψ corresponds
to the lower leg orientation along the positive z axis.   In both
Figs. 22a & b the plotted values represent the average of the
maximum torque values obtained from three tests for each subject.

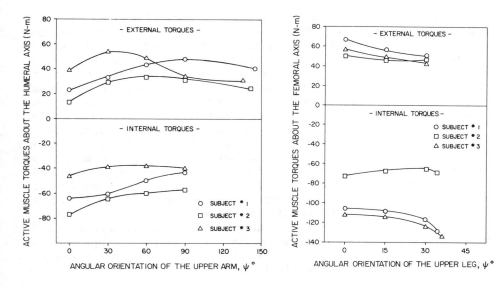

(a)   (b)

Fig. 22   Active muscle torques (a) about the upper arm axis for various internally rotated upper arm orientations (b) about the upper leg axis for various externally rotated upper leg orientations.

Note that the active muscle torque data presented in Figs. 22a & b correspond to only one specific orientation of the upper arm for Fig. 22a and the upper leg for Fig. 22b; by changing the orientation of the upper arm and the upper leg and repeating the torque tests, one can get a more complete description of the active muscle torque behavior about the humeral and femoral axes. The results presented in Figs. 22a & b were obtained from three healthy young male subjects with no special training to increase muscular strength. It is reasonable to expect that the values of the active muscle torques about long-bone axes depend on age, sex and, particularly, degree of training for muscular strength. More extensive data on the active muscle force and moment response of all major articulating joints can be found in references 26-29.

6.   CONCLUDING REMARKS

The research work presented in this chapter was performed on live subjects with some obvious limitations. The immediate application of these results is the development of more realistic joint models to be used with the articulated total-human-body models of the human body. Although the resistive force and moment values which are displayed by the figures of the previous section are relatively low, they provide sufficient data for extrapolation beyond the test regions. Near the boundaries of the test regions the critical item of interest is the rate of change of the slopes of curves. For example, if we represent the predominant moment component, M_y, of the knee joint shown in Fig. 16b by a sixth degree least squares polynomial, the value of M_y for an additional five degrees of knee flexion increases over five times of the maximum test value. Of course, extrapolated values corresponding to a very small change in extension angles for the locked joint conditions that occur at some joints, should easily reach to values which are an order of magnitude higher than those obtained from experiments, provided suitable expansion functions are introduced. One of the primary tasks of the joint modeling is the distribution of the resistive force and moments as forces on the bony structure and on various soft tissues associated with the joint. One can expect that the total number of unknowns, i.e., contact and soft tissue forces, will exceed the number of equations that can be written for each joint; thus, the problem becomes indeterminate. The solution of this indeterminate problem requires more research on the subject matter.

Although one can base the development of the joint models on data which are collected on human subjects by means of quasi-static testing of the joints, these joint models must somehow reflect dynamic and viscoelastic effects since their final application is on the articulated total-body model of the human body. It is a well established fact that biological materials display strain rate sensitivity of varying magnitudes. Thus, the force response of a ligament at a given strain level will be different at different rates of loading; in general, the higher the rate of loading, the higher the magnitude of force. There are only a very few studies reported in the literature which deal with strain rate effects on ligaments. One must investigate their applicability on the modeling task or at least get some indications about the type of modifications one can make on the quasi-static data so that they can be more suitably applied for dynamic situations.

Finally, substantially more experimental data and modeling efforts are needed on the long bone fractures and joint dislocations. Research must be conducted on cadavers as well as on primates. The strength and fracture data obtained from primates should be appropriately scaled to humans so that more advanced models which have the capability of predicting fractures and dislocations in long bones and major articulating joints can be developed.

ACKNOWLEDGEMENTS: The research work described herein was supported by the Aerospace Medical Research Laboratory of the U.S. Air Force, Dayton, Ohio. Tests on subjects were conducted in conformance with the Human Subject Program Guidelines established by the Ohio State University Human Subject Review Committee.

REFERENCES

1. McHenry, R.R.   Analysis of the Dynamics of Automobile Passenger-Restraint System. Proceedings of the 7th Stapp Car Crash Conference (Charles C. Thomas, Springfield, Ill., 1965).
2. Segal, D.J. Revised Computer Simulation of the Automobile Crash Victim.   Cornell Aeronautical Lab. Report No. VJ-2759-V-a, 1971.
3. Danforth, J.P. and C.D. Randall. Modified ROS Occupant Dynamics Simulation User Manual. Publication No. GMR-1254 (GM Research Labs, 1972).
4. Glancy, J.J. and S.E. Larsen. User Guide for Program SIMULA. Report TDR No. 72-23 (Dynamic Science, 1972).
5. Robbins, D.H., B.M. Bowman and R.O. Bennett. "The MVMA Two-Dimensional Crash Victim Simulations," Proceedings of the 18th Stapp Car Crash Conference (1974) 657.
6. Karnes, R.N., J.L. Tocher and D.W. Twigg. Prometheus—A Crash Victim Simulator.   Symposium on Aircraft Crashworthiness (1975).
7. Robbins, D.H., R.O. Bennett and B.M. Bowman. User Oriented Mathematical Crash Victim Simulator. Proceedings of the 16th Stapp Car Crash Conference (1972) 128.
8. Young, R.D. A Three-Dimensional Mathematical Model of an Automobile Passenger. Texas Transportation Institute Research Report 140-2 (1970).
9. Huston, R.L., R.E. Hessel and C.E. Passerello. A Three-Dimensional Vehicle-Man Model for Collision and High Accelera-tion Studies. SAE Paper No. 740275 (1974).
10. Bartz, J.A. A Three-Dimensional Computer Simulation of a Motor Vehicle Crash Victim - Phase I - Development of the Computer Program. CAL Report No. VJ-2978-V-1, PB 204172 (1971).
11. Bartz, J.A. and F.E. Butler. A Three-Dimensional Computer Simulation of a Motor Vehicle Crash Victim, Phase 2 - Valida-tion of the Model. Calspan Technical Report No. VJ-2978-V-2 (1972).
12. Fleck, J.T., F.E. Butler and S.L. Vogel. An Improved Three-Dimensional Computer Simulation of Motor Vehicle Crash Victims. Calspan Final Technical Report No. AQ-5180-L-1 (1974).
13. King, A.I. and C.C. Chou. Mathematical Modeling, Simulation and Experimental Testing of Biomechanical Crash Response. Journal of Biomechanics 9 (1976) 301-317.

14. Engin, A.E.   Mechanics of the Knee Joint: Guidelines for Osteotomy in Osteoarthritis.   In: Orthopaedic Mechanics: Procedures and Devices (Edited by D.N. Ghista and R. Roaf, Academic Press, London, England) 55–98.

15. Barnett, C.H., D.V. Davies and M.A. Mac Conaill.   Joints, Their Structure and Mechanics.   (Charles C. Thomas Publishers, Springfield, Ill., 1949).

16. Steindler, A.   Kinesiology of the Human Body.   (Thomas, Springfield, 1964) 62.

17. Mac Conaill, M.A.   Joint Movement.   Physiotherapy 50 (1964) 359.

18. Dempster, S.T.   The Anthropometry of Body Motion.   Annals New York Academy of Sciences 63 (1955) 559.

19. Chasles, M.   Bull. Sci. Math. 14 (1830) 321.

20. Skreiner, M.   Study of the Geometry and the Kinematics of Instantaneous Spatial Motion.   Journal of Mechanisms 1 (1966) 115.

21. Klein, F.   Geometry (Translated by E.R. Hednick and C.A. Noble No. S151, Dover Publications, Inc., New York, N.Y., 1939).

22. Bocher, M.   Introduction to Higher Algebra.   No. S1238 (Dover Publications, Inc., New York, N.Y., 1964).

23. Engin, A.E.   On the Biomechanics of Major Articulating Human Joints.   NATO ASI-Progress in Biomechanics (Edited by N. Akkas, Sijthoff & Noordhoff International Publishers, Netherlands, 1979) 157–188.

24. Engin, A.E.   Measurement of Resistive Torques in Major Human Joints.   AMRL Report No. AMRL-TR-79-4 (1979).

25. Engin, A.E. and R.D. Peindl.   Two Devices Developed for Kinematic and Force Data Collection in Biomechanics—Application to Human Shoulder Complex.   In: Developments in Theoretical and Applied Mechanics, Vol. 10, 35–50 (Edited by J.E. Stoneking, The University of Tennessee Press, 1980).

26. Engin, A.E. and L. Kazarian.   Active Muscle Force and Moment Response of the Human Arm and Shoulder.   Aviation, Space and Environmental Medicine 52 (1981) 523–530.

27. Engin, A.E.   Active Muscle Force and Moments in Major Human Joints.   Proceedings of the VIIth International IRCOBI Conference, Koln, Germany (1982) 156–165.

28. Engin, A.E.   Isometric Muscle Force Response of the Human Lower Limb.   Aviation, Space and Environmental Medicine 54 (1983) 52–57.

29. Engin, A.E.   Response of the Human Shoulder to External Forces.   Biomechanics VIII-A (Edited by H. Matsui and K. Kobayashi, Human Kinetics Publishers, Champaign, Illinois, 1983) 125–131.

KINEMATICS OF THE HUMAN KNEE JOINT

R. Huiskes, R. van Dijk, A. de Lange, H. J. Woltring and Th. J. G. van Rens

Biomechanics Section, Lab. Exp. Orthopaedics, University of Nijmegen, 6500 HB Nijmegen, The Netherlands

1. INTRODUCTION

The human knee joint is probably one of the most complicated joint structures from a kinematics point of view, and certainly more complex than any technical joint design known. Viewed as a mechanical system it consists of two relatively irregular bearing surfaces, the tibial and femoral condyles, covered with articular cartilage. Interposed between these relatively rigid structures are the compliant menisci. The bones are connected by collageneous fibers organised in a capsule and several ligaments, of which the two cruciate ligaments and the two collateral ligaments are the most important (Figs. 1 and 2). The principal motion of the joint is flexion, although a considerable amount of rotation around the

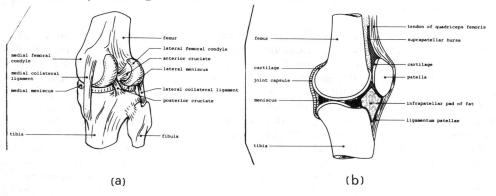

(a)   (b)

Fig. 1 (a) The knee joint viewed from postero-medially, without muscles and joint capsule; (b) a sagittal section; the terminology for some joint structures is indicated (reproduced from Ref. 46).

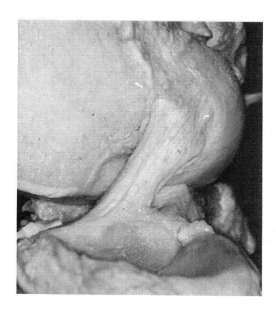

Fig. 2 The anterior cruciate ligament viewed medially; the medial
femoral condyle is excised. The three-dimensional fiber structure
of this ligament is easily recognized (reproduced from Ref. 3).

longitudinal tibial axis, called exo-endorotation, is also possible
when the joint is not in full extension. The most important extensor muscle group of the knee, the quadriceps, is connected to the
patella, which slides over a frontal femoral articulating surface.
The patella, in turn, is connected to the tibia by the patellar
tendon, thereby increasing the lever arm of the quadriceps with
respect to the joint (1,2).

Kinematics is the study of motion without taking the cause of
the motion into account. However, the actual kinematic behavior of
the knee joint, i.e. the motion patterns of the bones relative to
each other, varies depending on the muscle loads. Hence, a kinematic analysis of the knee can either be an analysis of joint
motion in specific functions (e.g. walking, running, stair climbing, etc.), or an analysis of the motion feasibilities, and the
freedom of motion characteristics of the joint. In this brief
introduction we will confine ourselves to the latter aspect. Where
knee motion analysis during specific functions is concerned, most
work has been done in the area of gait of normal and pathological
subjects (e.g. 4,5).

Analyzing the motion patterns of the knee joint, and determining how these are influenced by the characteristics of the articu-

lar surface geometry, the menisci, and the ligamentous structures is certainly of great interest. First of all, this knowledge is essential for fundamental concepts, i.e. kinematic joint models, on which functional analyses, such as gait analysis, must be based (6). Secondly, understanding the kinematics of the joint in terms of objective, quantitative concepts must be the basis for further dynamic analyses. Finally, but most important of course, is the need for more precise, quantitative data about normal and patho- logical knee joint behavior in fields such as orthopaedic surgery, rehabilitation, sports, and ergonomics.

In clinical orthopaedics, for example, the knee is a frequent subject of treatment. Most often occurring knee disorders are arthrosis, and traumatic ligament and meniscus lesions. In methods of diagnosis and treatment of such cases, a sound understanding of knee joint kinematics is important. A treatment of severe arthro- sis, for instance, is replacement of the joint by a prosthesis. The kinematic characteristics of the prosthetic device in relation to the remaining joint structures and the normal properties of the intact joint play a major role in a successful procedure (e.g. 7). In ligament trauma, the severity of the lesions must be assessed by objective diagnostic methods, which are partly based on evaluations of the kinematic behavior of the joint (e.g. 8,9). Severe lesions require surgery and ligament repair or replacement, procedures for which understanding of the ligament functions in joint kinematics is essential (e.g. 10). Not surprisingly, therefore, the knee joint motion patterns have been subject to studies for a long time (e.g. 11-15).

2.   DEFINITION OF THE PROBLEM

To describe joint motion, the femur and the tibia are fitted with Cartesian coordinate systems, E_X and E_x, respectively. We assume that the tibia moves with respect to the femur, and we refer to E_X and E_x as the "space-fixed" and the "body-fixed" systems, respectively. In the fully extended position of the joint, both systems coincide (Fig. 3). The reference systems are chosen such that translations and rotations more-or-less correspond with the accepted anatomical terminology. The X-axis points from lateral to medial, the Y-axis runs axially, pointing from distal to proximal, the Z-axis from posterior to anterior. The XY-plane is the frontal plane, the XZ-plane the horizontal plane, and the YZ-plane the sagittal plane.

Following the principles of rigid body kinematics (e.g. 16,17) the position of a point in the body-fixed system, $\underline{x} = (x, y, z)^T$, $\underline{X} = (X, Y, Z)^T$ by using

$$\underline{X} = [R]\underline{x} + \underline{d} \tag{1}$$

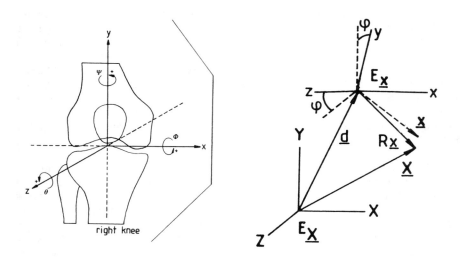

Fig. 3 Cartesian (body-fixed) coordinate system E_x attached to the tibia, right-handed for a right knee, left-handed for a left knee. In full extension of the knee this coordinate system coincides with the femoral (space-fixed) system E_X. Rotations about the x-axis (ϕ, flexion), y-axis (ψ, exo-endorotation) and z-axis (θ, ab-adduction) are indicated; the x-axis points medially, the z-axis anteriorly.

Fig. 4 An arbitrary finite motion step of E_x with respect to E_X is characterized by a transaltion $\underline{d}$ and subsequent rotations of E_X in the translated position about the x-, y-, and z-axes, respectively. Here, only one rotation (ϕ) is assumed.

where $\underline{d} = (d_X, d_Y, d_Z)^T$ denotes the position vector of the origin of E_x with respect to E_X, and [R] denotes the orientation matrix of E_x with respect to E_X. The orientation matrix [R] depends on three independent variables, commonly referred to as Euler angles. If E_x and E_X coincide in one position of the joint, then a subsequent position can be described as a translation $\underline{d}$ of the origin of E_x with respect to E_X, and subsequent rotations of E_x around the coordinate axes, expressed by [R], which is also referred to as the rotation matrix.

The rotation angles chosen is rather arbitrary, although the choice determines their anatomical significance. Here we use rotations about the x-axis (ϕ), y-axis (ψ) and z-axis (θ) of the body-fixed, tibial reference system (Figs. 3 and 4). The representation of these Euler angles in the rotation matrix is sequence dependent (16,17). Generally, as will be discussed later, these

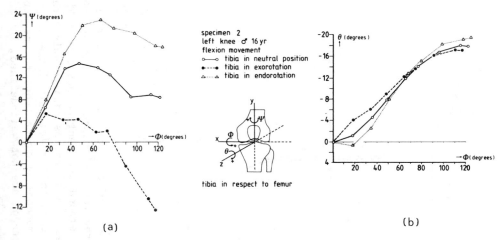

(a)   (b)

Fig. 5 Three step-by-step motion pathways in flexion of a knee joint specimen, measured with the roentgenstereophotogrammetric system: (a) exo-endorotation as function of flexion, and (b) ab-adduction as function of flexion (reproduced from Ref. 3).

rotations represent flexion-extension (ϕ, flexion positive), exo-endorotation (ψ, endorotation positive), and ab-adduction (θ, adduction positive).

The measurement, modeling and interpretation of joint motion in terms of the above kinematic parameters are complicated by number of problems and practical difficulties, which are inherent to the irregular biological nature of the structure or to the character of the descriptive parameters.

Firstly, although the knee joint has two major degrees of freedom (flexion-extension and exo-endorotation), kinematic coupling with other rotations and translations occurs to a significant degree. Figure 5.a shows the exo-endorotation (ψ) of a knee joint moved from full extension to 120 degrees of flexion (ϕ) along three different "pathways"; a graph which illustrates the two primary degrees of freedom. Figure 5.b shows, for the same motions, the ab-adduction rotation (θ) as a function of flexion. Apparently, although there is no significant <u>freedom</u> of rotation about the ab-adduction axis, there <u>is</u> rotation, coupled with the flexion and exo-endorotation motions. This coupling effect occurs in other rotations and translations as well.

A second problem is associated with the compliance of the joint restraints. The ligaments which, together with the articulating surfaces are the primary restraints of joint motion, have highly non-linear load-displacement characteristics. This has two

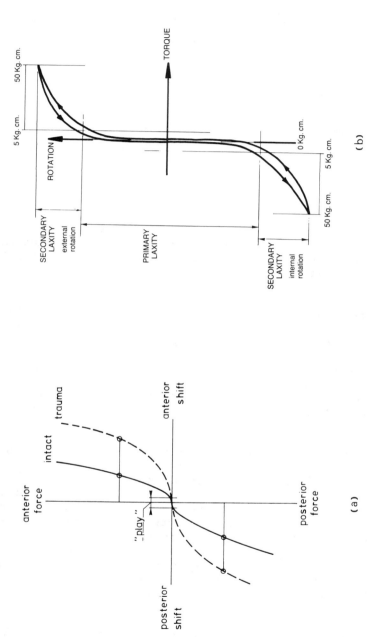

(a)

(b)

Fig. 6 Due to the non-linear compliance of the ligaments, force-displacement and moment-rotation relations have non-linear characteristics. (a) progressively increasing resistance is found against anterior and posterior forces, with only small resistance (play) around the neutral position. The amount of play may be very small or even non-existent in some knees, but increases considerably after ligament lesions; (b) the exo-endorotation displays freedom of motion in a relatively large range, limited by progressively increasing resistance against rotational moments (torques); due to the non-linear character of the resisting elements, the limits of motion freedom are not well-defined.

important consequences. Firstly, very small forces and moments will generate a certain amount of "play", small rotations about the ab-adduction axis and translations in the antero-posterior (d_z), the medio-laterial (d_x), and the longitudinal (d_y) directions (e.g. 18). This "play" is most distinguishable in the A-P-direction, a shift which is often referred to as the "A-P-drawer" (Fig. 6.a). This lack of rigid restraints implies that the joint has actually six degrees of freedom, and that its designation as a two degree-of-freedom mechanism by considering the primary motions only, is rather an arbitrary one. A second consequence of the ligament laxity under relatively small loading conditions concerns the limits of exo-endorotation (Fig. 6.b). As the resistance to increased rotation builds up progressively, these limits are rather arbitrary, and depend on the applied torque. Hence, not only the actual motion of the joint, but also its degrees of freedom depend, to a certain extent, on the external loads. Quite often the terms "primary" and "secondary" laxity are used, as depicted in Fig. 6.b, with arbitrary limits, to describe joint motion.

A third, but major difficulty is that virtually no method exists to relate the coordinate systems to the local anatomy of the

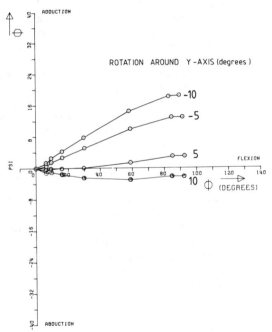

Fig. 7 Ab-adduction as a function of flexion for a specific motion pathway of one joint specimen. Different curves are obtained when the rotation angles are expressed in different body-fixed reference systems where the axes system is rotated −5, −10, +5, and +10 degrees about the y-axis (compare with Fig. 3).

bones in a precise and consistent manner. This particularly com-
plicates a detailed comparison between motion characteristics of
different joints. An illustration of the extent of this problem is
shown in Fig. 7. As in Fig. 5.b, this graph presents the ab-adduction rotation (θ) as a function of flexion (ϕ) for a knee joint
specimen. All four curves represent the same motion pathway, but
for different body-fixed reference systems, where the axes system
is rotated +5, -5, +10, and -10 degrees about the y-axis (compare
with Fig. 3). Evidently, the orientation of the coordinate system
with respect to the joint anatomy can have a significant influence
on the motion curves obtained.

A fourth difficulty lies in the interpretation of kinematic
motion parameters in anatomical terms. While exo-endorotation of
the tibia is, rotation about the body-fixed y-axis, flexion-
extension is rotation about the space-fixed X-axis. The latter
coincides with the x-axis in full extension, but not in flexion.
Hence, the flexion angle ϕ represents flexion in the anatomical
sense only if the flexion position of the tibia with respect to the
femur refers to the fully extended position. The ab-adduction
rotation is, in an anatomical sense, not well-defined; the use of
the z-axis or the Z-axis would be defendable. The arbitrary
character of the "anatomical" ab-adduction axis has resulted in
many controversies in the literature, in particular where knee
motion patterns in higher flexion angles were concerned (3).

A linkage system to be used as a reference which more closely
corresponds with the anatomical terminology, a so-called gyroscopic
system, has been suggested (19,20). This system is defined on the
X-axis, the y-axis, and a third floating axis perpendicular to the
first two. This linkage system, which is neither body-fixed nor
space-fixed, is not orthogonal. However, in addition to its
anatomical nature it also has the advantage that the rotation
matrix describing the motion is sequence independent.

The kinematic parameters defined in any one system can be easily transformed to another one. It has been suggested (21) to
relate reference systems to well-defined bony landmarks, so that
all coordinate systems can then be related to an anatomical one.
However, apart from the fact that bony landmarks are not easily
identified in a precise reproducible fashion, there remains the
problem of defining "anatomical" coordinate systems for joints in
an unambiguous way.

3.   EXPERIMENTAL METHODS AND MODELING TOOLS

A large number of methods have been proposed in the literature
to measure knee joint motion both in vivo and in vitro (e.g.
22,23). Many of these techniques rely on the assumption of planar

(flexion-extension) motion (e.g. 9). In general, experimental techniques can be divided into two, analog and digital. In the first case an instrumented linkage mechanism may be fixed to the bones, which moves in parallel with the joint; the motion of the linkage system is then monitored and transformed to the joint coordinate system. Well-known examples of such mechanisms are simple planar goniometers measuring flexion-extension only, the triaxial goniometer (24) monitoring the three joint rotations, and six degrees-of-freedom linkage mechanisms measuring the complete joint motion (25,26).

Use of the digital method implies measuring relative joint positions after finite motion steps. If the positions of three non-collinear landmarks i (i = 1, 2, 3) are measured before (x) and after ($\underline{X}_i$) a finite motion, then

$$\underline{X}_i = [R]\underline{x}_i + \underline{d} \qquad (i = 1, 2, 3) \tag{2}$$

gives a set of equations from which the three Euler angles and the translation components describing the change of position can be evaluated. The finite motion methods are based on this principle. Lacking well defined bony landmarks, object points are usually attached as landmarks to the limbs or the bones, although anatomical points have also been used. To register the coordinates of object points, different methods such as cinematography, sonic digitizing, photogrammetry, and optoelectronics can be used (22,23).

An experimental system for studies of the skeleton based on roentgenstereophotogrammetry was developed by Selvik (17), and this technique is used to measure and describe joint motion in vitro at the biomechanics laboratory in Nijmegen (3,27,28,29,30). Object points are small tantalum pellets, 0.5 to 1.0 mm in diameter, inserted in the bones. The object is imaged in successive positions on two roentgenograms, which are measured on a 2-D coordinate digitizer. The roentgenograms include the images of a calibration cage with markers of known 3-D positions. Using principles of analytical stereophotogrammetry (17), the 3-D locations of the object points are reconstructed by a computer program, based on the 2-D evaluations of the roentgenograms.

An essential feature of the subsequent calculations of the kinematic parameters describing the relative change in position is the redundancy of the landmark system. If a bone contains n tantalum pellets (n $\geqslant$ 3), the kinematic parameters [R] and $\underline{d}$ are evaluated by minimizing

$$\sum_{i=1}^{n} (\underline{X}_i - [R]\underline{x}_i - \underline{d})^2 \tag{3}$$

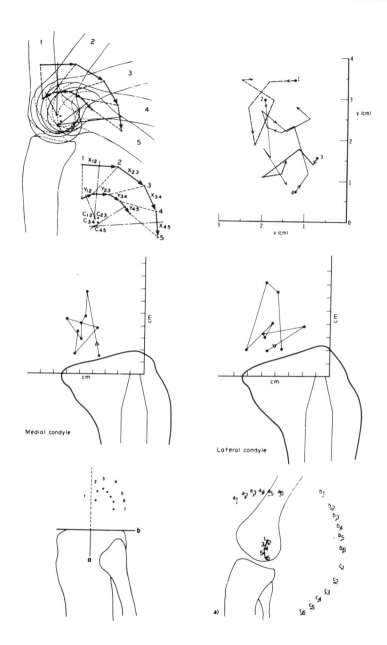

Fig. 8 "Instant center of rotation" pathways as evaluated in planar and quasi-planar knee joint kinematic studies, usually calculated from sequential lateral roentgeongrams (adapted from Refs. 9 (top left), 36 (top right), 38 (middle), 37 (bottom left), and 34 (bottom right); reproduced from Ref. 3).

which is solved using a non-linear least square method (17). The
redundancy of the markers ensures a higher accuracy in the kinematic parameters, depending on the number of markers implanted.

A well-known method to describe changes in relative positions
between rigid bodies, as an alternative to Euler angles and 'translation vectors, is the use of the so-called helical axis, or screw
axis (16,17). From Eqn. 2 it follows that when a point q undergoes
a translation

$$\underline{d}_q = \underline{X}_q - \underline{x}_q = [R]\underline{x}_q - \underline{x}_q + \underline{d} \tag{4}$$

This implies that all points on the line $\underline{x}_q = \underline{x}_s + \gamma\underline{n}$ $(-\infty < \gamma < \infty)$
undergo the same translation if $[R]\underline{n} = \underline{n}$, which is satisfied for an
eigenvector of $[R]$. These points lie on the helical axis, identi-
fied by the unit direction vector $\underline{n}$ and the position vector $\underline{x}_s$.
The motion of the two bones relative to each other can now be
characterized by a rotation   about, and a translation t along this
axis. The helical axis parameters $\underline{x}_s$, $\underline{n}$, a and t can be evaluated
from the rotation matrix $[R]$ and translation vector $\underline{d}$ by using
several different methods (e.g. 17,31).

For planar motions the helical axis is perpendicular to the
plane of motion and hence can be characterized by a point, which is
called the "instant center of rotation", and represents a point
about which a finite rotation takes place (Fig. 8).

An example of subsequent helical axes in knee flexion is shown
in Fig. 9.a. Each axis describes a flexion step of approximately
15 degrees. An attractive aspect of the helical axis representation is its illustrative quality, giving a more direct impression
of joint motion as compared to the abstract Euler angles and translation vector representation. Another advantage is the invariance
of the helical axis position for the chosen coordinate systems,
although the axes must eventually be related to the joint anatomy
for visual interpretation.

The helical axis method is a versatile tool to represent a
specific joint motion, but not so much to describe the freedom of
motion in multi degrees-of-freedom joints. Fig. 9.b, for example,
shows the successive helical axes for the same knee of Fig. 9.a,
but this time flexed along another pathway (exorotation; compare
with Fig. 5). The apparent discrepancy between the two bundles of
axes cannot readily be interpreted physically.

The helical axis position is also strongly influenced by other
slight differences in motion characteristics, as for instance
"play" and, for the same reason, by stochastic measurement errors
in the motion assessment (i.e. the calculated 3-D positions of
object landmarks).

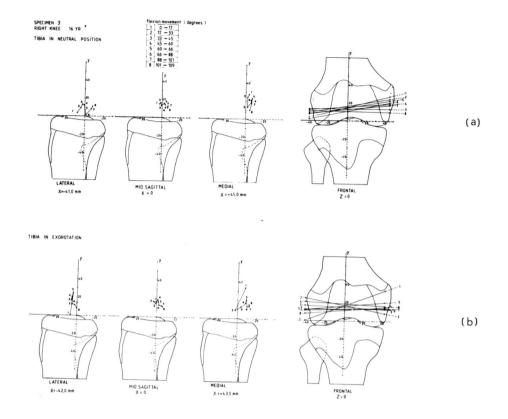

Fig. 9 Helical axes for sequential flexion steps of a knee joint specimen shown in a frontal projection (right), and the piercing points of these areas with the lateral, mid-sagittal and medial planes (left); (a) for a neutral pathway (compare with Fig. 5), and (b) for a pathway more towards exorotation (reproduced from Ref. 3).

It was shown in a theoretical analysis (32), assuming an isotropic object landmark distribution, that the error propagation in the helical axis position and direction (represented by $\underline{x}_s$ and $\underline{n}$) strongly depends on the distance between the helical axis and the center of gravity of the landmark distribution. Therefore, the object points should be chosen or placed such as to surround the anticipated axis. When both the distance of helical axis to landmark center of gravity, and the helical rotation are small ($|a| \ll 1$ rad), it can be shown (32) that the propagation of a landmark position standard error   per coordinate in the helical axis parameters follows from

$$\sigma_a = \frac{\sigma}{\rho}\sqrt{2/n} \quad , \quad \sigma_t \simeq \sigma\sqrt{2/n} \quad , \quad \sigma_{\underline{n}} \simeq 2\sigma/\rho a\sqrt{n} \quad ,$$

$$\sigma_{\underline{x}_s} \simeq 2\sigma/a\sqrt{n} \tag{5}$$

where ρ is the effective landmark distribution radius, n the number of landmarks, σ_a and σ_t the standard errors in the helical rotation and the helical shift t, respectively, $\sigma_{\underline{n}}$ the direction standard error of $\underline{n}$, and $\sigma_{\underline{x}_s}$ the standard error in $\underline{x}_s$. These theoretical results have been confirmed in wrist joint kinematic measurements (30), and are in agreement with error analyses of the instant center of rotation for planar motions (33,34). Evidently, besides placing the landmarks around the anticipated helical axis, the width of the landmark distribution (2ρ) and the number of landmarks (n) must be as large as possible to ensure accurate results. Most importantly, however, the rotation step must not be too small.

The last aspect of error propagation leads to a controversy in the helical axis concept. The helical axis represents a model, describing the change in position of a rigid body as a pure rotation around, and a translation along the axis. The smaller the motion step, the better this model will describe the real motion pattern, but the less accurately the axis can be determined. In the knee joint motion evaluation of Fig. 9, six tantalum landmarks were applied in a distribution with an effective radius of about 10 mm. Given, for example, the standard error of the 3-D landmark position evaluation of approximately 50 μm, the standard direction error of $\underline{n}$ will vary according to the above formula, and will take values between 1.3 and 13 degrees corresponding to a helical rotation variation from 10 to 1 degrees. Hence, improvement of the helical axis model towards representation of continuous motions is achieved only at the cost of a considerable loss in accuracy.

Returning now to the results shown in Fig. 9, which are typical for several joint specimens (3), it is evident that the knee motion is not a planar one. Comparing Fig. 9.a with Fig. 9.b also indicates that the motion is not unique. However, for a rough, first order approximation of knee motion, the assumption of a fixed, "best fitting" axis, as has been proposed earlier (35), would not be too unrealistic. Although this "optimal" axis should be slightly inclined both in the frontal and lateral planes (Fig. 9.a), it would probably be possible to assess its position by rough approximation from lateral X-rays, assuming planar motion and using the instant center of rotation concept. However, in view of the rather wildly scattered intersection points of the successive axes with the sagittal planes (Fig. 9), it seems rather useless to designate any realistic value to the patterns of such a planar instant center of rotation, specifically for diagnostic purposes. The large differences in instant-center-of-rotation patterns reported in the literature support this conclusion (Fig. 8).

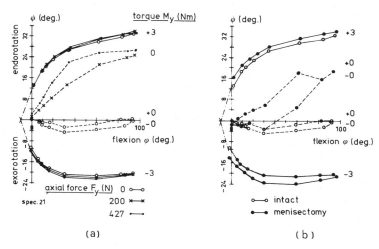

(a)   (b)

Fig. 10 Exo-endorotation as a function of flexion, as measured for
one knee specimen; (a) unloaded and loaded with several axial
forces and exo-endorotation moments; (b) unloaded and loaded with
an exo- and an endorotation moment, before and after menisectomy.

4.   THE EFFECTS OF KNEE STRUCTURAL ELEMENTS AND LOADING

The kinematic behavior of the knee in terms of freedom of
motion is determined by the geometrical and material properties of
the joint structures. To evaluate the influence of each structure
on the knee kinematics is important, particularly from a clinical
point of view. The actual motion of the knee joint in the performance of a certain task depends on the freedom of motion, as well
as on the external loads. In the remainder of this chapter some of
these effects will be discussed.

Figure 10 presents a number of curves, similar to those shown
in Fig. 5.a. Each curve represents an exo-endorotation movement,
ψ, as function of flexion, ϕ , determined for one knee joint specimen using the roentgensterephotogrammetric method discussed previously. In Fig. 10.a the effects of two kinds of loads are shown,
a torsional moment around the y-axis, M_y, and an axial compressive
force, F_y . When the joint is unloaded ($F_y = 0$, $M_y = \pm\ 0$), hardly
any exo- or endorotation occurs, but the precise motion path is
rather uncertain ($M_y = \pm\ 0$ refers to slight rotational shifts
applied at the first motion step). We will refer to these curves
($M_y = \pm\ 0$) as the "neutral" pathways. If endo- or exorotation
moments are applied the joint follows corresponding endo- and
exorotation pathways. The range of exo-endorotation motion arbitrarily measured here for applied torsional moments of −3 Nm and 3
Nm respectively, increases with flexion. It appears that this

freedom of motion is not influenced by an axial force (Fig. 10.a). The neutral curve, however, displays a considerable shift towards endorotation for increasing axial loads, as also shown in the figure. Besides these shifts, there is a definite "firmness" of these pathways in axially loaded cases: the motion is less arbitrary and is not affected by small torsional moments ($M_y = \pm 0$).

These shifts in the neutral curve due to an axial load may be caused by cartilage deformation and/or as a result of articular surface geometry.

The influence of the menisci on the exo-endorotation freedom of motion is illustrated in Fig. 10.b. The freedom region increases approximately by 5 to 10 per cent, under torsional moments of $M_y = \pm 3$ Nm, after removal of the menisci. The neutral curves are less "firm", and more strongly affected by small rotational shifts. Under axial loads, however, the original curves for the intact joint are almost reproduced. Hence, it appears that the influence of menisci on the kinematic behavior of the knee joint is not very pronounced. It must be remarked, however, that the meniscus has an important function in static and dynamic load transmission.

The effects of the axial and torsional loads, and those of meniscotomy on the kinematic characteristics discussed here are reproducible in other specimens as well. They are also in agreement with observations reported elsewhere (18, 40-43). However, due to the arbitrary nature of the imposed load-dependent exo-endorotation limits the terminology of the interpretations varies to some extent (e.g. 43).

A major role in knee motion characteristics has traditionally been attributed to the cruciate ligaments (e.g. 3,11,14,15,44,46). A well known concept for planar knee motion assumes the cruciates to act as rigid bars, kept taut by distraction forces generated due to articular contact (e.g. 15,44). The joint thus behaves as a four-bar-linkage mechanism, with an instant rotation center coinciding with the point of intersection of the ligaments. Essential in this concept is the close interaction between articular surface geometry and ligaments.

Evidently, however, the ligaments are relatively compliant 3-D structures rather than rigid line elements (Fig. 2), and the question is whether such a simple and therefore attractive model can be maintained in spatial motion concepts.

When the rotation matrix [R] and the translation vector $\underline{d}$ have been calculated for each relative knee joint attitude, the location of a femoral insertion point of a ligament, $\underline{X}_{fj}$, can be related to a tibial insertion point $\underline{x}_{tj}$, if these vectors are known in their

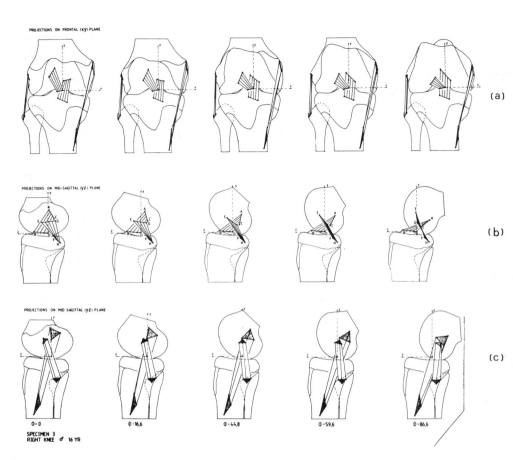

Fig. 11 Frontal (a) and sagittal (b,c) views of a knee joint specimen in successive flexion steps along a neutral pathway as shown in
Fig. 5.   The cruciate and collateral ligament insertion regions are
marked with two and three pellets, respectively.   This way the
geometrical changes of these ligaments can be interpreted visually
as represented by the line-elements (adapted from Ref. 3).

respective   coordinate   systems.   In   several   motion   evaluation
experiments the insertion regions of the cruciate and collateral
ligaments were marked with two and three tantalum pellets respectively, and the 3-D locations of these pellets were measured
(3,28).   As a result, a geometric configuration model of the ligaments and their deformation during joint motion are determined, as
shown in Fig. 11.   The flexion positions represented here correspond to a neutral, unloaded pathway, depicted in Fig. 5.

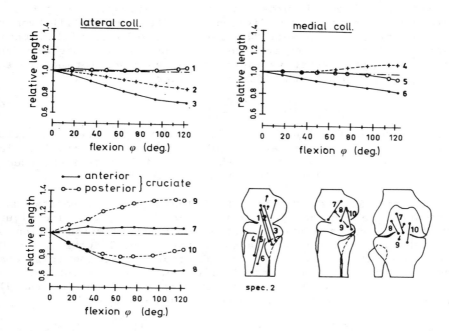

Fig. 12 Changes of the line-element lengths representing ligament bands of a knee joint specimen in flexion (neutral pathway). Lengths are expressed as a percentage of ligament lengths in full extension (adapted from Ref. 3).

The action of the cruciate ligaments as four-bar-linkage elements can be appreciated from Fig. 11.b. They appear to "pull" the femur posteriorly, controlling the sliding/rolling motion between the two articular surfaces. When combining these projections in the sagittal plane with those of the piercing points representing the helical axes of Fig. 9, it follows that the axes intersect the crossing regions of the ligaments in all positions (3).

The cruciates however, are relatively large in size, and their fibers follow different spatial courses in both the sagittal and frontal planes. It is therefore obvious that the various fibers play different roles at different knee joint positions, as also was demonstrated by anatomical observations (e.g. 3,14,46).

It is interesting to note that the collateral ligaments are also crossed in the sagittal plane (Fig. 11.c). However, unlike the cruciates, they uncross during flexion.

Although these pictures give a good impression of the geometrical complexity of the ligaments, their true contribution to
knee kinematics depends on the tension developed within their
fibers, which in turn relates to the length changes between the
insertions. This latter variable can be assessed for any chosen
line element defined by the insertion markers, from

$$L_j = |\underline{x}_{fj} - \underline{x}_{tj}| = |\underline{x}_{fj} - [R]\underline{x}_{tj} - \underline{d}| \tag{6}$$

where L_j denotes the length of a line element j between insertion
points $\underline{x}_{fj}$ and $\underline{x}_{tj}$ in a certain joint position determined by [R]
and $\underline{d}$. Defining L_{jo} as the length of j in full extension, then e_j
$= L_j/L_{jo}$ gives the relative length in the element j.

The relative length changes of ten ligament elements as a
function of the flexion angle ϕ are shown in Fig. 12. The figure
shows that there is a significant influence of flexion motion on
the length patterns. Increases and decreases of lengths up to 40%
occur. With the exception of the anterior parts, the collateral
ligaments seem to become untaut in flexion. The anterior parts of
the cruciates apparently increase in length (elements 7 and 9),
whereas the posterior parts decrease (elements 8 and 10).

As suggested by the curves of Fig. 12, the length changes of
the elements are extremely sensitive to the location of the chosen
insertion points. Nevertheless, the patterns shown for one joint
specimen are qualitatively reproducible in other specimens, particularly for the collateral ligaments (3,28). In addition, they
show only small changes when other pathways of flexion, discussed
earlier, are followed; again these changes are mildest in the
collateral ligaments (28).

Although the length patterns shown in Fig. 12 illustrate the
complexity of the ligament influences on the kinematic behavior of
the joint, it is difficult to interpret them in terms of restraints
against freedom of motion. Firstly, as illustrated in Fig. 2 not
all the collagen fibers in the ligaments follow a parallel course
from femoral to tibial insertion (e.g. 3,46). Therefore, when a
line element increases or decreases in length, the true fibers may
not follow the same pattern. Secondly, the relative length changes
are related to the initial length, and since it is unknown whether
a ligament is taut or relaxed in that state, the relative length
changes do not represent element strain. It is probably, for
example, that a ligament fiber represented by line element 9
(anterior part of the posterior cruciate) is relaxed in full extension, since a strain of 40% would generate a force close to its
tensile strength. Finally, effectiveness of a ligament band in
restraining a certain freedom of motion depends on its 3-dimen-
sional configuration. It is interesting to note, for example, that
element 9, which is probably subjected to the highest force, has in

flexion a course almost perpendicular to the joint surfaces (Figs. 11.a and b, line element E-F). Therefore, if indeed a high force is generated in this band of the posterior cruciate, then it would act only to compress the joint surfaces, without giving much resistance to motion in other directions.

5. KNEE JOINT MODELS

It should be evident from the above discussion that the human knee joint is a rather complex mechanical system. Kinematic analyses of its motion characteristics have increased the knowledge about its capabilities and performance, as have anatomical observations, functional gait analyses and experimental evaluations of properties to isolated knee joint structures. However, a complete understanding of the joint function, and in particular, the quantitative effects of the knee structural elements can only evolve if the available knowledge is combined in a mathematical concept, a model. We have already discussed a simple kinematic model, the four-bar-linkage mechanism (15,44), which describes the flexion-extension motion as influenced by the cruciate ligaments.

Although a model could be a simplified representation of reality, in order to be representative of the complex reality, it should include and account for the essential features of the real system. In that respect it seems obvious that a realistic knee joint model should be three dimensional and represent the compliance of the knee structures. That is it should include the external loads as well as the stiffness characteristics of the knee tissues. Such a model combines kinetic and kinematic effects. Two models of this kind have been proposed in the literature (47,48).

The model of Wismans (47) describes the articulating bones as three dimensional rigid surfaces, in contact at two points (medial and lateral condyles), and the ligamentous connections as line elements with non-linear elastic properties. The number of line elements is arbitrary in principle. In the model, the flexion angle is prescribed, as are the external forces and moments, with the exception of the flexion-extension moment. This leaves five degrees of freedom and one loading variable to be determined. Further unknowns are the locations of the contact points on the medial and lateral condyles (2 coordinates per condyle, 8 in total), the magnitudes of the two contact forces, and the forces in the ligament line elements. The latter are described by a priori known data about force-displacement characteristics of the ligaments, which leaves 16 unknown variables. These are evaluated by a system of 16 equations resulting from requirements of equilibrium (6 equations) and contact conditions (10 equations).

The menisci are neglected in this model, as is the compliance of the articular cartilage-bone complex. In addition, the validity of a multiple line element approximation of the ligaments is as yet unknown. The question is not, of course, if these assumptions are very accurate, but whether such an assembly of simplified descriptions can produce valid predictions of knee behavior. It is obvious that such a model must be validated extensively and only then it can be applied to circumstances for which it was developed. The menisci, for example, have shown to exert only minor influences on the normal knee joint kinematics in the experiment discussed in the previous section. However, if one or more knee structures, as ligaments, were deficient or ruptured, it is quite possible that the relative importance of the menisci could increase. A situation which could not be accounted for in this model.

Another problem of sophisticated and complex mathematical models of this kind is that they depend heavily on a priori known data on geometrical and material properties, e.g. quantitative mathematical descriptions of joint surfaces and ligament geometrical and elastic properties. The sensitivity of the model results on these properties must be in balance with the accuracy by which this data can be experimentally determined; the higher the sensitivity, the higher the requirements for accuracy. This again, emphasizes the need for continuing experimental efforts of increasing sophistication.

Acknowledgement:

The authors' research in this field was sponsored in part by Grant No. 90-90 of the Netherlands Organisation for the Advancement of Pure Research (ZWO).

We gratefully acknowledge the assistance of Dr. Göran Selvik (Dept. Anatomy, Univ. of Lund, Sweden) and Ir. Ton Hamer (Dept. Mech. Engrg., Eindhoven Univ. of Technology and Univ. of Limburg, The Netherlands) in the completion of the experimental equipment and software.

REFERENCES

1. Kapandji, I.A.   The Physiology of the Joints, vol. II (Churchill Livingstone, Edinburgh, London, New York, 1970).
2. Lanz, J. and W. Wachsmuth.   Praktische Anatomie, Bein und Statik (Springer Verlag, Berlin, Heidelberg, New York, 1972).
3. Dijk, R. van.   The Behaviour of the Cruciate Ligaments in the Human Knee.   Dissertation, University of Nijmegen, The Netherlands, 1983.

4. Crowninshield, R. and R.A. Brand. Kinematics and Kinetics of Gait, CRC Handbook of Engineering in Medicine and Biology, Section B: Instruments and Measurements (CRC-Press, West Palm Beach, FL, 1978) pp. 413-425.
5. Chao, E.Y., R.K. Laughman, E. Schneider and R.H. Stauffer. Normative Data of Knee Joint Motion and Ground Reaction Forces in Adult Level Walking. J. Biomechanics 16 (1983) pp. 219-233.
6. Cappozzo, A. Considerations on Clinical Gait Evaluation. Letter to the Editor, J. Biomechanics 16 (1983) p. 302.
7. Walker, P.S. Human Joints and their Artificial Replacement (Charles C. Thomas, Springfield, Illinois, 1977).
8. Jacobson, K. Gonylaxometry, Acta Orthop. Scand. Suppl. no. 194, 1981.
9. Frankel, V.H., A.H. Burstein, and D.C. Brooks. Biomechanics of Internal Derangement of the Knee. J. Bone Jt. Surg. 53-A (1971) pp. 945-963.
10. Hughston, J.C., J.R. Andrews, M.J. Cross, and A. Moschi. Classification of Knee Ligament Instabilities, Parts I and II. J. Bone Jt. Surg. 58-A (1976) pp. 159-179.
11. Weber, W. and E. Weber. Mechanik der Menschlichen Gehwerkzeuge, Part II, Ueber das Kniegelenk, Gottingen (1836) pp. 161-202.
12. Meyer, H. Mechanik des Kniegelenkes. Arch. Anat. Physiol und Wissensch. Medicin (1853) pp. 497-547.
13. Braune, W. and O. Fischer. Die Bewegungen des Kniegelenks. Abhandl. der Mathem. Phys. Classe der Konigl. Sachs. Gesellsch. der Wissensch. 17 (1891) pp. 77-150.
14. Fick, R. Anatomie und Mechanik der Gelenke (Gustav Fischer, Jena) Part I (1904), Part II (1910), Part III (1911).
15. Strasser, H. Lehrbuch der Muskel- und Gelenkmechanik (Julius Springer, Berlin, 1917).
16. Goldstein, H. Classical Mechanics (Addison-Wesley, Reading, MA, 1959).
17. Selvik, G. A Roentgen Stereophotogrammetric Method for the Study of the Kinematics of the Skeletal System. Dissertation, University of Lund, AV-Centralen, Lund, Sweden, 1974.
18. Markolf, K.L., J.S. Mensch, and H.C. Amstutz. Stiffness and Laxity of the Knee - The Contributions of the Supporting Structures. J. Bone Jt. Surg. 58-A (1976) pp. 583-593.
19. Suntay, W.J., E.S. Grood, F.R. Noyes, and D.L. Butler. A Coordinate System for Describing Joint Position, Advances in Bioengineering (ASME, New York, 1978) p. 59.
20. Chao, E.Y.S. and K.N. An. Perspectives in Measurements and Modeling of Musculo-Skeletal Joint Dynamics, Biomechanics: Principles and Applications (Edited by R. Huiskes, D. H. van Campen and J. R. de Wijn; Martinus Nijhoff, The Hague, Boston, London, 1982) pp. 1-18.

21. Lewis, J.L. and W.D. Lew. A Note on the Description of Articulating Joint Motion. J. Biomechanics 10 (1977) pp. 675-678.

22. Woltring, H.J. On Methodology in the Study of Human Movement, Human Motor Actions – Bernstein Reassessed (Edited by H.T.A. Whiting, North-Holland Publishing Company, Amsterdam, 1983) in press.

23. Kinzel, G.L. and L.J. Gutkowski. Joint Models, Degrees of Freedom, and Anatomical Motion Measurement. J. Biomech. Engrg. 105 (1983) pp. 55-62.

24. Chao, E.Y.S. Justification of Triaxial Goniometer for the Measurement of Joint Rotation. J. Biomechanics 13 (198) pp. 989-1006.

25. Kinzel, G.L., A.S. Hall, and B.M. Hillberry. Measurement of the Total Motion Between Two Body Segments, Part I – Analytical Development. J. Biomechanics 5 (1972) pp. 93-105.

26. Kinzel, G.L. et al. Measurement of the Total Motion Between Two Body Segments, Part II – Description and Application. J. Biomechanics 5 (1972) pp. 283-293.

27. Dijk, R. van, R. Huiskes, and G. Selvik. Roentgenstereophotogrammetric Methods for the Evaluation of the Three-Dimensional Kinematic Behaviour and Cruciate Ligament Length Patterns of the Human Knee Joint. J. Biomechanics 12 (1979) pp. 727-731.

28. Lange, A. de, R. van Dijk, R. Huiskes, G. Selvik, and Th. J. G. van Rens. The Application of Roentgenstereophotogrammetry for Evaluation of Knee-Joint Kinematics in vitro, Biomechanics: Principles and Applications (Edited by R. Huiskes, D.H. van Campen and J.R. de Wijn; Martinus Nijhoff, The Hague, Boston, London, 1982) pp. 177-184.

29. Lange, A. de, R. van Dijk, R. Huiskes, and Th. J.G. van Rens. Three-Dimensional Experimental Assessment of Knee Ligament Length Patterns in vitro, Proceedings 29th Annual ORS (Orthopaedic Research Society, Chicago, 1983) p. 10.

30. Lange, A. de, C. van Leeuwen, J. Kauer, R. Huiskes, and A. Huson. A 3-D Kinematic Evaluation of a Human Wrist-Joint Specimen, 4th General Meeting, European Society of Biomaterials, Leuven, Belgium, August 31 – September 2, 1983 (to be published in proceedings).

31. Spoor, C.W. and F.E. Veldpaus. Rigid Body Motion Calculated from Spatial Coordinates of Markers. J. Biomechanics 13 (1980) pp. 391-393.

32. Woltring, H.J., R. Huiskes, and A. de Lange. Measurement Error Influence on Helical Axis Accuracy in the Description of 3-D Finite Joint Movement in Biomechanics, 1983 Biomechanics Symposium (Edited by S.L. Woo and R.E. Mates, AMD-vol. 56, ASME, New York, 1983) pp. 19-22.

33. Panjabi, M.M., V.K. Goel, S.D. Walter, and S. Schick. Errors in the Center and Angle of Rotation of a Joint: An Experimental Study. J. Biomech. Engrg. 104 (1982) pp. 232-237.

34. Soudan, K., R. van Audekercke, and M. Martens. Methods, Difficulties and Inaccuracies in the Study of Human Joint Kinematics and Patho-Kinematics by the Instant Center Concept, Example: The Knee Joint. J. Biomechanics 12 (1979) pp. 27-33.

35. Lewis, J.L. and W.D. Lew. A Method for Locating an Optimal "Fixed" Axis of Rotation for the Human Knee Joint. J. Biomech. Engrg. 100 (1978) pp. 187-193.

36. Walker, P.S., H. Skoji, and M.J. Erkman. The Rotational Axis of the Knee and its Significance to Prosthesis Design. Clin. Orthop. Rel. Res. 89 (1972) pp. 160-170.

37. Smidt, G.L. Biomechanical Analysis of Knee Flexion and Extension. J. Biomechanics 6 (1973) pp. 79-92.

38. Harding, M.L. and M.E. Blakemore. The Instant Centre Pathway as a Parameter of Joint Motion - An Experimental Investigation of a Method of Assessment of Knee Ligament Injury and Repair. Engrg. in Medicine 9 (1980) pp. 195-200.

39. Nietert, M. Das Kniegelenk des Menschen als Biomechanisches Problem. Biomed. Tech. 22 (1977) pp. 13-21.

40. Ahmed, A.M., D.L. Burke, O. Szklar, and G.A. Fraser. An in vitro Study of the Role of the Menisci in the Passive Torsional Stability of the Knee, Proceedings 26th Annual ORS (Orthopaedic Research Society, Chicago, 1980).

41. Hsieh, H. and P. Walker. Stabilizing Mechanics of the Loaded and Unloaded Knee Joint. J. Bone Jt. Surg. 58-A (1976) pp. 87-93.

42. Levy, I.M., P.A. Torzilli, and R.F. Warren. The Effect of Medial Meniscectomy on Antero Posterior Knee Motion, Proceedings 28th Annual ORS (Orthopaedic Research Society, Chicago, 1982).

43. Wang, C.J. and P.S. Walker. Rotatory Laxity of the Human Knee Joint. J. Bone Jt. Surg. 56-A (1974) pp. 161-170.

44. Huson, A. Biomechanische Probleme des Kniegelenks. Orthopadie 3 (1974) pp. 119-126.

45. Shaw, J.A., M. Eng, and D.G. Murray. The Longitudinal Axis of the Knee and the Role of the Cruciate Ligaments in Controlling Transverse Rotation. J. Bone Jt. Surg. 56-A (1974) pp. 1603-1609.

46. Girgis, F.G., J.L. Marshall, and A.R.S. Monajen. The Cruciate Ligaments of the Knee Joint. Clin. Orthop. Rel. Res. 106 (1975) pp. 216-231.

47. Wismans, J. A Three-Dimensional Mathematical Model of the Human Knee Joint. Dissertation, Eindhoven University of Technology, The Netherlands, 1980.

48. Andriacchi, T.P., R.P. Mikosz, S.J. Hampton, and J.O. Galante. Model Studies of the Stiffness Characteristics of the Human Knee Joint. J. Biomechanics 16 (1983) pp. 23-29.

DYNAMIC MODELING OF HUMAN ARTICULATING JOINTS

A. E. Engin, N. Berme* and N. Akkas**

Department of Engineering Mechanics, *Mechanial Engineering Department, The Ohio State University, Columbus, Ohio   43210 U.S.A.
**Civil Engineering Department, The Middle East Technical University, Ankara, Turkey

1. INTRODUCTION

Realistically developed theoretical models of human joints play a significant role in understanding both normal and abnormal joint functions, as well as improving biodynamic response of multi-segmented total-human-body models. A substantial difficulty in theoretical modeling of human joints arises from the fact that the number of unknowns are usually far greater than the number of available equilibrium or dynamic equations. Thus, the problem is an indeterminate one. To deal with this indeterminate situation, optimization techniques have been employed in the past (1,2). However, the selection of objective functions appears to be arbitrary, and justification for such minimization criteria is indeed debatable. Another technique dealing with the indeterminate nature of the joint modeling considers the anatomical and physiological constraint conditions together with the equilibrium or dynamic equations. These constraint conditions include the fact that soft tissues only transmit tensile loads while the articulating surfaces can only be subjected to compression. Electromyographic data from the muscles crossing the joint also provide additional information for the joint modeling effort. The different techniques used by various researchers mainly vary on the method of applying these conditions. At one extreme all unknowns are included in the equilibrium or dynamic equations. A number of unknown forces are then assumed zero to make the system determinate so that the reduced set of equations can be solved. This process is repeated for all possible combinations of the unknowns, and the values of the joint forces are obtained after discarding the inadmissible solutions (3). At the other extreme, first the primary functions of all structures are identified and equations are simplified before they are solved (4). A combination of these two techniques was also used to solve several quasi-static joint modeling problems (5,6).

All models described in the previous paragraph are quasi-static models. That is the equilibrium equations together with the inertia terms are solved for a known kinematic configuration of the joint. Complexity of joint modeling becomes paramount when one considers a true dynamic analysis of an articulating joint structure possessing realistic articulating surface geometry and non-linear soft tissue behavior. Because of this extreme complexity, the multi-segmented models of the human body, thus far, have been employing simple geometric shapes for their joints.

Although in the literature (7), there are mathematical joint models that consider both the geometry of the joint surfaces and behavior of the joint ligaments, these models are quasi-static in nature, and employ the so-called inverse method. In the inverse method the ligament forces caused by a specified set of translations and rotations along the specified directions are determined by comparing the geometries of the initial and displaced configurations of the joint. Furthermore, in the inverse method utilized in (7) it is necessary to specify the external force required for the preferred equilibrium configuration. Such an approach is applicable only in a quasi-static analysis. In a dynamic analysis, on the other hand, the equilibrium configuration preferred by the joint is the unknown and the mathematical analysis itself is to provide that dynamic equilibrium configuration.

The main thrust of this chapter is the presentation of a mathematical modeling of an articulating joint defined by contact surfaces of two body segments which execute a relative dynamic motion within the constraints of ligament forces. Mathematical equations for the joint model are in the form of second-order nonlinear differential equations coupled with nonlinear algebraic constraint conditions. Solution of these differential equations by application of Newmark method of differential approximation and subsequent usage of Newton-Raphson iteration scheme will be discussed. The two-dimensional version of the dynamic joint model will be applied to human knee joint for several dynamic loading conditions on tibia. Results for the ligament and contact forces, contact point locations between the femur and tibia and the corresponding dynamic orientation of the tibia with respect to femur will be presented.

2.   FORMULATION OF THE THREE-DIMENSIONAL DYNAMIC JOINT MODEL

The articulating joint is modelled by two rigid body segments connected by nonlinear springs simulating the ligaments. It is

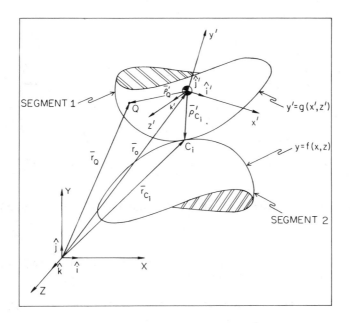

Fig. 1 A two-body segmented joint is illustrated in three dimensions, showing the position of a point, Q, attached to the moving
coordinate system (x',y',z').

assumed that one body segment is rigidly fixed while the second
body segment is undergoing a general three-dimensional dynamic
motion relative to the fixed one. The coefficients of friction
between the articulating surfaces are assumed to be negligible.
This is a valid assumption due to the presence of synovial fluid
between the articulating surfaces (8). Accordingly, the friction
force between the articulating surfaces will be neglected.

2.1 Representation of the Relative Positions

The position of the moving body segment 1 relative to fixed
body segment 2 is described by two coordinate systems as shown in
Fig. 1. The inertial coordinate system (x,y,z) with unit vectors
$\hat{i}$, $\hat{j}$ and $\hat{k}$ is connected to the fixed body segment and the coordinate system (x',y',z') with unit vectors $\hat{i}'$, $\hat{j}'$ and $\hat{k}'$ is attached
to the center of mass of the moving body segment. The (x',y',z')
coordinate system is also taken to be the principal axis system of
the moving body segment. The motion of the moving (x',y',z')
system relative to the fixed (x,y,z) system may be characterized by
six quantities: the translational movement of the origin of the

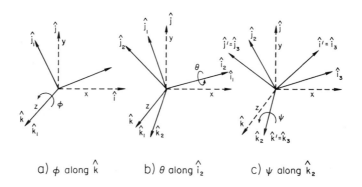

a) ϕ along $\hat{k}$ b) θ along $\hat{i}_2$ c) ψ along $\hat{k}_2$

Fig. 2 Successive rotations of ϕ, θ, and ψ, of the (x,y,z) coordinate system.

(x',y',z') system in the x, y, and z directions, and θ, ϕ, and ψ rotations with respect to the x, y, and z axes.

Let the position vector of the origin of the (x',y',z') system in the fixed system be given by (Fig. 1):

$$\underline{r}_o = x_o\hat{i} + y_o\hat{j} + z_o\hat{k} \quad . \tag{1}$$

Let the vector, $\underline{\rho}'_Q$, be the position vector of an arbitrary point, Q, on the moving body segment in the base $(\hat{i}',\hat{j}',\hat{k}')$. Let $\underline{r}_Q$ be the position vector of the same point in the base $(\hat{i},\hat{j},\hat{k})$. That is,

$$\underline{\rho}'_Q = x'_Q\hat{i}' + y'_Q\hat{j}' + z'_Q\hat{k}' \quad , \quad \underline{r}_Q = x_Q\hat{i} + y_Q\hat{j} + z_Q\hat{k} \quad . \tag{2}$$

Referring to Fig. 1, vectors $\underline{\rho}'_Q$ and $\underline{r}_Q$ have the following relationship:

$$\{r_Q\} = \{r_o\} + [T]^T\{\rho'_Q\}, \tag{3}$$

where [T] is a 3x3 orthogonal transformation matrix. The angular orientation of the (x',y',z') system with respect to the (x,y,z) system is specified by the nine components of the [T] matrix and can be written as a function of the three variables, θ, ϕ, and ψ:

$$T = T(\theta,\phi,\psi). \tag{4}$$

There are several systems of variables such as θ, ϕ, and ψ which can be used to specify T. At the present formulation the Euler angles are chosen.

The orientation of the moving coordinate system $(\hat{i}', \hat{j}', \hat{k}')$ is obtained from the fixed coordinate system $(\hat{i}, \hat{j}, \hat{k})$ by applying successive rotation angles, ϕ, θ, and ψ (Fig. 2). First, the $(\hat{i}, \hat{j}, \hat{k})$ system is rotated through an angle ϕ about the z-axis (Fig. 2a), which results in the intermediary system $(\hat{i}_1, \hat{j}, \hat{k}_1)$. The second rotation through an angle θ about the i_1-axis (Fig. 2b), produces the intermediary system $(\hat{i}_2, \hat{j}_2, \hat{k}_2)$, and the third rotation through an angle ψ about the k_2-axis (Fig. 2c), gives the final orientation of the moving $(\hat{i}', \hat{j}', \hat{k}')$ system relative to the fixed $(\hat{i}, \hat{j}, \hat{k})$ system. The orthogonal transformation matrix [T] resulting from above rotations is given by

$$[T] = \begin{bmatrix} \cos\phi\cos\psi & \cos\psi\sin\phi & \\ -\sin\psi\cos\theta\sin\phi & +\sin\psi\cos\theta\cos\phi & \sin\theta\sin\psi \\ & & \\ -\sin\psi\cos\phi & -\sin\psi\sin\phi & \\ -\cos\psi\cos\theta\sin\phi & +\cos\psi\cos\theta\cos\phi & \cos\psi\sin\theta \\ & & \\ \sin\phi\sin\theta & -\sin\theta\cos\phi & \cos\theta \end{bmatrix} \quad (5)$$

2.2 Joint Surfaces and Contact Conditions

Assuming rigid body contacts between the two body segments at points C (i=1,2) as shown in Fig. 1, let us represent the contact surfaces by smooth mathematical functions of the following form:

$$y = f(x,z) \quad , \quad y' = g(x',z') . \tag{6}$$

As implied in Eq.(6) y and y' represent the fixed and the moving surfaces, respectively. The position vectors of the contact points C_i(i=1,2) in the base $(\hat{i}, \hat{j}, \hat{k})$ is denoted by

$$\underline{r}_{c_i} = x_{c_i}\hat{i} + f(x_{c_i}, z_{c_i})\hat{j} + z_{c_i}\hat{k} \tag{7}$$

and the corresponding ones in the base (i',j',k) are given by

$$\underline{\rho}'_{c_i} = x'_{c_i}\hat{i}' + g(x'_{c_i}, z'_{c_i})\hat{j}' + z'_{c_i}\hat{k}' . \tag{8}$$

Then, at each contact point C_i, the following relationship must hold:

$$\{r_{c_i}\} = \{r_o\} + [T]^T\{\rho'_{c_i}\} .$$ (9)

This is a part of the geometric compatibility condition for the two contact surfaces. Furthermore, the unit normals to the surfaces of the moving and fixed body segments at the points of contacts must be colinear.

Let n_{c_i} $(i=1,2)$ be the unit normals to the fixed surface, $y = f(x,z)$, at the contact points, $C_i(i=1,2)$, then

$$n_{c_i} = \frac{1}{\sqrt{\det[G]}}\left(\frac{\partial r_{c_i}}{\partial x_{c_i}}\right) \times \left(\frac{\partial r_{c_i}}{\partial z_{c_i}}\right) \quad i=1,2$$ (10)

where r_{c_i} is given in Eq. 7 and the components of the matrix $[G]$ are determined by

$$G_{k\ell} = \left(\frac{\partial r_{c_i}}{\partial x^k}\cdot\frac{\partial r_{c_i}}{\partial x^\ell}\right) \quad i=1,2$$ (11)

with

$$x^1 = x_{c_i} , \quad x^2 = z_{c_i} , \quad x^3 = f(x_{c_i},z_{c_i}) .$$

Therefore, the components of matrix $[G_{k\ell}]$ may be expressed as

$$G_{xx} = \left(\frac{\partial x_{c_i}}{\partial x_{c_i}}\right)^2 + \left(\frac{\partial y_{c_i}}{\partial x_{c_i}}\right)^2 + \left(\frac{\partial z_{c_i}}{\partial x_{c_i}}\right)^2$$ (12a)

$$G_{zz} = \left(\frac{\partial x_{c_i}}{\partial z_{c_i}}\right)^2 + \left(\frac{\partial y_{c_i}}{\partial z_{c_i}}\right)^2 + \left(\frac{\partial z_{c_i}}{\partial z_{c_i}}\right)^2$$ (12b)

$$G_{xz} = G_{zx} = \left(\frac{\partial x_{c_i}}{\partial x_{c_i}}\right)\left(\frac{\partial x_{c_i}}{\partial z_{c_i}}\right) + \left(\frac{\partial y_{c_i}}{\partial x_{c_i}}\right)\left(\frac{\partial y_{c_i}}{\partial z_{c_i}}\right) + \left(\frac{\partial z_{c_i}}{\partial x_{c_i}}\right)\left(\frac{\partial z_{c_i}}{\partial z_{c_i}}\right)$$ (12c)

Since $(\partial z_{c_i}/\partial x_{c_i})=0$ and $(\partial x_{c_i}/\partial z_{c_i})=0$, then the components of matrix $[G_{k\ell}]$ reduce to

$$G_{xx} = 1 + \left(\frac{\partial f}{\partial x_{c_i}}\right)^2 \quad , \quad G_{zz} = 1 + \left(\frac{\partial f}{\partial z_{c_i}}\right)^2 \qquad (13a, b)$$

$$G_{xz} = G_{zx} = \left(\frac{\partial f}{\partial x_{c_i}}\right)\left(\frac{\partial f}{\partial z_{c_i}}\right). \qquad (13c)$$

From Eqs. 13, the det[G] can be written as

$$\det[G] = 1 + \left(\frac{\partial f}{\partial x_{c_i}}\right)^2 + \left(\frac{\partial f}{\partial z_{c_i}}\right)^2 \qquad (14)$$

and therefore the unit outward normals expressed in Eq. 10 will have the following form:

$$\hat{n}_{c_i} = \frac{\gamma}{\sqrt{1 + \left(\frac{\partial f}{\partial x_{c_i}}\right)^2 + \left(\frac{\partial f}{\partial z_{c_i}}\right)^2}}\left[\left(\frac{\partial f}{\partial x_{c_i}}\right)\hat{i} - \hat{j} + \left(\frac{\partial f}{\partial z_{c_i}}\right)\hat{k}\right], \quad (15)$$

where the parameter, γ, is chosen such that $\hat{n}_{c_i}$ represents the outward normal. Similarly, following the same procedure as outlined above $\hat{n}'_{c_i}$ (i=1,2), the unit outward normal to the moving surface, $y' = g(x',z')$, at contact points, C (i=1,2), and expressed in $(\hat{i}',\hat{j}',\hat{k}')$ system, can be written as

$$\hat{n}_{c_i} = \frac{\beta}{\sqrt{1 + \left(\frac{\partial g}{\partial x'_{c_i}}\right)^2 + \left(\frac{\partial g}{\partial z'_{c_i}}\right)^2}}\left[\left(\frac{\partial g}{\partial x'_{c_i}}\right)\hat{i}' - \hat{j}' + \left(\frac{\partial g}{\partial z'_{c_i}}\right)\hat{k}'\right], \quad (16)$$

where the parameter, β, is chosen such that $\hat{n}'_{c_i}$ represents the outward normal. Colinearity of unit normals at each contact point C_i(i=1,2), requires that

$$\{n_{c_i}\} = -[T]^T\{n'_{c_i}\} \quad . \qquad (17)$$

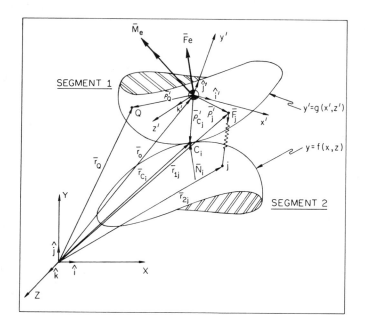

Fig. 3   Forces acting on the moving body segment of a two-body
segmented joint in three dimensions.

Note that colinearity condition can also be satisfied by requiring
that the cross product ($\hat{n}_{c_i} \times T^T \hat{n}'_{c_i}$) be zero.

2.3   Ligament and Contact Forces

During its motion the moving body segment is subjected to the
ligament forces, contact forces and the externally applied forces
and moments (Fig. 3). The contact forces and the ligament forces
are the unknowns of the problem and the external forces and moments
will be specified. These forces are discussed in some detail in
the following paragraphs.

The ligaments are modelled as nonlinear elastic springs. To
be more specific, for the major ligaments of the knee joint the
following force-elongation relationship can be assumed:

$$F_j = K_j(L_j - \ell_j)^2 \quad \text{for} \quad L_j > \ell_j . \tag{18a}$$

in which K_j is the spring constant, L_j and ℓ_j are, respectively, the current and initial lengths of the ligament j. The tensile force in the jth ligament, thus, designated by F_j. It is assumed that the ligaments cannot carry any compressive force; accordingly,

$$F_j = 0 \quad \text{for} \quad L_j < \ell_j \ . \tag{18b}$$

The stiffness values, K_j, are estimated according to the data available in the literature (9,10).

Let $(\underline{\rho}_j')_m$ be the position vector in the base $(\hat{i}',\hat{j}',\hat{k}')$ of the insertion point of the ligament, j, in the moving body segment. The position vector of the origin point of the same ligament, j, in the fixed body segment is denoted by $(\underline{r}_{2j})_f$ in the base $(\hat{i},\hat{j},\hat{k})$. Here the subscripts m and f outside the parenthesis imply "moving" and "fixed," respectively. The current length of the ligament is given by

$$L_j = \sqrt{[(\underline{r}_{2j})_f - \underline{r}_o - T^T(\underline{\rho}_j')_m] \cdot [(\underline{r}_{2j})_f - \underline{r}_o - T^T(\underline{\rho}_j')_m]}. \tag{19}$$

The unit vector, $\hat{\lambda}_j$, along the ligament, j, directed from the moving to the fixed body segment is

$$\hat{\lambda}_j = \frac{1}{L}[(\underline{r}_{2j})_f - \underline{r}_o - T^T(\underline{\rho}_j')_m]. \tag{20}$$

Thus, the axial force in the ligament, j, in its vectorial form, becomes

$$\underline{F}_j = F_j \hat{\lambda}_j \ , \tag{21}$$

where F_j is given by Eq. 18. Since the friction force between the moving and fixed body segment is neglected, the contact force will be in the direction of the normal to the surface at the point of contact. The contact forces, N_i, acting on the moving body segment is given by

$$\underline{N}_i = |N_i| [(n_{c_i})_x \hat{i} + (n_{c_i})_y \hat{j} + (n_{c_i})_z \hat{k}], \tag{22}$$

where $|N_i|$ are the unknown magnitudes of the contact forces and $(n_{c_i})_x$, $(n_{c_i})_y$, and $(n_{c_i})_z$ are the components of the unit normal $\hat{n}_{c_i}$, in the x, y, and z directions, respectively.

In general, the moving body segment of the joint is subjected to various external forces and moments whose resultants at the center of mass of the moving body segment are given as

$$\underline{F}_e = (F_e)_x \hat{i} + (F_e)_y \hat{j} + (F_e)_z \hat{k}, \quad \underline{M}_e = (M_e)_x \hat{i} + (M_e)_y \hat{j} + (M_e)_z \hat{k}. \tag{23}$$

2.4 Equations of Motion

The equations governing the forced motion of the moving body segment are

$$(F_e)_x + \sum_{i=1}^{q} |N_i|(n_{c_i})_x + \sum_{j=1}^{p} F_j(\lambda_j)_x = M\ddot{x}_0 \tag{24a}$$

$$(F_e)_y + \sum_{i=1}^{q} |N_i|(n_{c_i})_y + \sum_{j=1}^{p} F_j(\lambda_j)_y = M\ddot{y}_0 \tag{24b}$$

$$(F_e)_z + \sum_{i=1}^{q} |N_i|(n_{c_i})_z + \sum_{j=1}^{p} F_j(\lambda_j)_z = M\ddot{z}_0 \tag{24c}$$

$$\sum M_{x'x'} = I_{x'x'}\dot{\omega}_{x'} + (I_{z'z'} - I_{y'y'})\omega_{y'}\omega_{z'} \tag{25a}$$

$$\sum M_{y'y'} = I_{y'y'}\dot{\omega}_{y'} + (I_{x'x'} - I_{z'z'})\omega_{z'}\omega_{x'} \tag{25b}$$

$$\sum M_{z'z'} = I_{z'z'}\dot{\omega}_{z'} + (I_{y'y'} - I_{x'x'})\omega_{x'}\omega_{y'} \tag{25c}$$

where p and q represent the number of ligaments and the contact points, respectively. $I_{x'x'}$, $I_{y'y'}$, and $I_{z'z'}$ are the principal moments of inertia of the moving body segment about its centroidal principal axis system (x', y', z'), and $\omega_{x'}$, $\omega_{y'}$, and $\omega_{z'}$, are the components of the angular velocity vector which are given below in terms of the Euler angles:

$$\omega_{x'} = \dot{\theta}\cos\psi + \dot{\phi}\sin\theta\sin\psi, \quad \omega_{y'} = \dot{\theta}\sin\psi + \dot{\phi}\sin\theta\cos\psi, \quad \omega_{z'} = \dot{\phi}\cos\theta + \dot{\psi}. \tag{26}$$

The angular acceleration components, $\dot{\omega}_{x'}$, $\dot{\omega}_{y'}$, and $\dot{\omega}_{z'}$ are directly obtained from Eq. 26:

$$\dot{\omega}_{x'} = \ddot{\theta}\cos\psi - \dot{\psi}(\dot{\theta}\sin\psi - \dot{\phi}\cos\psi\sin\theta) + \ddot{\phi}\sin\theta\sin\psi + \dot{\phi}\dot{\theta}\cos\theta\sin\phi \tag{27a}$$

$$\dot{\omega}_{y'} = -\ddot{\theta}\sin\psi - \dot{\psi}(\dot{\theta}\cos\psi + \dot{\phi}\sin\psi\sin\theta) + \ddot{\phi}\sin\theta\cos\psi + \dot{\phi}\dot{\theta}\cos\theta\cos\psi \quad (27b)$$

$$\dot{\omega}_{z'} = \ddot{\phi}\cos\theta - \dot{\phi}\dot{\theta}\sin + \ddot{\psi}. \quad (27c)$$

Note that the moment components shown on the left-hand side of Eqs. 25 have the following terms:

$$\underline{M} = \underline{M}_e + \sum_{i=1}^{q} [T]^T (\underline{\rho}'_{c_i}) \times (|N_i|\underline{n}_{c_i}) + \sum_{j=1}^{p} [T]^T (\underline{\rho}'_j) \times (F_j\underline{\lambda}_j), \quad (28)$$

where $\underline{M}_e$ is applied external moment, and p and q again represent the number of ligaments and contact points, respectively.

Equations 24 and 25 form a set of six nonlinear second-order differential equations which, together with the contact conditions (9) and (17), form a set of 16 nonlinear equations (assuming two contact points, i.e., i=1,2) with 16 unknowns:
(a) θ, ϕ, and ψ, which determine the components of transformation matrix [T];
(b) x_o, y_o, and z_o: the components of position vector $\underline{r}_o$;
(c) x_{c_i}, z_{c_i}, x'_{c_i} and z'_{c_i} (i=1,2): the coordinates of contact points;
(d) $|N_i|$(i=1,2): the magnitudes of the contact forces.
The problem description is completed by assigning the initial conditions which are

$$\dot{x}_o = \dot{y}_o = \dot{z}_o = 0 \quad , \quad \dot{\omega}_x = \dot{\omega}_y = \dot{\omega}_z = 0 \quad (29)$$

along with specified values for x_o, y_o, z_o, θ, ϕ, and ψ at t=0. Before we describe the numerical procedure employed in the solution of the governing equations in the next section, the following observation must be made. During its motion the segment 1 is subjected to the ligament forces, contact forces and the externally applied forces and moments, Fig. 3. The contact force and the ligament forces are the unknowns of the problem and the external forces and moments are specified. At this time, the reader might wonder why the muscle forces are not included in the dynamic modeling of an articulating joint. If the model under consideration is intended to simulate events which take place during a very short time period such as 0.1 seconds, then it is sufficient to consider only the passive resistive forces at the model formulation. However, direct exclusion of the muscle forces from the model does not restrict its capabilities to have the effects of muscle forces to be included, if desired, as a part of the applied force and moment vector on the moving body segment.

3. NUMERICAL SOLUTION PROCEDURE

The governing equations of the initial value problem at hand are the six equations of motion (24) and (25), four contact conditions (9) and six geometric compatibility conditions (17). The main unknowns of the problem are x, y, z, θ, ϕ, ψ, x_{c_1}, z_{c_1}, x_{c_2}, z_{c_2}, x'_{c_1}, z'_{c_1}, x'_{c_2}, z'_{c_2}, N_1, and N_2. The problem is, thus, reduced to the solution of a set of simultaneous nonlinear differential and algebraic equations.

The first step in arriving at a numerical solution of these equations is the replacement of the time derivatives with a temporal operator; in the present work, the Newmark operators (11) are chosen for this purpose. For instance, x_0 is expressed in the following form:

$$\ddot{x}_0^t = \frac{4}{(\Delta t)^2}(x_0^t - x_0^{t-\Delta t}) - \frac{4}{\Delta t}\dot{x}_0^{t-\Delta t} - \ddot{x}_0^{t-\Delta t}, \quad \dot{x}_0^t = \dot{x}_0^{t-\Delta t} + \frac{\Delta t}{2}\ddot{x}_0^{t-\Delta t} + \frac{\Delta t}{2}\ddot{x}_0^t,$$

(30)

in which Δt is the time increment and the superscripts refer to the time stations. Similar expressions may be used for $\ddot{y}_0$, $\ddot{z}_0$, ϕ, θ, and ψ. In the application of Eqs. 30, the conditions at the previous time station $(t-\Delta t)$ are, of course, assumed to be known.

After the time derivatives in Eqs. 24 and 25 are replaced with the temporal operators defined, the governing equations take the form of a set of nonlinear algebraic equations. The solution of these equations is complicated by the fact that iteration or perturbation methods must be used. In this work, the Newton-Raphson (12) iteration process is used for the solution. To linearize the resulting set of simultaneous algebraic equations we assume

$$^k x_0^t = {}^{k-1}x_0^t + \Delta x_0$$

(31)

and similar expressions for the other variables are written. Here, the right superscripts denote the time station under consideration and the left superscripts denote the iteration number. At each iteration k the values of the variables at the previous $(k-1)$ iteration are assumed to be known. The delta quantities denote incremental values. Equation 31 and the corresponding ones for the other variables are substituted into the governing nonlinear algebraic equations and the higher order terms in the delta quantities are dropped. The set of n simultaneous algebraic (now linearized) equations can be put into the following matrix form

$$[K]\{\Delta\} = \{D\},$$

(32)

where [K] is an n x n coefficient matrix, {Δ} is a vector of incremental quantities, and {D} is a vector of known values.

The iteration process at a fixed time station continues until the delta quantities of all the variables become negligibly small. In the present work, a solution is accepted and iteration process is terminated when the delta quantities become less than or equal to 0.01% of the previous values of the corresponding variables. The converged solution of each variable is then used as the initial value for the next time step and the process is repeated for consecutive time steps.

The only problem that the Newton–Raphson process may present in the solution of dynamic problems is due to the fact that the period of the forced motion of the system may turn out to be quite short. In this case it becomes necessary to use very small time steps; otherwise, a significantly large number of iterations is required for convergence. The time increment used in the present work is t = 0.0001 sec.

Numerical procedure outlined above can be utilized for the solution of the three-dimensional joint model equations presented so far. However, because of the extreme complexity of these equations, in this chapter we will present only the numerical results of the two-dimensional version of our formulation applied to the dynamic model of the human knee joint. Detailed numerical solution and complete discussion of the previously developed knee joint models are given in (13).

4.   THE TWO-DIMENSIONAL DYNAMIC MODELS AND RESULTS

The two dimensional version of an articulating joint model which connects two body segments which are designated as segments 1 and 2 is shown in Figs. 4 and 5. An inertial coordinate system (x,y) with unit vectors î and ĵ is connected to the fixed body segment, while the coordinate system (x′,y′) with unit vectors î′ and ĵ′ is attached to the center of mass of the moving body segment 1. The motion of the moving (x′,y′) system relative to the fixed (x,y) system may be characterized by three quantities: the translational movement of the origin of the (x′,y′) system in the x- and y-directions, and its rotation, α, with respect to the fixed (x,y) system.

In a two-dimensional formulation the articulating contact surfaces can be represented by smooth mathematical functions of the following form:

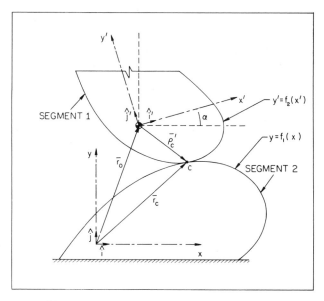

Fig. 4   The two-dimensional articulating joint model.

$$y = f_1(x) \text{ and } y' = f_2(x').$$ (33)

The colinearity of the normals at the contact point C, Eq. 17, takes the following form:

$$\sin\alpha\left[1 + \left(\frac{df_1}{dx}\right)_{x=x_c} \left(\frac{df_2}{dx'}\right)_{x'=x'_c}\right] \;-$$

$$\cos\alpha\left[\left(\frac{df_1}{dx}\right)_{x=x_c} \left(\frac{df_2}{dx'}\right)_{x'=x'_c}\right] = 0$$ (34)

Formulation of the ligament and contact forces are very similar to the three-dimensional case and the equations of motion (Eqs. 24, 25) reduce to the following set:

$$(F_e)_x + \gamma N(n_1)_x + \sum_{j=1}^{p} F_j(\lambda_j)_x = M\ddot{x}_o$$ (35a)

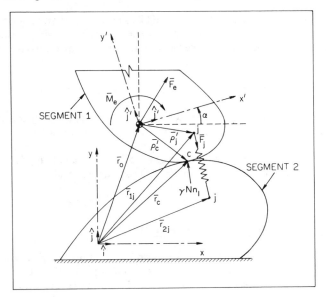

Fig. 5   Forces acting on the moving body segment of a two-body
segmented joint and relevant vectors for the contact point, C, and
ligament, j, are illustrated.

$$(F_e)_y + \gamma N(n_1)_y + \sum_{j=1}^{p} F_j(\lambda_j)_y = M\ddot{y}_o \qquad (35b)$$

$$M_e + (T\underline{\rho}'_c)x(\gamma N\underline{n}_1) + \sum_{j=1}^{p} (T\underline{\rho}'_j)x(F_j\lambda_j) = I_z\ddot{\alpha} \qquad (35c)$$

where p is the number of ligaments and the subscripts, x and y,
denote the components of the related quantities in the x and
y-directions. The mass of the moving body segment is denoted by M
and the dots denote derivatives with respect to time, t. The mass
moment of inertia of the moving body segment about the z-axis is I_z
and $\ddot{\alpha}$ designates its angular acceleration. $(F_e)_x$, $(F_e)_y$ and M_e are
the components in the base $(\hat{i},\hat{j})$ of the external force and moment,
respectively, which are applied to the center of mass of the moving
body segment. The problem description is completed by assigning
the initial conditions, which are:

$$\dot{x}_o = \dot{y}_o = \dot{\alpha} = 0 \qquad (36)$$

along with the specified values for x_o, y_o and α at t=0.

Three nonlinear second order differential equations, Eqs. 35a, b, and c, along with the geometric compatibility and contact conditions provide the necessary relationships to determine the following unknowns:

(a) x_o and y_o; the components of vector r_o,

(b) x_c and x_c'; the x and x'-coordinates of the contact point, C, in the base (i,j) and (i',j'), respectively,

(c) α; the orientation angle of the moving (x',y') system relative to the fixed (x,y) system, and

(d) N; the magnitude of the contact force.

4.1 Numerical Results and Discussion

The human knee joint is chosen for the application of the mathematical formulation presented in this chapter. Detailed discussions of various anatomical and functional aspects of the human knee joint can be found in (14,15). The first task in obtaining numerical results is determination of the functions $f_1(x)$ and $f_2(x')$ from a radiograph of the lateral view of a human knee joint. A number of points on the two-dimensional profiles of the femoral and tibial articulating surfaces were utilized to obtain quartic and quadratic polynomials, respectively:

$$f_1(x) = 0.04014 - 0.247621x - 6.889185x^2 - 270.4456x^3 - 8589.942x^4$$

$$f_2(x') = 0.213373 - 0.0456051x' + 1.073446x'^2. \tag{37}$$

The numerical results to be presented are only for an external force acting on the tibia (Fig. 6) without the presence of an external moment. It is assumed that the force is always perpendicular to the longitudinal axis of the tibia (y' axis) and passes through its center of mass. Let this force be denoted by $F_e(t)$. A parametric study of the effect of various combinations of moment and force acting simultaneously on the response of the knee joint may prove to be rewarding.

However, for the present work we will only consider an external force and believe that this will be sufficient to illustrate the capabilities of the model. The effect of the shape of the forcing function on the knee joint response will be studied by considering the following two functions for $F_e(t)$:

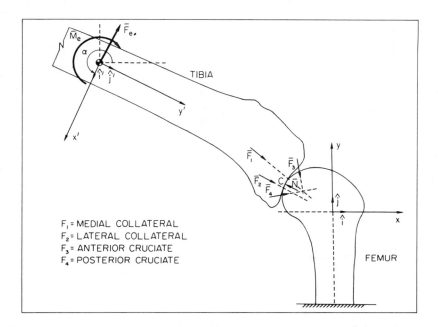

Fig. 6 Forces acting on the moving tibia are shown for the two-dimensional model of the knee joint.

$$F_e(t) = A[H(t) - H(t-t_0)], \tag{38}$$

which is a rectangular pulse of duration t_0, and amplitude A; and

$$F_e(t) = Ae^{-4.73(t/t_0)^2}\sin(\frac{\pi t}{t_0}), \tag{39}$$

which is an exponentially decaying sinusoidal pulse of duration t_0, and amplitude A. A dynamic loading in the form of Eq. 38 is extremely difficult to simulate experimentally; however, the study of these two functions will hopefully be helpful in understanding the effect of rise time of the dynamic load on the joint response. Equation 39 is a more realistic forcing function and it has been previously used as a typical representation of the dynamic load in head impact analysis (16).

The following are obtained as a function of time from a computer program developed for the two-dimensional model; the

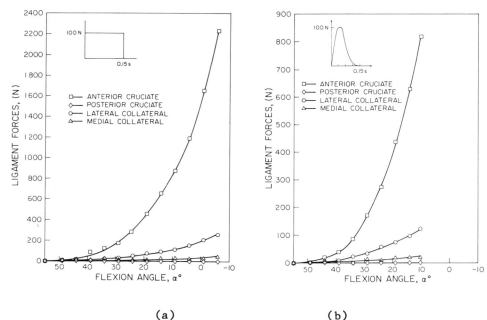

(a)   (b)
Fig. 7 Ligament forces as functions of flexion angle, for an externally applied (a) rectangular and (b) exponentially decaying sinusoidal pulses of 100N amplitude and 0.15 second duration.

coordinates x_o, y_o of the center of mass tibia; the flexion angle α; the coordinates x_c and x_c' of the contact point in (x,y) and (x',y') coordinate systems, respectively; the magnitude, N, of the contact force; the elongations of the ligaments and the ligament forces, F_j . Before the application of the external force, the flexion angle of the knee is chosen to be about 55° for which the ligaments of the joint are in nearly unstretched state.

The effect of pulse duration on the response of the knee joint motion is studied by taking t_o =0.05, 0.10, and 0.15 seconds for both rectangular and exponentially decaying sinusoidal pulses. The effect of pulse amplitude, A, is also examined by taking A=20, 60, 100, 140, 180N for both types of pulses. In principle, it is possible to plot the numerical results in numerous ways. However, because of the space limitations only some representative results will be presented.

Ligament forces as functions of flexion angle of the knee joint for the two previously described forcing functions are presented in Figs. 7a and b. Results indicate that when the knee joint is extended by a dynamic application of a pulse on the tibia, lateral collateral, medial collateral and anterior cruciate

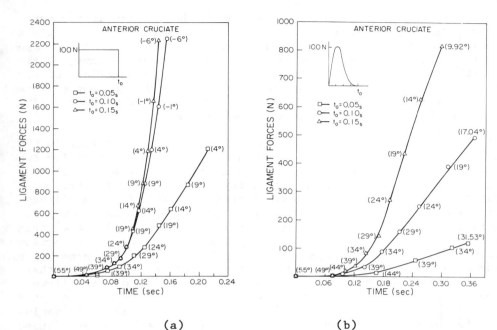

(a) (b)

Fig. 8 Anterior cruciate ligament force as a function of time for externally applied (a) rectangular and (b) exponentially decaying sinusoidal pulses of 100N amplitude and durations of 0.05, 0.10 and 0.15 seconds.

ligaments are elongated while the posterior cruciate ligament is shortened. The load carried by the anterior cruciate ligament is substantially higher than those of the lateral collateral and medial collateral ligaments. The variation of the lengths of ligaments and the forces carried by them during normal knee motion has been the subject of various studies reported in the literature and in these studies several different opinions and conclusions have been expressed in regard to the biomechanical role and function of various ligaments of the knee joint. The function of the anterior cruciate as depicted in the dynamic knee-model is to resist anterior displacement of the tibia.

The present dynamic model also predicts that the medial and lateral collateral ligaments offer very little resistance in the flexion-extension motion of the knee joint. The major role of these ligaments is to offer varus-valgus and partial internal-external rotational stability. The model shows that as the knee joint is extended under influence of a dynamic load the lateral collateral and medial collateral ligaments elongate at different magnitudes.

The model shows good agreement with the quasi-static experimental investigations reported in the literature. It is important
to note that the dynamic model presented here is an idealized
representation of a very complex anatomical structure; thus, static
experimental studies may not support some of the predictions of the
model. Additional disagreements may also be due to approximate
locations of the attachment sites of the ligaments in particular,
and two-dimensional nature of the model in general.

In Figs. 8a and b a few representative plots of forces in the
anterior cruciate ligament are shown as a function of time for two
different forcing functions with varying pulse durations. Although
not presented here, similar curves may be obtained for other pulse
durations and pulse magnitudes. Generally, for a fixed amplitude,
the shorter the pulse duration, the sooner the tibia reaches its
turning point (i.e., direction of motion reverses) and for a given
pulse duration, the smaller the amplitude, the sooner the turning
point is reached. In Figs. 7, 8 and 9 the values in parentheses
indicate the flexion angles at the corresponding times. Note that,
for illustrative purposes up to 6° of hyperextension was allowed.
Generally, one expects only 1 to 3° of hyperextension to be anatomically tolerable beyond which joint failure becomes unavoidable.
In Fig. 9, contact forces as a function of time are plotted. These
forces are in response to the different forcing functions with
varying amplitudes and pulse durations. Note that the magnitudes
of the anterior cruciate ligament and the corresponding contact
forces in response to a particular forcing function are comparable.
Finally, femoral and tibial contact point locations as a function
of flexion angle are plotted in Figs. 10 a and b. In these figures
the values in the parentheses indicate the total elapsed time of
the motion since its initiation. The difference between the curves
representing the femoral and tibial contact points may be attributed to the combined rolling and sliding motion of the tibia on the
femur.

5.   SUMMARY AND CONCLUDING REMARKS

The research work discussed and presented in this chapter can
be summarized in the following paragraphs:

1. A three-dimensional mathematical dynamic model of a general
two-body-segmented articulating joint has been formulated in order
to describe the relative motion between the segments and the
various forces produced at the joint.

2. The two-dimensional version of this formulation has been
applied to the human knee joint to study the relative dynamic
motion between femur and tibia and the forces in the joint. The

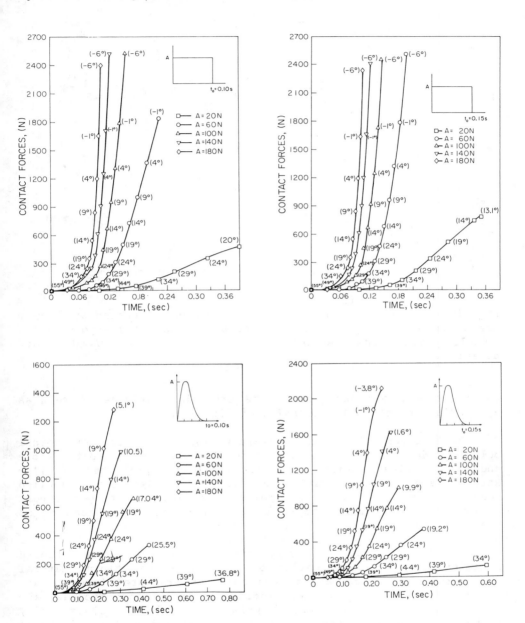

Fig. 9 Contact forces as a function of time for externally applied rectangular and exponentially decaying sinusoidal pulses of 20N, 60N, 100N, 140N and 180N amplitudes for 0.10 and 0.15 second durations.

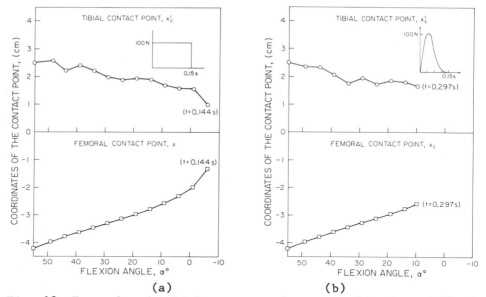

Fig. 10 Femoral and tibial contact points as a function of flexion
angle for externally applied (a) rectangular and (b) exponentially
decaying sinusoidal pulses of 100N amplitude and 0.10 second
duration.

model includes the geometry of the articular surfaces as well as
appropriate constitutive behavior of ligaments.

3. A rectangular and an exponentially decaying sinusoidal
pulses of duration, t , and amplitude, A, were applied to the tibia
and the numerical results from this model were presented to illustrate the effects of duration and shape of the dynamically applied
loads on the response of the joint. Special attention has been
given to the ligament and contact forces, and the location of
contact points.

4. The model predicts that when the knee joint is extended
dynamically, by an application of a pulse on the tibia, lateral
collateral, medial collateral and anterior cruciate ligaments are
elongated while the posterior cruciate ligament is shortened. The
load carried by the anterior cruciate ligament is substantially
higher than those of the lateral collateral and medial collateral
ligaments.

5. With this mathematical model the influence of the variations of initial strain of the ligaments and their attachment
sites (i.e. insertions and origins) on the response of the model
can be determined and a parametric study addressing to these points

may reveal the sensitivity of the model to the variations of the coordinates of the insertions and origins of the ligaments.

6. In a similar way the mathematical models of the other major articulating joints can be developed. However, a special attention should be given in modeling of the ligaments. Some ligaments, particularly the thick band or large cord-like ligaments, have complex behavior, with various portions behaving differently under given conditions or configurations. These are described in the literature as, in the case of the broad ligaments of the hip joint, having anterio_ and posterior fibers, or medial and lateral components. The mathematical model should include additional elastic elements to reflect the contributions of various fibers of the ligaments. Unfortunately proper experimental data to determine the constitutive behavior of these thick band or broad ligaments do not exist.

It is appropriate to make several concluding remarks on the numerical techniques tried in the course of obtaining the solution for the governing equations of the dynamic joint model. In the first method, the second-order differential equations were transformed to a set of nonlinear algebraic equations by substituting for the differential elements, their equivalent backward difference approximations. In this case, it was impossible to obtain a converging solution due to the highly nonlinear nature of these equations. In the second method, the flexion angle, α, of the moving tibia and contact point coordinates, x_c and x_c' were obtained from the simultaneous solution of the nonlinear contact and geometric compatibility conditions. Knowing α, $\ddot{\alpha}$ was obtained via backward difference method and then the normal force, N, was determined from one of the equations of motion. The other two second-order nonlinear differential equations which were in terms of x_0 and y_0 were written as a set of four first order differential equations by direct substitutions. Runge-Kutta method was applied to these equations and solutions for x_0, y_0 and their time derivatives were obtained. Using the new values of x_0 and y_0, a new value of α and contact point coordinates were obtained and the entire procedure was repeated for the next time step. Although mathematically all the geometric constraints and governing equations of motion were satisfied, the results obtained using this second method were not in agreement with the actual physical geometry and the anatomy of the joint. This was concluded to be due to the solution technique which was not solving all the equations simultaneously, and during the solution process it was forcing some of the variables to accept values which were mathematically correct but physically unacceptable. Finally, the Newton-Raphson iteration process along with Newmark method of differential approximation was chosen as the method of solution which yielded accurate and stable solutions for the model.

ACKNOWLEDGEMENTS: The research work described herein was supported by the Mathematics and Analysis Branch of the Aerospace Medical Research Laboratory at Wright-Patterson Air Force Base under Contract No. F33615-78-C-510 to the senior author. The authors also acknowledge assistance of Manssour H. Moeinzadeh, one of the graduate students of the Senior author, in various aspects of the research, especially, in computer programming to obtain the numerical results.

REFERENCES

1. Seirek, A. and R.J. Arvikar. A Mathematical Model for Evaluation of Forces in Lower Extremities of the Musculo-Skeletal System. Journal of Biomechanics 6 (1973) 313.

2. Seirek, A. and R.J. Arvikar. The Prediction of Muscular Load Sharing and Joint Forces in the Lower Extremities During Walking. Journal of Biomechanics 8 (1975) 89-102.

3. Chao, E.Y., J.D. Opgrande and F.E. Axmear. Three-Dimensional Force Analysis of Finger Joints in Selected Isometric Hand Functions. Journal of Biomechanics 9 (1976) 387-397.

4. Paul, J.P. Forces Transmitted by Joints in the Human Body. Inst. Mech. Engrs. Proc. 181 (1967).

5. Berme, N., J.P. Paul and W.K. Purves. A Biomechanical Analysis of the Metacarpo-Phalangeal Joint. Journal of Biomechanics 10 (1977) 409-412.

6. Berme, N. Forces Transmitted by the Finger and Thumb Joints in Selected Hand Functions. Proc. First Meeting of the European Society of Biomechanics (Ed. by Burny, F., Acta Orthopaedica Belgica, 1978) 157-165.

7. Wismans, J., F. Veldpaus, J. Janssen, A. Huson and P. Struben. A Three-Dimensional Mathematical Model of the Knee-Joint. Journal of Biomechanics 13 (1980) 677-686.

8. Radin, E.L. and I.L. Paul. A Consolidated Concept of Joint Lubrication. Journal of Bone and Joint Surgery 54A (1972) 607-616.

9. Trent, P.S., P.S. Walker and B. Wolf. Ligament Length Patterns, Strength and Rotational Axes of the Knee Joint. Clin. Orthoped. Related Res. 117 (1976) 263-270.

10. Kennedy, J.C., R.J. Hawkins, R.B. Willis and K.D. Danylchuk. Tension Studies of Human Knee Joint Ligaments. Journal of Bone and Joint Surgery 58A (1976) 350-355.

11. Bathe, K.J. and E.L. Wilson. Numerical Methods in Finite Element Analysis (Englewood Cliffs, New Jersey: Prentice-Hall, 1976).

12. Kao, R. A Comparison of Newton-Raphson Methods and Incremental Procedures for Geometrically Nonlinear Analysis. Computers and Structures 4 (1974) 1091-1097.

13. Engin, A.E. and M.H. Moeinzadeh. Modeling of Human Joint Structures. AF AMRL-TR-81-117 (1981).
14. Engin, A.E. and M.S. Korde. Biomechanics of Normal and Abnormal Knee Joint. Journal of Biomechanics 7 (1974) 325-334.
15. Engin, A.E. Mechanics of the Knee Joint: Guidelines for Osteotomy in Osteoarthritis. In: Orthopaedic Mechanics: Procedures and Devices, Ed. by D.N. Ghista and R. Roaf (London, England: Academic Press, 1978) 55-98.
16. Engin, A.E. and N. Akkas. Application of a Fluid-Filled Spherical Sandwich Shell as a Biodynamic Head Injury Model for Primates. Aviation, Space and Environmental Medicine 49 (1978) 120-124.

LUBRICATION OF JOINTS

J. P. Renaudeaux

Laboratoire Mecanique des Fluides
Bat. 502 - Campus Universitaire
91405 Orsay, France

Lubrication is the action of attenuating friction between two bodies by interposing a fluid between them. Joint lubrication depends on the nature, form, and rheological properties of articular surfaces, as well as the lubricant, and the combined movement and forces--a set of parameters which are not yet completely determined. The mechanism of lubrication, therefore, has not yet revealed all its secrets. Nevertheless, the laws of mechanics, associated with experiments on representative models, allow to formulate a reasonable hypothesis on the important factors governing proper functioning of joints.

1. THE SYNOVIAL FLUID

Hyaluronate, a complex of macromolecules of hyaluronic acid and proteins, and water are the main components of synovial fluid. The hyaluronate confers to this liquid complex mechanical properties, close to the qualities of polymers, which depend on the nature of the applied stresses and cannot be completely described by a simple and general mathematical law.

1.1 Synovial Fluid is Non-Newtonian

1.1.1 Viscosity is a function of shear rate. Experimental tests show that the apparent viscosity μ of healthy synovial fluid is a function of shear rate (Fig. 1). At rest ($\gamma = 0$) and for $\gamma < 10^{-2}$ s^{-1}, synovial fluid behaves as a gel whose viscosity approaches 10 Pa.s [1].

When γ increases from 10^{-2} s^{-1} to 10^{3} s^{-1}, μ is a decreasing function of the shear rate [1,2]; when γ becomes larger than 10^{3} s^{-1}, the viscosity approaches a limit within the range 1 to 5×10^{-3}

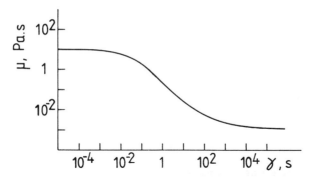

Fig. 1 typical relationship between apparent viscosity and shear rate of synovial fluid.

Pa.s. Zeidler et al. (1) also observes the existence of normal stresses large enough to be measurable. Caygill and West (2) who studied synovial fluids from knees for shear rates between 73.5 and 735 s^{-1} proposed the power law as a model

$$\mu = \mu_\infty + A^{-2/3}$$

and determined the coefficients μ_∞ and A to be

$$0.001 \leq \mu_\infty \leq 0.007 \text{ Pa.s}$$

$$0.49 \leq A \leq 2.3 \quad (S.I.)$$

Lai et al. (3) took Caygill and West's experimental results for one of the synovial fluid samples. Firstly, he assigned the power coefficient to be $-2/3$, and secondly allowed it to adjust itself to obtain the following two relations

$$\mu = 0.007 + 0.99\,\gamma^{-2/3}$$

and $\mu = 0.0105 + 1.664\,\gamma^{-0.793}$

Both of these describe the experimental values well. Lai et al. also found that the measurements of the Ogston and Stanier (4) on bovine synovial fluid can be well represented by the Powell-Eyring law when the shear rate varies from 1 to 50 s^{-1}

$$\mu = 0.0133 + (0.235 - 0.0133)\,\frac{\sin^{-1}(0.921\,\gamma)}{0.921\,\gamma}$$

1.1.2 Viscosity depends on physical and chemical properties. Caygill and West (2) observed that rheumatoid and diluted synovial fluid have a more nearly Newtonian behaviour than healthy synovial fluid (the coefficient A is smaller). They attributed this fact to the lower molecular weight of hyaluronate proteins found in inflammatory arthritis, but did correlate the two phenomena. In fact, the non-Newtonian characteristic of synovial fluid is due to the hyaluronate whose properties can vary in the following different ways: molecular weight, concentration in hyaluronic acid or in proteins, as well as interaction between acid and proteins.

1.2 Synovial Fluid is Viscoelastic

The viscoelastic behaviour of synovial fluid has been demonstrated by experiments on viscosimeters in oscillating motion. Assuming the linear viscoelastic theory, Amadere et al. (5) determined the variations of the complex modulus of viscosity $\mu^* = \mu' - i\mu''$ as a function of the shear rate for a frequency of 2 Hz. From a comparative study on 176 patients he observed, confirming the results of Balazs and Gibbs (6) and Zeidler et al. (1), that the elastic coefficient μ' and the viscous coefficient μ'' are of the same order of magnitude, and both constant up to a shear rate of 10 s^{-1} and decreasing for higher shear rates. The elastic component is higher than the viscous one in subjects with meniscus defects. Only subjects with seropositive rheumatoid arthritis have a constant viscosity and do not present a detectable elasticity. The calculation of the normal stresses induced by the viscoelastic properties of synovial fluid shows that these stresses do not exceed 500 Pa for a healthy young fluid and are weaker for the other fluids (3).

2. THE ARTICULAR CARTILAGE

Cartilage is a diphasic material: the solid phase is composed of collagen fibres (45 to 60% of the dry weight) and cells (1 to 20% of the dry weight); the liquid phase, which forms 60 to 80% of the total weight, is composed of water which is partially bonded and partially free. The degree of freedom is a function of the glycosaminoglycans in the ground substance. The main parameters for the lubrication are surface topography, softness and permeability.

2.1 The Surface of Cartilage

Studies do not permit to conclude whether the cartilage is smooth or not. The results depend on the methods adopted. Visually or using transmission electron microscopy, the cartilage seems to be smooth (7,8), rugosities appear to be in the range of 0.025 μm to 0.3 μm. On the contrary, the scanning electron microscopy shows the surface as very ruguous (9-11). Measurements with stylus indicate an elevation between peaks and valleys of 2.5 μm.

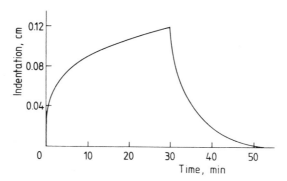

Fig. 2 A typical indentation deformation of cartilage as a function of time. Load is applied at time zero, and removed at t = 30 min.

2.2   Experimental Measurement of Deformation of Cartilage

During the movement of joints, cartilage is submitted to pressure normal to the surface and tensile stresses parallel to it. As cartilage is a composite material, its tensile and compressive mechanical properties are different. In the same way, as the cartilage is anisotropic, its mechanical properties are direction dependent.

2.2.1 Mechanical properties in compression. Compressive and indentation tests show that, under a constant load, cartilage exhibits an instantaneous deformation followed by a time-dependent creep phase during 30 to 60 minutes (Fig. 2). When the load is removed, there is also an immediate recovery, followed by a time-dependent recuperation (12-14).

The observed indentation-time curves are often interpreted as viscoelasticity. However only a few studies (15,16) have been carried out to model this behaviour. Among these, Hayes et al. (17) proposed the following creep function

$$f(t) = \frac{1}{E_o} + \sum_{i=1}^{R} \frac{1}{E_i} \left[1 - \exp \left(-\frac{E_i}{\mu_i}t \right) \right]$$

Kempson et al. (12) calculated the compressive stiffness of the human femoral head cartilage in terms of the creep modulus at two seconds after application of the load and found that it varies between 1.92 and 14.4 MPa. He observed that the stiffness varies topographically in a ratio 3:1, and that an arthrosic cartilage is softer than a healthy one. The creep modulus is a linear increasing function of the amount of glycosaminoglycans and decreases when permeability increases, but seems independent of the collagen content.

2.2.2 Mechanical properties in tension.   Tensile tests have been carried out by Kempson (18) and Woo et al. (19) on samples cut parallel to the surface. Kempson's main results are, a) the stiffness decreases from the surface to the deep zone and depends strongly on the orientation of the sample, b) the stiffness increases with the amount of collagen fibres and c) depends very little on the amount of proteoglycans. Woo et al.'s results agree with those of Kempson, but they insist on the important contraction of cartilage due to loss of fluid. Woo et al. proposes Fung's law (2) as a constitutive equation for cartilage

$$\sigma = A \ [\exp \ (B\epsilon) - 1]$$

where A varies from 1 to 3   MPa, and B from 1.65 to 3.5.

2.3   The Permeability of Cartilage

First measurements on permeability K have been made by McCutchen (14)   and Maroudas (21).   Both have applied a pressure difference of 1 bar and waited for the stabilization of the flow rate for a long time. Maroudas' measurements have allowed to demonstrate that the permeability normal to the surface decreases generally with increasing depth (K = 3 to $9\text{x}10^{-19}$ m^2 near the surface and K = 1 to 2.5x 10^{-19} m^2 near the bone). For some samples permeability has a maximum value below the surface. These values agree with those of McCutchen, who gives a mean permeability of $5.8\text{x}10^{-19}$ m^2. The mean tangential permeability is equal to the normal one. Cartilage globially behaves isotropically (2).

Permeability decreases when the density of fixed charges increases (21).

Permeability is a decreasing function of pressure, which can be formulated by the empirical law (22) when p varies from 0.5 to 15 bars

$$K = K_{\infty} + B/p,$$

where $0.3\text{x}10^{-19} \leq K_{\infty} \leq 0.9\text{x}10^{-19}$ m^2, and $3.5\text{x}10^{-14} \leq B \leq 15\text{x}10^{-14}$ N^{-1}.

Permeability is also a function of the applied mechanical stresses (23).

2.4 Cartilage is a Poroelastic Material

2.4.1 The concept. The obvious creep curves of cartilage have conducted numerous authors to qualify this material as viscoelastic, while recognizing that fluid transfer takes place when stresses are applied. This concept is replaced more and more by that of poroelasticity, which has been introduced for the first time by McCutchen. The poroelasticity theory called consolidation theory had been developed by Biot (24) in 1941.

In the viscoelastic theory, the elastic and viscous properties are attributed to the entire material. In the poroelastic theory, elastic effects come from the solid matrix while viscous effects are the consequence of the fluid flow.

2.4.2   Comparison between viscoelasticity and poroelasticity. Biot's theory demonstrates that the mean deformation m of a sample of cartilage subjected, at time t = 0, to a pressure step p obeys the relation

$$\epsilon_m = \frac{p}{2E} \left\{ 1 - \frac{8}{\pi^2} \sum_{n=0}^{\infty} \frac{1}{(2n+1)^2} \exp\left[-\frac{KE}{\mu e^2} (2n+1)^2 \pi^2 t \right] \right\},$$

where E is the elastic modulus and e the thickness. The corresponding creep function is

$$f_p(t) = \frac{1}{2E} \left\{ 1 - \frac{8}{\pi^2} \sum_{n=0}^{\infty} \frac{1}{(2n+1)^2} \exp\left[-\frac{KE}{\mu e^2} (2n+1)^2 \pi^2 t \right] \right\}.$$

The creep function of a viscoelastic body depends on the chosen constitutive equation. For example, with the generalized Kelvin model it is:

$$f_v(t) = \frac{1}{E_o} + \sum_{i=1}^{R} \frac{1}{E_i} \left\{ 1 - \exp\left[-\frac{E_i}{\mu_i} t \right] \right\}.$$

Functions $f_v(t)$ and $f_p(t)$ are both sums of exponentials. They have consequently the same aptitude to adjust or not to adjust an experimental curve. These functions are equivalent if $E_o = \infty$. If $E_o \neq \infty$, the viscoelastic creep function takes the value $1/E_o$ at t = 0 and allows to account for the instantaneous deformation. This possibility does not seem to appear in the poroelastic model, since $f_p(0) = 0$. Nevertheless, a more careful study of this equation shows that its time derivative $f_p'(0)$ is infinite at initial stage. It follows that a poroelastic material may exhibit a finite deformation in a very short time after the application of the pressure. However, at the present, no experimental confirmation exists.

The coefficients E_i and μ_i, of the function f_v, respectively have the dimensions of elastic modulus and viscosity, but they have no separate particular physical sense. The coefficients K, E, e and μ, of the function f_p, respectively represent the permeability, elastic modulus, the thickness of the cartilage, and the viscosity of the fluid.

If the final poroelastic deformation (at infinite time) depends only on the ratio of pressure to elastic modulus (p/E), then the values of the deformation soon after the load application are dominated by the parameter $\lambda = KE/\mu e^2$. Deformations are naturally a function of the elastic modulus, but also of the permeability, the viscosity and the thickness. Therefore, the diagnosis established from the deformation of cartilage should be interpreted in terms of variations of λ and not E_i. Among others, Kempson (18) found that two seconds after loading, the deformation varies in a ratio 1:3 as a function of the position and concludes that the creep modulus is a function of the sample's place in the joint. The analysis of the parameter λ shows that this can effectively be the case, but that more probably the thickness of the cartilage is not constant and is responsible for the variations of deformation.

3.   FRICTION AND LUBRICATIONS

If a body A, which exerts a load F on a body B has to slide on it, it is necessary to apply a force F' in the direction of the movement to overcome the friction (Fig. 3). The friction coefficient C_f is defined as the ratio F'/F.

When the friction is dry, the order of magnitude of C_f is between 1 and 3. To lower the friction it is possible a) to separate the surfaces completely by a fluid film; friction coefficient then becomes 0.01-0.001 and lubrication is called fluid lubrication, or b) to cover the surfaces by a thin skin which stays bonded such as soap or graphite; friction coefficient is then between 0.05 and 0.1 and lubrication is called boundary lubrication.

The friction coefficient for joints is measured to be between 0.003 and 0.02, depending on the technique and author.

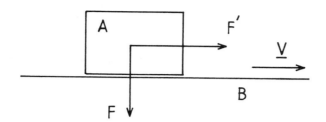

Fig. 3 Friction coefficient C_f = F'/F.

Fluid lubrication is characterized by the movement of the fluid separating the solids. The criterion of choice of the lubricant is its viscosity. In the boundary lubrication however, a layer of fluid is adsorbed at the wall and the criterion of choice is its oiliness, i.e. a set of physical and chemical properties which lower the friction.

4.   BOUNDARY LUBRICATION

4.1 Synovial Fluid is an Oily Lubricant

This is demonstrated by comparing the friction coefficient of synovial fluid with that of other natural or artificial fluids obtained in the same experimental conditions. In his experiments, Linn (25) tested lubrication by measuring, in vitro, the coefficient of friction of dog ankles during continuous oscillation at 40 cycles per minute under a constant load (200 N). He found a friction coefficient of 0.0044 when lubricated by synovial fluid and 0.0099 with buffered saline. In the same way, Radin et al. (26) found that the coefficient of friction is lower with synovial fluid than with other artificial lubricants.

Linn and Radin (27) observed that the friction coefficient is a decreasing function of frequency, as that can be in boundary lubrication, but is also a decreasing function of the load. This latter result cannot be explained by boundary lubrication alone.

4.2 Friction Coefficient is Time Dependent

Radin et al. (26) noticed that the friction decreases during the first 15 to 20 minutes of moving and stabilizes afterwards. Reimann et al. (28) observed the same diminution in the case of shear oscillations between a rubber plate and a parallel glass plate lubricated with synovial fluid, but states that this effect is less important when synovial fluid is replaced by serum.

Unsworth et al. (29) experimented with a pendulum and found that the friction coefficient decreases only when the apparatus is statically loaded. When the load is suddenly applied, the friction coefficient increases at the beginning and decreases afterwards.

The lowering of the friction coefficient is attributed to the time taken by synovial fluid to be adsorbed. In these experiments and particularly in Reimann et al.'s experiments, the main mechanism is very probably boundary lubrication. Nevertheless, it would be hazardous to transpose these conclusions to the walking mechanism. If load and velocity have physiological intensities they are not constant and, as shown in Unsworth et al.'s experiments, results are different when the load is dynamic.

4.3 The Role of Viscosity

The non-Newtonian properties of synovial fluid are due to hyaluronic acid. A partial digestion of the mucin by hyaluronidase makes the fluid Newtonian, but does not modify the friction coefficient (27). A complete digestion of the mucin increases C_f appreciably, which however stays lower than that obtained with saline solutions.

The dilution of synovial fluid in more than three parts of serum decreases the viscosity without deteriorating its lubricating ability.

All these properties indicate that the synovial fluid lubricates well and that this quality does not depend on the viscosity in the experiments described. Synovial fluid is then a good oily lubricant.

4.4 Physical and Chemical Effects

The friction coefficient of synovial fluid whose mucin is treated with trypsine increase up to values close to those obtained with saline solutions. Thypsin destroys the protein fraction but has no effect on the velocity (27).

Changes in pH, molarity, concentration in heparin or formalin affect the coefficient of friction and modify the deformability of cartilage.

The factor responsible for the experimentally observed ability to lubricate seems to be the proteic fraction of synovial fluid, associated with the aptitude of the cartilage to deform.

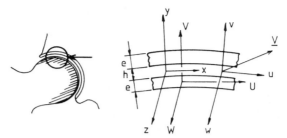

Fig. 4 Schematization of the joint.

5. THE EQUATIONS OF FLUID LUBRICATION

As load is time dependent, the study of the joint lubrication is that of a non-Newtonian fluid flowing between two ruguous, soft and porous walls of finite thickness. The mechanical problem is too complex to have a rigorous mathematical solution. The examination of the equations and the order of magnitude of the variables permit however to make realistic assumptions and to grasp the prevailing mechanisms.

5.1 Description of the Problem

Hip joint can be schematized by two surfaces in the form of rigid half spheres of closed radii, covered by a thickness e of cartilage and separated by a variable gap h in which synovial fluid flows (Fig. 4). The components of the fluid velocity V are u, v, w and relative displacements of each point of cartilage are U, V, W.

5.2 Equations and First Simplifications

The fundamental law of mechanics applied to the fluid is:

$$\rho \frac{d\underline{V}}{dt} = \rho\underline{F} + \underline{T} \tag{1}$$

where, $\rho\underline{F}$ represents the body forces and $\underline{T}$ the surface forces. The expression of $\underline{T}$ depends on the rheological properties of the fluid. Assuming the body forces to be negligible and the fluid to be incompressible and Newtonian, Eqn. 1 becomes

$$\rho\left(\frac{\partial u}{\partial t} + u\frac{\partial u}{\partial x} + v\frac{\partial u}{\partial y} + w\frac{\partial u}{\partial z}\right) = -\frac{\partial p}{\partial x} + \left(\frac{\partial^2 u}{\partial x^2} + \frac{\partial^2 u}{\partial y^2} + \frac{\partial^2 u}{\partial z^2}\right) \tag{2}$$

$$\rho\left(\frac{\partial v}{\partial t} + u\frac{\partial v}{\partial x} + v\frac{\partial v}{\partial y} + w\frac{\partial v}{\partial z}\right) = -\frac{\partial p}{\partial y} + \left(\frac{\partial^2 v}{\partial x^2} + \frac{\partial^2 v}{\partial y^2} + \frac{\partial^2 v}{\partial z^2}\right) \tag{3}$$

$$\rho\left(\frac{\partial w}{\partial t} + u\frac{\partial w}{\partial x} + v\frac{\partial w}{\partial y} + w\frac{\partial w}{\partial z}\right) = -\frac{\partial p}{\partial z} + \left(\frac{\partial^2 w}{\partial x^2} + \frac{\partial^2 w}{\partial y^2} + \frac{\partial^2 w}{\partial z^2}\right) \tag{4}$$

The assumption of Newtonian fluid is justifiable only when the shear rate is higher than 10^3 s^{-1}, and this condition has to be verified for each configuration.

The fundamental law applied to the cartilage neglecting the gravity forces is:

$$\frac{\partial \sigma_{xx}}{\partial x} + \frac{\partial \sigma_{xy}}{\partial y} + \frac{\partial \sigma_{xz}}{\partial z} - \frac{\partial p}{\partial x} = \frac{d^2 U}{dt^2} \tag{5}$$

$$\frac{\partial \sigma_{xy}}{\partial x} + \frac{\partial \sigma_{yy}}{\partial y} + \frac{\partial \sigma_{yz}}{\partial z} - \frac{\partial p}{\partial y} = \frac{d^2 V}{dt^2} \tag{6}$$

$$\frac{\partial \sigma_{xz}}{\partial x} + \frac{\partial \sigma_{yz}}{\partial y} + \frac{\partial \sigma_{zz}}{\partial z} - \frac{\partial p}{\partial z} = \frac{d^2 W}{dt^2} \tag{7}$$

If the matrix is supposed to be isotropic and obeys the law of linear elasticity, the stress-strain relation is the Hooke's law

$$\sigma_{ij} = 2 G \left(\epsilon_{ij} + \frac{\nu}{1-2\nu} \epsilon_{kk} \delta_{ij}\right) \tag{8}$$

with $G = \dfrac{E}{2(1+\nu)}$ and $\epsilon_{ij} = \dfrac{1}{2}\left(\dfrac{\partial U_i}{\partial x_j} + \dfrac{\partial U_j}{\partial x_i}\right)$

The assumption of linear elasticity is an approximation valid for small deformations. Isotropic hypothesis is unvalidated by Kempson (18). There is, in fact, a ratio of two between deformations of samples in two perpendicular directions. An isotropic model can be developed by taking different elastic moduli in the three directions.

5.3 Non-Dimensional Equations

The dimensional parameters (Fig. 5) of the joint are the radius R, the thickness e of the cartilage and h of the fluid film, the period T or the frequency $\omega = 2\pi/T$, the elastic modulus E and the permeability K of the cartilage, the viscosity μ of the fluid, the load F, and the angle of rotation θ. The following dimensionless variables can be defined as:

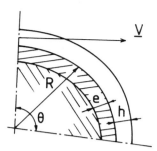

Fig. 5 Dimensional parameters.

$$x_+ = \frac{x}{R\theta} \; , \; y_+ = \frac{y}{H} \; , \; z_+ = \frac{z}{R\theta} \; , \; U_+ = \frac{U}{R\omega} \; , \; V_+ = \frac{V}{h\omega} \; , \; W_+ = \frac{W}{R\omega}$$

$$t_+ = \omega t \; , \; P_+ = P\frac{R^2\theta}{F} \; , \; U_+ = \frac{U}{R\theta} \; , \; V_+ = \frac{V}{e} \; , \; W_+ = \frac{W}{R\theta} \; , \; y_{++} = \frac{y}{e}$$

Fluid variables fluctuate about unity; U , V , W have the same order of magnitude but small compared to one. The input of these new variables in the Eqns. (2-4) gives

$$SW_o^2\theta\left[\theta\frac{\partial u_+}{\partial t_+} + u_+\frac{\partial u_+}{\partial x_+} + \theta v_+\frac{\partial u_+}{\partial y_+} + w_+\frac{\partial u_+}{\partial z_+}\right] = -\frac{\partial P_+}{\partial x_+}$$

$$+ S\left[\frac{\partial^2 u_+}{\partial x_+^2} + \frac{R^2\theta^2}{h_+^2}\frac{\partial^2 u_+}{\partial y_+^2} + \frac{\partial^2 u_+}{\partial z_+^2}\right] \tag{9}$$

$$SW_o^2\frac{h^2\theta}{R^2}\left[\frac{\partial v_+}{\partial t_+} + \frac{u_+}{\theta}\frac{\partial v_+}{\partial x_+} + v\frac{\partial v_+}{\partial y_+} + \frac{w_+}{\theta} + \frac{\partial v_+}{\partial z_+}\right] = -\frac{\partial P_+}{\partial y_+}$$

$$+ S\left[\frac{h^2}{R^2\theta}\frac{\partial^2 v_+}{\partial x_+^2} + \theta\frac{\partial^2 v_+}{\partial y_+^2} + \frac{h^2}{R^2\theta}\frac{\partial^2 v_+}{\partial z_+^2}\right] \tag{10}$$

$$SW_o^2\theta\left[\theta\frac{\partial w_+}{\partial t_+} + u_+\frac{\partial w_+}{\partial x_+} + \theta v_+\frac{\partial w_+}{\partial y_+} + w_+\frac{\partial w_+}{\partial z_+}\right] = -\frac{\partial P_+}{\partial z_+}$$

$$+ S\left[\frac{\partial^2 w_+}{\partial x_+^2} + \frac{R^2\theta^2}{h_+^2}\frac{\partial^2 w_+}{\partial y_+^2} + \frac{\partial^2 w_+}{\partial z_+^2}\right]. \tag{11}$$

Two dimensionless numbers appear: the Sommerfeld number $S = \mu\omega R^2/F$ and the Womersley number $W_o^2 = \rho R^2\omega/\mu$.

Likewise the three equations for cartilage after having introduced Hooke's law in Eqns. 5-7 are:

$$\xi_1\left\{\frac{(1-\nu)}{(1-2\nu)}\left[\frac{\partial^2 U_+}{\partial x_+^2} + \frac{\partial^2 V_+}{\partial x_+ \partial y_{++}} + \frac{\partial^2 W_+}{\partial x_+ \partial z_+}\right] + \frac{R^2\theta^2}{2e^2}\frac{\partial^2 U_+}{\partial y_{++}^2} + \frac{1}{2}\frac{\partial^2 U_+}{\partial z_+^2}\right\}$$

$$= \frac{\partial p_+}{\partial x_+} + \xi_2\frac{d^2 U}{dt^2} \tag{12}$$

$$\xi_1\left\{\frac{(1-\nu)}{(1-2\nu)}\left[\frac{\partial^2 V_+}{\partial y_{++}^2} + \frac{\partial^2 W_+}{\partial y_{++}\partial z_+} + \frac{\partial^2 U_+}{\partial x_+ \partial y_{++}}\right] + \frac{e^2}{2R^2\theta^2}\left[\frac{\partial^2 V_+}{\partial z_+^2} + \frac{\partial^2 V_+}{\partial x_+^2}\right]\right\}$$

$$= \frac{\partial p_+}{\partial y_{++}} + \xi_2\frac{e^2}{R^2\theta^2}\frac{d^2 V}{dt^2} \tag{13}$$

$$\xi_1\left\{\frac{(1-\nu)}{(1-2\nu)}\left[\frac{\partial^2 W_+}{\partial z_+^2} + \frac{\partial^2 U_+}{\partial x_+ \partial z_+} + \frac{\partial^2 V_+}{\partial z_+ \partial y_{++}}\right] + \frac{R^2\theta^2}{2e^2}\frac{\partial^2 W_+}{\partial y_{++}^2} + \frac{1}{2}\frac{\partial^2 W_+}{\partial x_+^2}\right\}$$

$$= \frac{\partial p_+}{\partial z_+} + \xi_2\frac{d^2 W}{dt^2} \tag{14}$$

and also two dimensionless numbers appear

$$\xi_1 = \frac{2GR^2\theta}{F} \quad \text{and} \quad \xi_2 = \frac{\rho R^4\omega^2\theta^3}{F}$$

5.4 Analysis of the Equations and Simplifications

The following orders of magnitude can be retained for the hip joint

$R = 2\times10^{-2}$ m $T = 1$ s $F = 2\times10^3$ N

$e = 2\times10^{-3}$ m $\theta = 1$ radian $G = 10^6$ N/m^2

$h = 10^{-5}$ m $\mu = 4\times10^{-3}$ Pa.s $\rho = 10^3$ kg/m^3.

The values of the dimensionless numbers are then:

$$S = 5\times10^{-9} \qquad W^2 = 6\times10^2 \qquad \xi_1 = 4\times10^{-1} \qquad \xi_2 = 3\times10^{-6}$$

$$SW_o^2 = 3\times10^{-6} \qquad R^2/h^2 = 4\times10^6 \qquad R^2/e^2 = 100.$$

As R^2/h^2 is very large compared to one and SW_o^2 is very small compared to SR^2/h^2, the equations of fluid movement reduce to

$$0 = -\frac{\partial P_+}{\partial x_+} + \frac{R^2\theta^2 S}{h^2}\frac{\partial^2 U_+}{\partial y_+^2} \qquad (15)$$

$$0 = -\frac{\partial P_+}{\partial y_+} \qquad (16)$$

$$0 = -\frac{\partial P_+}{\partial z_+} + \frac{R^2\theta^2 S}{h^2}\frac{\partial^2 W_+}{\partial y_+^2} \qquad (17)$$

Or in dimensional form

$$0 = -\frac{\partial p}{\partial x} + \frac{\partial^2 u}{\partial y^2} \qquad (18)$$

$$0 = -\frac{\partial p}{\partial y} + \frac{\partial^2 w}{\partial y^2} \qquad (19)$$

$$p = p(x,z,t); \quad u = (y,t); \quad w = (y,t).$$

These results allow two important conclusions: a) the approximation of quasi-stationary movement may be applied to the hip joint lubrication, b) the Eqns. 18 and 19 are those used by Reynolds, and therefore his lubrication theory can be applied, at any given instant in time, to the movement of the joint fluid.

Similarly, as ξ_2 is small compared to ξ_1, the Eqns. 12-14 reduce to

$$\xi_1\frac{R^2\theta}{2e^2}\frac{\partial^2 U_+}{\partial y_{++}^2} = \frac{\partial P_+}{\partial x_+}, \qquad (20)$$

$$\xi_1\frac{R^2\theta}{2e^2}\frac{\partial^2 W_+}{\partial y_{++}^2} = \frac{\partial P_+}{\partial z_+}, \qquad (21)$$

or in dimensional form

$$G \frac{\partial^2 U}{\partial y^2} = \frac{\partial p}{\partial x} \tag{22}$$

$$G \frac{\partial^2 W}{\partial y^2} = \frac{\partial p}{\partial z} \tag{23}$$

$$p = p(x,z,t); \quad U = U(y,t); \quad W = W(y,t).$$

The equations of elastotatic may therefore be applied, to the cartilage, at a given instant in time.

5.5 Reynolds Equation

The integration of Eqns. 18 and 19 combined with the continuity equation allows the classical lubrication law known as Reynolds equation to be obtained.

$$\frac{\partial}{\partial x}\left\{\left[\frac{h_1^3 - h_2^3}{12\mu} + \frac{h_1 h_2 (h_2 - h_1)}{4\mu}\right]\frac{\partial p}{\partial x}\right\} + \frac{\partial}{\partial z}\left\{\left[\frac{h_1^3 - h_2^3}{12} + \frac{h_1 h_2 (h_2 - h_1)}{4}\right]\frac{\partial p}{\partial z}\right\}$$

$$= v_1 - v_2 + \frac{1}{2}(h_1 - h_2)\left[\frac{\partial}{\partial x}(u_1 + u_2) + \frac{\partial}{\partial z}(w_1 + w_2)\right]$$

$$+ \frac{1}{2}\left[(u_2 - u_1)\frac{\partial}{\partial x}(h_1 + h_2) + (w_2 - w_1)\frac{\partial}{\partial z}(h_1 + h_2)\right] \tag{24}$$

In this formula, $u_1(x,z,t)$, $v_1(x,z,t)$, $w_1(x,z,t)$ are the components of the fluid velocity at the point $h_1(x,z,t)$ or the cartilage surface, and u_2, v_2, w_2 are those at point h_2. By hypothesis, these velocities are equal to the corresponding components of the cartilage deformation velocities and to the fluid velocities at the surface of the porous medium.

Reynolds equation, valid for describing the joint lubrication, is not analytically integrable without making other assumptions which would be incompatible with joint anatomy. Nevertheless, it is of extreme consequence because it permits to explain why the pressure generated in the fluid (represented by the left-hand terms of the equation) results from the three complementary actions (represented by the right-hand terms):

a) the squeeze action: $v_1 - v_2$,

b) the hydrodynamic action: $\frac{1}{2}\left[(u_2 - u_1)\frac{\partial}{\partial x}(h_1 + h_2) + \right.$

$$+(w_2-w_1)\frac{\partial}{\partial z}(h_1+h_2)\Big]$$

c)   the elastic action: $\frac{1}{2}(h_1-h_2)\left[\frac{\partial}{\partial x}(u_1+u_2)+\frac{\partial}{\partial z}(w_1+w_2)\right]$

The influence of these effects depends on the order of magnitude of the terms, which now has to be studied.

6.   HYDRODYNAMIC LUBRICATION

The lubrication is hydrodynamic if the pressure is generated by:

$$\frac{1}{2}\left[(u_2-u_1)\frac{\partial}{\partial x}(h_1+h_2) + (w_2-w_1)\frac{\partial}{\partial z}(h_1+h_2)\right]$$

and if the two other terms of the right-hand side of Reynolds equation have a negligible contribution.   The calculation of the film thickness is possible in some configurations.   In the case of two cylinders of radii R_1, R_2 and length L, Dowson et al. (30) indicated that the minimum thickness h that obeys the law is

$$\frac{h}{R'} = 4.9\ \mu\ \frac{(u_1+u_2)}{F}\ L \tag{25}$$

where $R' = R_1 R_2/(R_1+R_2)$ is the equivalent radius, which is in the range of 10 to 50 cm (31).

By taking a slide velocity of 6×10^{-2} m/s, a load F = 2000 N, a length L = 0.1 m and a viscosity $\mu = 4\times10^{-3}$ Pa.s, the film thickness would be between 6×10^{-3} μm and 30×10^{-3} μm, which is much smaller than the surface rugosity.   It therefore follows that the hydrodynamic effect is insufficient to generate high enough a pressure to separate the surfaces.

7.   ELASTOHYDRODYNAMIC LUBRICATION

This term is used to describe the lubrication resulting from the combined action of fluid and wall deformability in permanent movement (30).

The relationship of Eqn. 25 should be replaced by the expression

$$\frac{h}{R'} = 1.35 \left[\frac{2\mu(u_1+u_2)L}{ER'} \right]^{1/2} \tag{26}$$

by taking E = 6 MPa, h is obtained between 1 μm and 6 μm, and is of the same order of magnitude as the surface rugosities.

Elastohydrodynamic effect is important. However, due to the approximate nature of the calculations and the lack of physiological experimentation, it is not possible to conclude if this type of lubrication is sufficient to permit a complete separation of the surfaces.

8. SQUEEZE LUBRICATION AND POROELASTICITY

When there is no slide velocity, Reynolds equation reduces to

$$\frac{\partial}{\partial x} \left\{ \left[\frac{h_1^3-h_2^3}{12\mu} + \frac{h_1 h_2(h_2-h_1)}{4\mu} \right] \frac{\partial p}{\partial x} \right\} + \frac{\partial}{\partial z} \left\{ \left[\frac{h_1^3-h_2^3}{12\mu} \right. \right.$$
$$\left. \left. + \frac{h_1 h_2(h_2-h_1)}{4\mu} \right] \frac{\partial p}{\partial z} \right\} = v_1 - v_2 .$$

The velocity $v_1 - v_2$ can be considered as the algebraic sum of two contributions: a) the squeeze velocity of cartilage, assumed rigid and non-porous, and b) the velocity of the fluid in or out of the cartilage.

8.1 Squeeze Lubrication

8.1.1 Cartilage is assumed rigid and impermeable. The squeeze time, defined as the time necessary for the surfaces to approach from a gap h to a gap h, can be calculated in some simple configurations (32). In the case of two spheres of radii R and R , the calculation gives, when $R_1 - R_2 = 10^{-3}$ m, a time of 4×10^{-4} s for a final thickness of 10^{-5} m. This time is very small compared to the characteristic time of increasing pressure (0.2 s). Squeeze effect with rigid walls, therefore, is quite insufficient to ensure joint lubrication.

Taking the non-Newtonian effect into account this type of lubrication cannot significantly modify the result (33).

8.1.2 Cartilage is supposed rigid or very slightly deformable and permeable, fluid is non-Newtonian. Squeeze time measured for cartilage lubricated with synovial fluid is very much longer than for rubber of the same dimensions (34). Walker et al. (34) stated that the main difference between the two materials is the permeability of the cartilage. It is large enough to allow water to flow

through pores, but constitutes an impassable barrier for the large
hyaluronate molecules. Walker et al. therefore proposed an original mechanism, the boosted lubrication. Under the pressure, water
and electrolytes infiltrate into cartilage; synovial fluid concentrates in the gap and forms a viscous gel which is very difficult
to expel.

Dowson et al. (35) developed a theoretical analysis, based on
the hypothesis that the concentration in hyaluronic acid is
inversely proportional to the film thickness. Their calculation
demonstrated that squeeze time is then multiplied by a factor six.
This duration is still insufficient to lubricate.

8.2 Cartilage is Supposed Poroelastic, Fluid is Newtonian

The increase of squeeze time observed by Walker et al. has
another explanation, given by McCutchen (36) as far back as 1959.
Under pressure cartilage deforms, exudes fluid in the loaded areas
and supplies the film between the walls.

McCutchen's theory, called weeping lubrication, is based on
the following observations: a) the friction coefficient is lower
with synthetic porous materials than with non-porous ones, but it
increases with time, b) during movement, there is substantial
outward seepage in the loaded areas (detected by dyeing a particular volume of liquid), and c) when measuring friction coefficient,
it is necessary to wait a certain time between two experiments to
have reproducible results. This time is necessary for the cartilage to resoak fluid.

8.2.1 Influence of elasticity on squeeze time. Elasticity considerably extends squeeze time. Gaman et al. (37), studying the
approach between a rigid sphere and a soft plane plate of finite
thickness, measured a squeeze time for a gap of 25 μm 1000 to 10000
times that with a rigid plate. He noticed that minimum gap does
not occur in center of the contact area, but on a circle of radius
r. This wad creates a headloss which reduces the outflow and
increases the time. It is the consequence of the elastohydrodynamic pressure distribution (different from the elastic one), which
gives a uniform contact, and therefore exists for every form of
surface.

If elasticity increases the time by 1000, the preceding value
of 4×10^{-4} s is replaced by 0.4 s, and becomes comparable with the
physiological time.

8.2.2 Influence of the porosity. Cartilage is poroelastic and not
only elastic. The permeability modifies the pressure distribution
at its surface to present more uniformity. This effect, which

leads to a reduction in the squeeze time, has never been quantified, but should be low.

Poroelasticity permits a fluid flow at the surface of cartilage. The flow is the algebraic sum of the displacement created by
deformation of cartilage and the flow through cartilage due to
pressure differences.

Deformation involves an exudation with a velocity v_e when
pressure increases, and an adsorption when pressure decreases (Fig.
6). Fluid flow through cartilage obeys Darcy's law. Fluid fil-
trates with a velocity v_i from loaded to unloaded areas. Poroelasticity increases squeeze time when the resulting velocity $v_e - v_i$
supplies the film, and takes a negative part otherwise.

The measurement of the amount of fluid wrung out from cartilage samples submitted to a pressure step, shows that Darcy's flow
is negligible compared to exudation flow for physiological times.
Both flows become comparable only after a long time, and the amount
of exuded fluid creates a film thickness between 6 and 40 μm 0.1s
after load application (38).

Poroelasticity thus brings a contribution to the film supply
and delays the squeeze time during walking.

9. CONCLUSION

In spite of the extreme complexity of the problem and of the
doubt still existing on some anatomical or physiological magnitudes, it is possible to assure that the very low friction coefficient occurring during walking results mainly from softness of the
cartilage and the accompanying fluid exudation.

The very good lubricant qualities of synovial fluid probably
relay the fluid lubrication in the two following cases: a) load is
extreme: the film becomes too thin, proteins assume boundary
lubrication, b) at the beginning of the movement, fluid lubrication
is not yet developed but, as the shear rate is very low, synovial
fluid forms a gel which prevents the joint binding.

10. LUBRICATION OF PROSTHESES

10.1 The Mechanism

a) The examination of removed prostheses after implantation
indicates that fluid is present in the cavity and wear debris
exist.

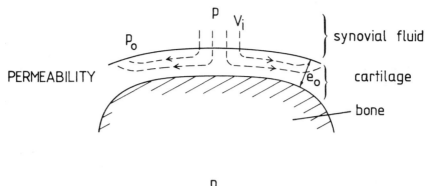

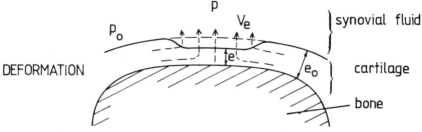

Fig. 6 Flow through cartilage (see text).

b) The experiments on simulators give a friction coefficient of 0.15 for the metal-metal prostheses and of 0.05 for the metal-plastic prostheses.

c) The study of the lubrication of normal joints establishes that a wall deformation is necessary to lubricate efficiently.

All these arguments permit to think that boundary lubrication occurs during a part of the cycle and that dry friction can be expected under some conditions. A very important improvement will occur only after the creation of new biomaterials which will have at least a soft and if possible porous superficial layer, or which will have a specific extremely low friction coefficient.

10.2 Friction and its Sequels

Friction is at the origin of several mechanical problems. a) It produces wear debris and inflammatory diseases as well as limiting the life of prostheses. b) It transmits shear stresses which can cause loosening.

Although wear is generated by friction, there is no general law connecting one to the other.

10.3 Conditions to Reduce Friction

a) Dry friction mainly depends on the nature of the materials used. Low friction occurs with such materials as polyethylene.

b) Friction is reduced when surfaces are polished.

c) Low friction is obtained by maintaining at least a partial fluid film. As the film life is longer if pressure is lower, it follows that the largest and most congruent prostheses surfaces reduce friction.

10.4 Conditions to Reduce Wear

a) Wear mainly depends on the nature of materials. It decreases when their hardness increases. Plastic prostheses have a high wear rate of 100 to 400 μm per year (39).

b) Wear depends on the dimensions of the pieces. For Weightman (40), in the case of plastic-metal prostheses, two eventualities are to be considered. If wear debris can create a danger, the femoral head diameter should be very small to minimize debris volume; if the femoral head risks to wear through the cup, its diameter should be the half of cup diameter, which itself should be as large as possible.

10.5 Conclusion

The criteria of improvement of wear and friction are different and sometimes opposite. It is thus not possible to describe an ideal model of prosthesis. Qualities and defects of each device must be separately discussed.

REFERENCES

1. Zeidler, H., Altman, S., John, B., Gaffga, R., Kulicke, M. Rheologie pathologischen Gelenkflussigkeiten: weitere Ergebnisse zum Viskoelastizitat. Rheol. Acta, 1979, 18, 191.
2. Caygill, J.C., West, G.H. The rheological behaviour of synovial fluid and its possible relation to joint lubrication. Med. Biol. Engng., 1969, 7, 507-516.
3. Lai, W.M., Kuei, S.C., Mow, V.C., Rheological equations for synovial fluids. J. Biomech. Engng., 1978, 100, 169-186.
4. Ogston, A.G., Stanier, J.E. On the state of hyaluronic acid in synovial fluid. Biochemical J., 1950, 46, 364-376.

5. Amadpre, I., Chmiel, H., Laschner, W. Viscoelasticity of normal and pathological synovial fluid. Biorheol., 1979, 16, 179.

6. Balazs, E.A., Gibbs, D.A. Biological function of hyaluronic acid in: Balazs, E.A., Chemistry and molecular biology of the intercellular matrix. Academic Press, 1970, 3, 1241-1253.

7. Davies, D.V., Barnett, C.H., Cochrane, W., Palfrey, A.J. Electron microscopy of articular cartilage. Annals of Rheumatic Diseases, 1962, 21, 11a.

8. Weiss, C., Rosenberg, L., Helfet, A.J. An ultrastructural study of normal young adult human articular cartilage. J. Bone Jt. Surg., 1968, 50A, 633-674.

9. Walker, P.S., Sikorski, J., Dowson, D., Longfeld, M.D., Wright, V., Buckley, T. Behaviour of synovial fluid on surfaces of articular cartilage. A scanning electron microscope study. Ann. Rheum. Diseases, 1969, 28, 1-14.

10. McCall, J. Scanning electron microscopy of articular surfaces. Lancet, 1968, 2, 1194.

11. Clarke, I.C. The microevaluation of articular surface contours. Annals of Biomed. Engng., 1972, 1, 31-43.

12. Kempson, G.E., Freeman, M.A.R., Swanson, S.A.V. The determination of a creep modulus for articular cartilage from indentation tests on the human femoral head. J. Biomechanics, 1971, 4, 239-250.

13. Parsons, J.R., Black, J. Mechanical behaviour of articular cartilage: quantitative changes with alteration of ionic environment. J. Biomechanics, 1979, 12, 765-773.

14. McCutchen, C.W. The frictional properties of animal joints. Wear, 1962, 5, 1-17.

15. Fantuzzo, D.G., Graziatti, G. A mathematical model for articular cartilage. Digest of the 7th Int. Conf. on Med. and Biol. Engng., Stockholm, 1967.

16. Coletti, J.M., Akeson, W.H., Woo, J.L.Y. A comparison of the physical behaviour of normal articular cartilage and the arthroplasty surface. J. Bone Jt. Surg., 1972, 54A, 147.

17. Hayes, W.C., Keer, L.M., Herrmann, G., Mockros, L.F. A mathematical analysis for indentation tests in articular cartilage. J. Biomechanics, 1972, 5, 541-552.

18. Kempson, G.E. The tensile properties of articular cartilage and their relevance to the development of osteo arthroses. Proc. of 12th Cong. of the Int. Soc. of Orthop. Surg. and Traumat., Tel Aviv, 1972, 44-58.

19. Woo, L.Y., Lubock, P., Gomez, M.A., Jemmott, G.F., Kuei, S.C., Akeson, W.H. Large deformation nonhomogeneous and directional properties. J. Biomechanics, 1979, 12, 437-446.

20. Fung, Y.C. Elasticity of soft tissues in simple elongation. Am. J. Physiol., 1967, 213, 1532-1544.

21. Maroudas, A. Physico-chemical properties of articular cartilage in: Freeman, M.A.R., Adult articular cartilage. Pitman medical, Ondon, 1973.

22. Renaudeaux, J.P. Hydromechanical properties of articular cartilage and joint lubrication. Proc. of the 3rd Int. Conf. on Mech. in Med. and Biol. Compiegne, 1982, 89-90.

23. Mansour, J.M., Mow, V.C. The permeability of articular cartilage under compressive strain at high pressures. J. Bone Jt. Surg., 1976, 58, 4, 509-516.

24. Biot, M.A. General theory of three dimensional consolidation. J. Appl. Physics, 1941, 12, 155-164.

25. Linn, F.C. Lubrication of animal joints: II the mechanism. J. Biomechanics, 1968, 193-205.

26. Radin, E.L., Paul, I.L., Weisser, P.A. Joint lubrication with artificial lubricants. Arthr. Rheumat., 1971, 14, 1, 126-129.

27. Linn, F.C., Radin, E.L. Lubrication of animal joints: III the effect of certain chemical alterations of the cartilage and lubricant. Arthritis and Rheumatism, 1968, 11, 5, 674-682.

28. Reimann, I., Stougaard, J., Northeved, a., Johnsen, S.J. Demonstration of boundary lubrication by synovial fluid. Acta Orthop. Scand., 1975, 46, 1-10.

29. Unsworth, A., Dowson, D., Wright, V., Koshal, D. The frictional behaviour of human synovial joints: I Natural joints. J. Lub. Technol., 1975, 369-376.

30. Dowson, D., Higginson, G.R., Archard, J.F., Crook, A.W. Elastohydrodynamic lubrication, Pergamon Press, 1966.

31. Mow, V.C., Lai, W.M. Mechanics of animal joints. Ann. REv. Fluid Mech., 1979, 11, 247-288.

32. Moore, D.F. A review of squeeze films. Wear, 1965, 8, 245-263.

33. McCutchen, C.W. Answer to analysis of "boosted lubrication in human joints," J. Mech. Engng. Sci., 1972, 14, 3.

34. Walker, P.S., Dowson, D., Longfeld, M.D., Wright V. "Boosted lubrication" in synovial joints by fluid entrapment and enrichment. Ann. Rheum. Diseases, 1968, 27, 512-520.

35. Dowson, D., Unsworth, A., Wright, V. Analysis of "boosted lubrication" in human joints. J. Mech. Engng. Sci., 1970, 12, 5, 364-369.

36. McCutchen, C.W. Mechanism of animal joints. Sponge hydrostatic and weeping bearings. Nature, 1959, 184, 1284-1285.

37. Gaman, I.D.C., Higginson, G.R., Norman, R. Fluid entrapment by a soft surface layer. Wear, 1974, 28, 345-352.

38. Renaudeaux, J.P. How the cartilage can lubricate the joints. Proc. of the World Cong. on Med. Phys. and Biomed. Engng., Hambourg, 1982.

39. McKellop, H., Clarke, I., Markolf, K., Amstutz, H. Friction and wear properties of polymer, metal and ceramic prosthetic joint materials evaluated on a multichannel screening device. J. Biomed. Mat. Res., 1981, 15, 619-653.

40. Weightman, B. Friction, lubrication and wear in: Swanson, S.A.V., Freeman, M.A.R., The scientific basis of joint replacement. Pitman medical, London, 1977.

BIOMECHANICS OF MUSCLES

K.M.C. Da Silva

Department of Physiology, Instituto Gulbenkian de Ciencia, Oeiras, Portugal

1. INTRODUCTION

The skeletal muscles are the source of power for the mechanical peripherals of the Central Nervous System (CNS) and they play a major role in relating a person to the world around him. Our understanding of the mechanisms through which the central control of the skeletal muscles makes possible the highly coordinated movements performed by the human being still is very limited. In this chapter this problem is approached by considering the skeletal muscles as being constituted by parallel and/or series combinations of basic one-degree-of-freedom neuromuscular assemblages, mechanoeffector units, whose structure is defined. The mechanical properties of a muscle are thus determined by those of its constituent units as well as by the way they are combined in it. The laws of combination of the mechanoeffector units are such that the whole muscle has the same formal structure, albeit with different component values, as a single mechanoeffector unit. This fact is taken advantage of to check the performance of a theoretical model against published data. This discussion is confined to the dynamical response to small perturbations around a quiescent working point so that linear approximations to the functional relationships which define the mechanoeffector unit may be used. Its dynamical performance is simulated numerically using published data on the characteristics of muscles and sensors and the capacity of the model to meet requirements of a) precision, b) stability, c) speed of response, and d) insensitivity to external loading. Use is made of neuronal corrective filters to improve the assemblage design and a configuration is reached which fits the known overall characteristics of its natural counterparts.

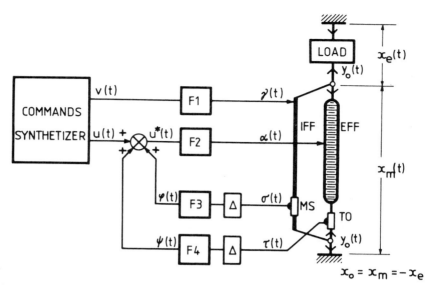

Fig. 1 Mechanoeffector Unit Control Assemblage. EFF–extrafusal
muscle fibres; IFF–intrafusal (muscle spindle) muscle fibres;
MS–muscle spindle sensor; TO–Golgi tendon organ; F_1, F_2, F_3, F_4
–correcting filters located in the CNS; Δ–propagation delays in the
nerve links. Small signal variables: u and v – muscle and fusimotor commands; a and γ – muscle and fusimotor efferent commands;
and r–afferent signals; ϕ and ψ–corrected afferent signals; x_m and
x_e–motor and load lengths (or strains); x_0–assemblage output length
(or strain); y_0–force developed by (or stress in) the mechanoeffector unit assemblage.

2.   MECHANOEFFECTOR UNIT CONTROL ASSEMBLAGE

     Fig. 1 illustrates the simplest, i.e. one-degree-of-freedom
mechanoeffector control assemblage. The state of the assemblage is
defined by the variables $x_0(t)$, its overall length, and $y_0(t)$, the
force it exerts on its insertions. Information about these two
variables is continuously fedback to the control centres by the
muscle spindle (MS) and the Golgi tendon organ (TO), which monitor
$x_0(t)$ and $y_0(t)$, respectively. The feedback relationships for the
sensorial outputs are those which have been found to be most suitable for the optimization of the control assemblage. The two
feedback arrangements have reasonable experimental support and both
have, separately or together, been considered in the past by other
authors (1): the length feedback from the MS is negative as a
result of the differential assemblage of this sensor and the force
feedback from the TO is positive. The filters F_1 to F_4 are correcting neuronal networks, supposedly located at spinal cord level,
which make the optimization of this control assemblage possible.

If feedback loops involving higher CNS areas are not considered, the only propagation delays to be taken into account are
those occurring in the peripheral nerves which can be adequately
represented by a delay in the afferent pathways. The commands
synthetizer represents an indiscriminated area of the cerebral
cortex which has the responsibility for learning, storing and
issuing the commands involved in the control of the assemblage.

The model represented in Fig. 1 as the basic mechanoeffector
unit is acceptable from a theoretical point of view in so far as
the performance of the extrafusal fibres is conditioned by the
information supplied by the muscle spindles and the tendon organs
respectively on their common length and on the force they develop
together. The functional structure shown in Fig. 1 and the way the
different mechanoeffector units in a given muscle are related to
each other are more delicate issues however.

Experimental evidence from muscles of the cat (2-5) and of the
mouse (6) shows that the muscle spindles and the tendon organs are
associated in the same regions of the muscle and, although their
numbers in a given muscle differ, their anatomical correlation
strongly suggests the existence of such control assemblages. These
however, must not be confused with the concept of motor unit (7,
8), a fact which is made obvious by comparing, for example, the 280
motor units in the medial gastrocnenius of the cat (9, 10) with the
number (around 60) of its spindle and tendon organ receptors (3).
These facts have long been recognized (11, 12). The circumstances
that a) in a given muscle the two types of sensors are represented
in different numbers, b) appreciable portions of the muscle have
little sensory representation, and c) the number of sensors per
unit volume varies from muscle to muscle, points to complex
arrangements in the functional architecture of the muscle but in no
way opposes the concept of the mechanoeffector unit being its basic
building block. Motor units have in fact been found to share
territories and each motor unit to extend through a large fraction
of the muscle volume (4, 13). These two factors could explain why
the sensors are able to concentrate in the region of the muscle
where, possibly, they can monitor its performance better, and the
remaining regions of the muscle are populated by peripheral fibres
of the motor units. The difference in the innervation ratios of
slow and fast muscles (14) also gives support to the notion that it
is the mechanoeffector unit, and not the motor unit, which constitutes the functional building block of the muscle. It is, however,
obvious that the validity of this concept can only be decided on
experimental grounds and this work is still waiting to be done.

The second major difficulty associated with the model of Fig.
1, and one which follows from what has been said above, is how to
obtain the characteristics of its components when the published
experimental data refer to complete muscles, and the

mechanoreceptors are only occasionally characterized individually. What we have done to enable us to do our numerical simulations was to take advantage of the fact that a muscle is itself a one-degree-of-freedom machine and identify the entire muscle with the set of the extrafusal muscle fibres. The super-mechanoeffector unit which thus results proved to be sufficiently realistic to make it worthwhile investigating its mechanical performance.

The feedback relationships adopted in Fig. 1 for the two sensorial pathways have different status; the length feedback from the muscle spindle is in agreement with the generally accepted view on the matter, whereas the positive nature of the tendon organ feedback differs from what is generally accepted (4), (15, 16). We have adopted this solution for the following reasons: a) the positive sign for the force feedback is the correct equivalent for the negative sign for the length feedback, and only then they both act congruently towards reducing the mechanoeffector unit output elastance, b) the influence of the tendon organ is greatly enhanced and its singular role comes out very clearly, and c) the proper integration of synergistic and antagonistic muscle systems depends on the existence of feedback linkages from the force sensors which are positive relative to the former and negative relative to the latter, so that correct sharing of the loads can be achieved. The experimental evidence seems to contradict (17-19) or hardly support (20) these theoretical considerations but the fact is that adequate experimental approach is still not available for satisfactorily estimating the gain and influence of the sensorial feedback pathways (21). Furthermore, the fact that the muscles are three-dimensional bodies in which the mechanical arrangement of the tendons is quite complex (11, 12) makes realistic interpretation of their functional relationship to the contraction of the associated muscle fibres difficult. Finally, even if experimental methods are devised which prove conclusively the negative nature of the tendon organ fedback linkage, the conclusions of the present work are not altered in their essence except for the fact that then the tendon organ is shown to loose its prominent role.

3.   MECHANOEFFECTOR UNIT TRANSFER RELATIONSHIPS

The relationships between the Laplace transforms of the mechanoeffector unit output length $x_o(s)$ and output force $y_o(s)$, the commands $u(s)$ and $v(s)$ and the load disturbances $y_e(s)$ are obtained from the characteristics of the unit components and of the load and from the feedback relationships shown in Fig. 1.

3.1 Characterization of the Components and the Load

The diagram of Fig. 2 shows the equivalent small-signal model of a muscle fibre (22). According to this model, the Laplace

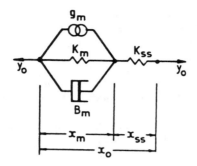

Fig. 2 Small-signal linear model of the skeletal muscle fibre.
Variables: x-lengths (or strains); y-forces (or stresses);
g_m -active-state equivalent force generator.   Parameters:
K-stiffness coefficients; B-viscosity coefficient.   Indices:
ss-series component; m-muscle or active component.

transform of the output force, y_o, is related to those of the
muscle length, x_o, and the force generator, g_m, as follows:

$$y_o(s) = \frac{a_2}{s+a_3} \, g_m(s) + B_m \cdot (s+a_1) \cdot x_o(s) \tag{1}$$

where s is the Laplace variable, $a_1 = K_m/B_m$, $a_2 = K_{ss}/B_m$ and $a_3 = (K_{ss} + K_m)/B_m$ are characteristic parameters, K_{ss} and K_m are respectively the series and parallel stiffness coefficients and B_m the
viscosity coefficient; x_o is taken as positive when the muscle
stretches.   The force generator is the output of the single-pole
low-pass "active state" filter which is stimulated by the motor
action potentials, and outputs a noisy estimate of the frequency of
the input pulses.   The relationship between the input and the
output of this filter is the following:

$$g_m(s) = C_m \cdot \frac{\beta}{s+\beta} \cdot a(s) \tag{2}$$

where β is the active-state decay rate constant, a the motor excitation frequency and C_m the frequency-to-force conversion
factor.   Substituting Eqn. 2 into Eqn. 1 we get the following relationship between the Laplace transforms of variables x_o, y_o and a:

$$y_o(s) = C(s) \cdot a(s) + Y_g(s) \cdot x_o(s) \tag{3}$$

where,

$$C(s) = C_m \cdot \frac{a_2 \cdot \beta}{(s+\beta)\,(s+a_3)} \text{ and } Y_g(s) = K_{ss} \cdot \frac{s+a_1}{s+a_3} \tag{4}$$

are the complex frequency-to-force conversion factor, and the muscle admittance or stiffness operator, respectively.

Transfer functions for the mechanoreceptors in the unit were also deduced from the literature:

$$r(s) = G_{t'} \cdot \frac{s+b_t}{s+a_t} \cdot y_o(s) = A_T(s) \cdot y_o(s) \tag{5}$$

for the tendon organ (23-25), and

$$r(s) = A_s(s) \cdot x_o(s) + B_s(s) \cdot y(s) \tag{6}$$

where,

$$A_s(s) = G_s \cdot \frac{s+b_s}{s+a_s} \text{ and } B_s = d_s \cdot \frac{\beta}{(s+a_s)(s+\beta)} \tag{7}$$

for the muscle spindle (26-30). The coefficients G_t and G_s, which are not frequency but amplitude dependent, represent conversion gains and display saturation characteristics. The values quoted for them are measured near the origin of these characteristics.

Finally, the load will be constituted, in the general case, by elastic (K_e), viscous (B_e) and inertial (mass) (M_e) components in parallel with a disturbing force generator, y_e. The input-output relationship for the load will then be:

$$y_o(s) = Y_e(s) \cdot x_e(s) + y_e(s) \tag{8}$$

where $Y_e(s) = M_e \cdot s^2 + B_e \cdot s + K_e$ is the stiffness (admittance operator of the load and $x_e = -x_o$.

3.2 Transfer and Output Elastance Relationships

The variables in the forward and feedback pathways of Fig. 1 are related as follows:

$$Y(s) = F_1(s) \cdot v(s)$$

$$a(s) = F_2(s) \cdot u^*(s)$$

$$\phi(s) = F_3(s) \cdot \sigma(s) = A_S^*(s) \cdot x_o(s) + B_S^*(s) \cdot Y(s)$$

$$\psi(s) = F_4(s) \cdot r(s) = A_T^*(s) \cdot y_o(s) \tag{9}$$

where s is the Laplace variable, and

$$A_S^*(s) = e^{-\Delta s} \cdot F_3(s) \cdot A_S(s); \quad B_S^*(s) = e^{-\Delta s} \cdot F_3(s) \cdot B_S(s)$$

$$\text{and } A_T^*(s) = e^{-\Delta s} \cdot F_4(s) \cdot A_T(s) \tag{10}$$

A_S, A_T and B_S are the complex operators defined in Eqns. 5 and 7, F_1, F_2, F_3 and F_4 are the transfer functions of the filters and Δ is the propagation delay in the afferent pathway from the sensors to the spinal cord circuitry. The feedback relationship as defined in Fig. 1 is the following:

$$u^*(s) = u(s) + \phi(s) + \psi(s) \tag{11}$$

From Eqns. 3–11 the following relationship between $x_o(s)$, the commands u(s) and v(s) and the load disturbances results:

$$x_o(s) = \frac{G(s)}{1 + G(s) \cdot H(s)} \left[u(s) + B_S^{**}(s) \cdot v(s) \right] + Z_o(s) \cdot Y_e(s) \tag{12}$$

where,

$$B_S^{**}(s) = F_1(s) \cdot B_S^*(s); \quad C^*(s) = C(s) \cdot F_2(s);$$

$$G(s) = \frac{C^*(s)}{Y_e(s) + Y_g(s)}; \tag{13}$$

$$H(s) = A_S^*(s) - A_T^*(s) \cdot Y_e(s) \tag{14}$$

and where,

$$Z_o(s) = \frac{1}{Y_e(s) + Y_g(s)} \cdot \frac{1 - C^*(s) \cdot A_T^*(s)}{1 + G(s) \cdot H(s)} \tag{15}$$

is the output elastance of the mechanoeffector unit. The assemblage output force $y_o(s)$ may be expressed in terms of u(s), v(s) and $x_o(s)$ as follows:

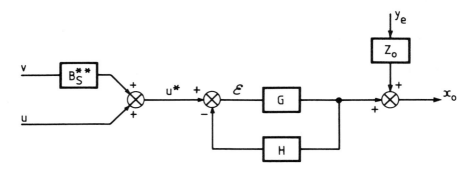

Fig. 3 Block diagram representation of the mechanoeffector unit. $u^* = (u + B_S^{**} \cdot v)$ is the combined (α, γ) command, $\epsilon = (1/1{+}GH) u^*$ the servo error signal and $x_o = (1/1{+}GH) \cdot u^* + Z_o \cdot y_e$ the output length.

$$y_o(s) = \frac{C^*(s)}{1 - C^*(s) \cdot A_T^*(s)} \cdot \left[u(s) + B_S^{**}(s) \cdot v(s) \right] -$$

$$\frac{Y_g(s) + C^*(s) \cdot A_S^*(s)}{1 - C^*(s) \cdot A_T^*(s)} \cdot x_o(s) \tag{16}$$

and, from this relationship, the muscle admittance or stiffness operator, $Y^*(s)$, as altered by the feedback, is given by:

$$Y_g^*(s) = -\frac{\partial y_o}{\partial x_o}(s) = \frac{Y_g(s) + C^*(s) \cdot A_S^*(s)}{1 - C^*(s) \cdot A_T^*(s)} \tag{17}$$

3.3 Interpretation of the Transfer and Output Elastance Relationships

Eqn. 12, which corresponds to the block diagram representation of the mechanoeffector unit shown in Fig. 3, embodies two main results. The first of these results consists in showing clearly that the command for the intrafusal fibres and the command for the extrafusal muscle fibres are closely tied up in the factor $(u + B_S^{**} \cdot v)$ and that they are therefore undistinguishable from a servomechanism point of view. Indeed, if the characteristics of the muscle spindle sensor (MS) allowed it to cover the full range of the mechanoeffector unit lengths, there should be no need for the v-command. As it is, the MS has a very narrow operating window and therefore the intrafusal muscle fibres have to be biased so as to locate that window in the region of muscle lengths which is to be monitored. Thus the need for a v-command may be looked upon as the price which has to be paid to compensate for the limitations of the technology with which the neuromuscular machines are built. There may however, exist a valuable merit in this arrangement: as it is explained later, the v-command could provide the very means for achieving an increased speed of response from the mechanoeffector unit without incurring in excessive overshoots. Secondly, Eqn. 12 also shows quite clearly how the mechanoeffector unit length x_o is made up of two components, one which is proportional to the command $u^* = (u+B_s^{**} \cdot v)$ and another which is due to the loading forces y_e applied to the unit. The first of these components is explicitly under the control of the usual stretch-reflex servo system whereas the second component, apparently independent of that servo system, is in fact also conditioned by it through its influence on Z_o as Eqn. 12 testifies. The precision of the mechanoeffector unit performance is controlled by the first of these two components and quantified by an error variable $\epsilon(s)$ which is the difference, measured in the absence of disturbing forces ($y_e = 0$), between the input command u^* and the command equivalent $\bar{u} = H \cdot x_o$ of the output length x_o; the corresponding design parameter is the steady state error $\epsilon(o)$ which, in percentual terms, is thus equal to $\epsilon^*(o)$ $= \epsilon(o)/u^*(o) = \left[1 + G(o) \cdot H(o)\right]^{-1}$. The presence of loading forces y_e introduces a second source of error in the performance, error which is minimized by minimizing Z_o.

Eqn. 15, in turn, reveals the singular role which is open to the tendon organ to play with regards to the output elastance of the system: whenever A_T^* is such that $A_T^*(s) \cdot C^*(s) = 1$ the assemblage will become infinitely stiff $\left[Z_o(s) = 0; Y_o(s) = \infty\right]$. Of course, infinite stiffness (which, in practical terms, means that the muscle displays a large value of dynamic output stiffness) can only occur if the feedback from the tendon organ is taken positively as we have done in Fig. 1.

4.   NEURAL FILTERING OF THE MECHANOEFFECTOR UNIT PATHWAYS

The existence of neural filters in the afferent and efferent pathways of the mechanoeffector unit could influence markedly its overall mechanical performance. The nature of these filters is not known and therefore we can only conjecture about their most likely characteristics and investigate how they would influence the mechanoeffector unit.

4.1 Afferent Pathways

The open-loop gain GH(s) may be written, if we ignore the delay Δ, as follows:

$$GH(s) = F_2(s) . \frac{a_2\beta}{(s+\beta)} . \frac{F_3(s).A_S^*(s)-F_4(s).A_T^*(s).(M_e s^2 +B_e s+K_e)}{(M_e s^2+B_z s+K_e) (s+a_3) + K_{ss} . (s+a_1)} \quad (18)$$

whose value for s = +j∞:

$$GH(j\infty) = a_2 \beta \lim_{s=j\infty} \frac{F_2(s) . F_4(s) . A_T^*(s)}{s^2} \quad (19)$$

shows that the tendon organ conditions the high frequency region of GH(jω). The value of Eqn. 14 for s = 0 is given by:

$$GH(o) = F_2(o) . a_2 . \frac{F_3(o) . A_S^*(o)-K_e . F_4(o) . A_T^*(o)}{a_2 K_e + a_1 K_{ss}} \quad (20)$$

and because the term F_3. A_S^* predominates over the term $K_e.F_4.A_T^*$, the low frequency region of GH(jω) is controlled by the muscle spindle feedback.

The filter transfer functions which are considered for F_3 and F_4 are suggested by Eqn. 18 and are of the form F(s) = k.E(s) where k is a scalar gain factor and E(s) a rational function of s. The eight filtering situations which are investigated are given in Table 1.

Situation	1	2	3	4	5	6	7	8
$E_3(s)$	1		W_S^{-1}		$(\frac{s+\beta}{\beta})$		$(\frac{s+\beta}{\beta}).W_S^{-1}$	
$E_4(s)$	1	W_T^{-1}	1	W_T^{-1}	$(\frac{s+\beta}{\beta})$	$(\frac{s+\beta}{\beta}).W_T^{-1}$	$(\frac{s+\beta}{\beta})$	$(\frac{s+\beta}{\beta}).W_T^{-1}$

$$W_S(s) = \frac{s+b_s}{s+a_s} \quad ; \quad W_T(s) = \frac{s+b_t}{s+a_a} \quad ;$$

Table 1   Filtering situations considered for the afferent pathways

The following points regarding this choice of filters deserve being commented: a) The inclusion of the factor (s+β)/β in both E_3 and E_4 is determined by the desire to remove the corresponding pole s = −β from GH. This result could be achieved by incorporating the factor (s+β)/β in F_2 instead, a solution which may seem more natural since this pole reflects a property of the muscle itself. Such a solution however, has the inconvenience of increasing the bandwidth of the muscle response and making it less dumped. Therefore, the system becomes more prone to oscillation: this fact reduces k_s and therefore leads to excessive position errors. The solution we have adopted, on the other hand, does not suffer from this shortcoming: b) The transfer functions $E(s) = W^{-1}$, where $W(s)$ is the transfer function of the respective sensor, corresponding to what we have called match-filtering; c) The match-filtering of the spindle has as a consequence that the Laplace transform of the spindle sensor output signal becomes,

$$\phi(s) = k_s \left[G_s \cdot (\frac{s+\beta}{\beta}) \cdot x_o(s) + F_1(s) \cdot (\frac{d_s}{s+b_s}) \cdot v(s) \right] \qquad (21)$$

That is, $\phi(t)$ is proportional to the derivative of $x_o(t)$ by the factor $(s+\beta)$, due to the extrafusal fibres, and is the same for both primary and secondary spindle afferents. This means, therefore, that there is no functional difference between the primary and the secondary spindle assemblages.

4.2 Efferent Pathways

From Eqns. 1, 2, 3 and 13 we may write $C^*(s) = F_2(s)$. $(a_2 \cdot \beta \cdot C_m)/(s+\beta)(s+a_3)$ where filter F_2 is of the general form $F_2(s) = k_2 \cdot E_2(s)$ and three different cases are considered for $E_2(s)$, namely, $E_2(s) = 1$, $E_2(s) = s+\beta/\beta$ and $E_2(s) = (s+a_3)/(s+p)$. The first value of $E_2(s)$ is used in filtering situations 1 to 8, the second in filtering situation 9 and the third in filtering situation 10.

The afferent signal $\phi(s)$ from the spindle has two components, one proportional to $x_o(s)$ and another proportional to $v(s)$, both of which are shaped by filter $F_3(s)$ according to Eqn. 9. The form of filter $F_3(s)$ which is chosen to optimize the characteristics of the systems has the inconvenience of introducing a pole $s = -b_s$ in the term $B_s^{**}(s) \cdot v(s)$, as shown in Eqn. 21. The pole degrades severely the contribution of this term to $\phi(t)$. This situation is obviated if we make $F_1(s)$ equal to:

$$F_1(s) = k_1 \cdot (s+b_s) \qquad (22)$$

This way the output from the spindle sensor responds quickly to the gammma-command and gradually reduces to zero as the target length is approached. The value of the scalar gain k_1 is obtained by postulating that in the absence of a disturbing load ($y_e = 0$) and for a step command ($u + B_s^{**} \cdot v$), the output signal $\phi(t)$ from the

spindle sensor tends to zero as the target length is reached.
Thus, from Eqns. 9, 12, 13 and 14 and calling U = mod u and V = mod
(B_S^{**} . v) we have, by the final value theorem:

$$\lim_{t=\infty} \phi(t) = V - (U+V) \cdot \lim_{s=0} \left[\frac{A_S^*(s) \cdot G(s)}{1 + G(s) \cdot H(s)} \right] = 0 \qquad (23)$$

Hence:

$$\text{mod } (B_S^{**} \cdot v) = \frac{M_o}{1-M_o} \cdot \text{mod } u \qquad (24)$$

where,

$$M_o = \lim_{s=0} \left[\frac{A_S^* G}{1+G \cdot H} \right] \qquad (25)$$

From the above the values of V = V(U) and of k_1 may be deduced.

5.   NUMERICAL SIMULATION OF THE MECHANOEFFECTOR UNIT RESPONSE

      In order to be able to simulate numerically the dynamical
performance of the mechanoeffector unit we need to know the characteristics of its components.   The parameters of the extrafusal
muscle fibres were taken as being those which could be deduced from
the data available in the literature (31-35) for whole muscles and
correspond to a fast skeletal muscle biased at a working point on
its isometric length-tension characteristics defined by a length
L/L_o = 0.9 and an excitation a/a_{max} = 0.29; L_o and a_{max} being its
rest length and its maximum rate of stimulation, respectively.
These parameters, expressed in S.I. units are the following: L_o =
26 mm; a_{max} = 110 s^{-1} ; K_m = 1.15 N/mm; K_{ss} = 5 N/mm; B_m = 78 N.s/m
and C_m = 0.13 N.s. The values of these parameters vary widely with
the working point and so does the mechanoeffector unit performance.
The tendon organ parameters where obtained from the literature
(23-25) as being b_t = 0.9 s^{-1} and G_t = 4s^{-1}.kN^{-1}. The muscle
spindle parameters a_s, b_s, d_s and G_s were deduced (26-30) as being
respectively equal to 20 s^{-1}, 1.3 s^{-1}, 0.40 s^{-1} and 64 s^{-1}.mm^{-1} for
a fast muscle (external intercostal) and 12.5 s^{-1} , 0.9 s^{-1}, 0.44s^{-1}
and 62 s^{-1} .mm^{-1} for a slow muscle (soleus). The load which has
been used in the present simulation has the following parameters:
K_e = 1 N/mm, B_e = 98 N.s/m and M_e = 0.5 kg.

      The influence of filters F_3 and F_4 on the characteristics of
the system and the possibility of using this influence to simplify
the description of the system and to improve its performance are

now going to be investigated. We ignore for the moment the influence of F_1 in the fusimotor pathway assuming that the commands synthesizer takes care of the driving requirements of this pathway. We shall analyze later the merits of adequately compensating for the characteristics of the intrafusal fibres. To simplify the analysis we begin by considering F_2 reduced to its simplest form, namely, $F_2 = k_2$ where k_2 is a scalar. Later we will consider the merits of using F_2 to eliminate poles $s = -\beta$ and $s = (K_m + K_{ss})/B_m$. The filter transfer functions we are going to investigate are those defined in Table 1. We will refer to all cases where the filter transfer function contains the reciprocal of the corresponding sensor transfer function "match-filtering." The relative virtues of these filtering situations are studied in the frequency domain through the Nyquist diagram. The system output elastance $Z_0(j\omega)$ and transmission gain

$$T(j\omega) = \frac{x_o}{(u + B_S^{**} v)} (j\omega)$$

are studied in the time domain with the aid of the response to a unit step in the $(u + B_S^{**} v)$ command. The results which follow were obtained for a fast skeletal muscle whose characteristics, together with those of the sensors and of the load were given previously. The influence of the propagation delays is ignored unless otherwise stated and k_2 is taken to be equal to 0.04.

5.1 Nyquist Diagram

Eqn. 18 provides the means for the computation of the Nyquist diagram of the mechanoeffector unit, and several cases of this diagram are illustrated in Fig. 4. They describe a position servomechanism of the type zero, i.e., with no pole at the origin of its open loop transfer function and therefore with a finite position error. According to Eqns. 19 and 20 the high and low frequency regions of the Nyquist diagram are predominantly controlled by the tendon organ and by the muscle spindle sensor, respectively. The influence of the two feedback gains k_t and k_s is identical for all the filtering arrangements which were studied: the phase and gain margins decrease when either gain increases and the steady-state error increases when k_t increases or k_s decreases. Fig. 4 compares filtering situation 1 with 2, 3, 5 and 8. The former corresponds to assembling the mechanoeffector unit from its component parts as described in the literature. The latter group correspond, respectively, to match-filter the tendon organ, to match-filter the muscle spindle, to eliminate the influence of the pole $s = -\beta$ of $G(s)$ in both feedback pathway, and to the match-filtering of both sensors with simultaneous elimination of the influence of $(s+\beta)$. The match-filtering of the tendon organ has little effect on the

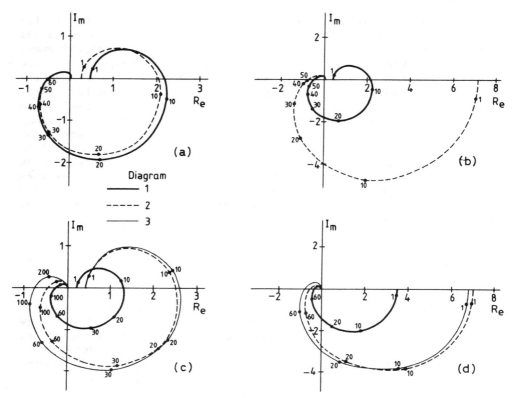

Fig. 4 Nyquist diagrams for different filtering arrangements: a) influence of match—filtering the tendon organ; Diagram 1 corresponds to condition 1 and Diagram 2 to condition 2; $k_t^* = 2$ and $k_s^* = 50$ for both diagrams; b) influence of match—filtering the muscle spindle; Diagram 1 corresponds to condition 1 and Diagram 2 to condition 3; $k_t^* = 2$ and $k_s^* = 50$ for both diagrams; c) influence of filtering $(s+\beta)$ in both feedback loops (condition 5); and d) influence of filtering condition 8.   The gains are the same for cases (c) and (d): Diagram 1 corresponds to $k_t^* = 0.05$ and $k_s^* = 1$, Diagram 2 to $k_t = 0.05$ and $k_s = 2$ and Diagram 3 to $k_t^* = 0.15$ and k_s^* = 2.   Numbers along the diagrams represent values of the angular frequency ω.

Nyquist diagram. Its merits reside simply in the simplification it brings to $A_T^*(s)$ which is thus reduced to $(s+\beta)(1/\beta).k_t$. The match—filtering of the muscle spindle similarly simplifies the description of the system by making $A_s^*(s) = (s+\beta)(1/\beta).k_t$ but at the same time markedly improves the low frequency region of the diagram. The compensation for the pole $(s+\beta)$ in $G(s)$ by the introduction of a zero $s = -\beta$ in both $E_3(s)$ and $E_4(s)$ has the merit of simplifying the transfer function of the system, but has the adverse

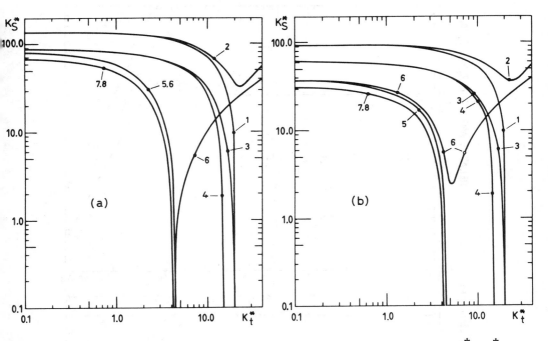

Fig. 5 Boundaries of stability: the regions of the plane (k_t^*, k_s^*) defined by each boundary and the coordinate axes represent domains of stable (k_t^*, k_s^*) designs; a) for a propagation delay $\Delta = 0.0$ ms, and b) a typical return (afferent and efferent) delay of $\Delta = 5.0$ ms. The numbers 1 to 8 indicate the corresponding filtering situation (Table 1). The scale factors for both k_s^* and k_t^* are 1 for boundaries 1 to 4, and 10 for boundaries 5 to 8.

consequence of reducing its response speed drastically. However, the simultaneous match-filtering of the tendon organ (situations 6 or 8) completely compensates for this adverse effect and restores the proper performance of the system.

The feedback loop gains k_s and k_t or, the compound gains $k_s^* = k_2 \cdot k_s$ and $k_t^* = k_2 \cdot k_t$, are conveniently related to the stability of the system through the boundaries of stability, defined as the loci in the (k_t^*, k_s^*) plane for which the relationship $GH(j\omega) = -1$ holds. Such boundaries are illustrated in Fig. 5 for the eight filtering situations described in Table 1 and for the muscle, sensor and load parameters given above. Fig. 5 shows that the values of the k_t^* and k_s^* for the filtering situations 5 to 8, i.e., those for which the influence of the $\beta/(s+\beta)$ factor $G(s)$ is eliminated through $E_3(s)$ and $E_4(s)$, are one order of magnitude smaller than those corresponding to situations 1 to 4. This fact reflects

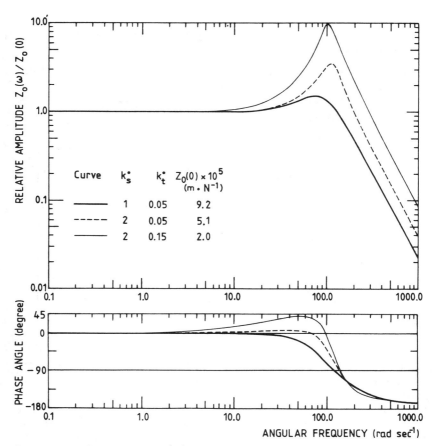

Fig. 6 Output elastance $Z_o(\omega)$ corresponding to filtering situation 8, $k_2 = 0.04$, and sets of k_t^* and k_s^* gains are indicated.

the presence of the additional low frequency gain introduced by the compensating zero in $E_3(s)$ and $E_4(s)$. Fig. 5 also illustrates how the domains of stability in the (k_t^*, k_s^*) plane are reduced by the propagation delay in the feedback pathway. The delay, which is supposed to be the same in both pathways, rotates each point in the Nyquist diagram in a clockwise direction and by an amount directly proportional to the corresponding frequency. The main consequence of the delay is to reduce the values of k_s^*, and therefore has adverse effects on both the position error and the output elastance of the system.

5.2 Output Elastance

The output elastance of the system is illustrated for three sets of (k_t^*, k_s^*) values and for situation 8 in Fig. 6. The values of Z which are obtained are in reasonable agreement with the experimental data (Z_0 = 0.1 mm/N) for the cat gastrocnemius muscle (15), although situation 8 leads to smaller values and to a more uniform variation of $Z_0(\omega)$ with the frequency than situation 1 does. The increase of either k_t^* or k_s^* tends to create a resonance peak at the high frequency end of the pass-band. The negative length-feedback from the spindle and the positive force-feedback from the tendon organ both tend to reduce the output elastance. The tendon organ feedback is however a more efficient mechanism for the performance of this task because the product $C^*A_T^*$ can be made very close to unify for very small values of k_t^*. For higher values of k_t^*, on the other hand, the output elastance becomes negative and the mechanoeffector unit becomes unstable in the sense that it will tend to reinforce the action of the forces applied to it isntead of resisting them. The value of k_t^* for which $C^*A_T^*(0)$ is equal to unity, is the critical value of k_t^*, and is equal to 150.87, 5.72, 6.03 and 0.229 for filtering situations 1 and 3, 2 and 4, 5 and 7 and 6 and 8, respectively.

5.3 Transmission Gain and Step Response

The transmission gain as a function of the frequency has been computed for several sets of (k_t^*, k_s^*) and for all the eight filtering situations considered in Table 1. The $T(\omega)$ plots correspond to a single pole low-pass filter and filtering situation 8 provides the best response over the entire frequency range, although the transmission gain is then almost one order of magnitude smaller than that of the corresponding cases for situation 1. The increase in the values of k_t^* and k_s^* tends, in all situations, to introduce a resonance peak at the end of the pass band. The excitation needed for a 20% (5mm) steady-state contraction of the muscle shows values between 3,000 and 18,000 Hz, which is six times higher for the cases of situation 8 than for corresponding values in situation 1. To understand these values of the excitation, it must be remembered that the muscle has at the order of 200 motor units (4) each capable of being excited at a maximum frequency of 110 Hz, thus resulting for the whole muscle a maximum excitation frequency of approximately 22,0000 Hz. It should be pointed out that the linear approximation used so far does not apply to large excursions in the muscle length; we use the values of excitation computed above as a simple measure of its real value.

The response $x_0(t)$ to a step in the (u + B_s^{**} . v) command were calculated by numerical inversion (36) of Eqn. 12 for the case when y_e = 0 and for the different filtering situations. The response displayed by the mechanoeffector unit in all cases corresponds to that of a single pole low-pass filter. Filtering situation 8 was shown to improve the value of the rise time by an order of magnitude with regard to that of situation 1, and to bring it to within the range of the known experimental data (37). This fact adds credibility to the corresponding filtering arrangements. It should be pointed out that this improvement is almost exclusively due to the filtering of the muscle spindle sensor. Compensation of pole s = $-\beta$, alone, in fact worsens the performance of the system and leads to rise times of the order of several seconds for the same load and muscle biasing conditions. The match-filtering of the tendon organ has practically no influence on the value of the rise time. The values of the gain factors k_t^* and k_s^* also do not have any appreciable influence on the response rise time, but they both cause oscillations when their increase brings the system closer to instability. The transmission delay has a very similar effect.

5.4 Merits of Filtering

Table 2 gives the figures of merit for several situation 1 and situation 8 mechanoeffector assemblage designs. It can be seen from it that the designs corresponding to the filtering situation 8 possess the following advantages relative to those corresponding to the filtering situation 1: a) the position error and the rise time are smaller (about one fifth and one tenth respectively, b) the low frequency output elastance is smaller (one tenth), and c) the bandwidth is about ten times greater. On the other hand, the low frequency transmission gain T(o) is about five times smaller in the case of filtering situation 8. Consequently, the excitation needed to achieve a given shortening of the muscle is five times larger in this case, although it still corresponds to reasonable values of the excitation. None of the designs of Table 2 displays either a peak in $T(\omega)$ or an overshoot in $x_0(t)$. The most important result embodied in Table 2 is the fact that the designs corresponding to situation 8 display characteristics which are in closer agreement with the available experimental data on neuromuscular performance. Table 2 therefore illustrates how the adequate filtering of the feedback pathways not only simplifies the system description but could provide the very means which are needed for the achievement of the desired performance characteristics.

5.5 Filtering Efferent Pathways

We have so far ignored both efferent pathways, and in particular assumed that the commands issued to the muscle spindle were automatically matched to the transmission characteristics $B_s^*(s)$ of the v-link. Since $\gamma = F_1 \cdot v$, this is indeed what Eqn. 22 means: the command to the intrafusal fibres is proportional to both the desired change in length and its desired rate of change. Only in this way will be muscle spindle not be cheated of a major potential advantage, namely, that of supplying a feedback signal which responds quickly to the gamma command and which goes to zero when the target length is approached. In this way fast responses of the mechanoeffector can be achieved without incurring in appreciable overshooting. In order to guarantee that the variational value of

Figures of Merit	Situation 1			Situation 8		
	$k_t^* = 2$	2	5	$k_t^* = 0.05$	0.10	0.20
	$k_s^* = 50$	80	60	$k_s^* = 2$	2	1
$\varepsilon^*(o)^{(*)}$ (Z)	68.6	57.6	64.9	12.5	12.6	24.2
$T(o) \times 10^6$ $^{(**)}$ (m.pps^{-1})	1.53	1.29	1.45	0.28	0.28	0.54
$3d_b$ Bandwidth (rad.sec^{-1})	2.5	2.3	2.6	25	26	28
Exc. $\times 10^{-3}$ (0.005m) (pps)	3.3	3.9	3.4	17.9	17.9	9.26
$Z_o(o) \times 10^5$ (m.N^{-1})	35.3	29.7	32.7	5.1	3.7	1.6
Max $\dfrac{Z_o(\omega)}{Z_o(o)}$	1.6	1.7	1.4	3.2	5.4	16.2
Rise time $^{(***)}$ (msec)	900	870	770	80	80	90

(*)   Steady state position error: $\varepsilon^*(o) = [1 + G(o).H(o)]^{-1}$
(**)   Steady state transmission gain: $T(o) = G(o). \varepsilon^*(o)$
(***)   Time taken by the step response to go from 10% to 90% of the final value.

Table 2   The comparison of figures of merit for situation 1 and 8 designs ($k_2 = 0.04$).

ϕ assumes its minimum value when the target length is reached the modulus of (B_S^{**} . v) must have the value defined by Eqn. 24. The corresponding time variation of $\phi(t)$ for situation 8, $k_s^* = 1.0$ and $k_t^* = 0.05$ is shown in Fig. 7(a). It should be noticed that Eqn. 24 is only satisfied for a particular set of muscle and load characteristics. If these change or if the load disturbance y_e is not zero, $\phi(t)$ will not tend to zero although it will tend to values in the vicinity of zero. When the fusimotor command is not matched to

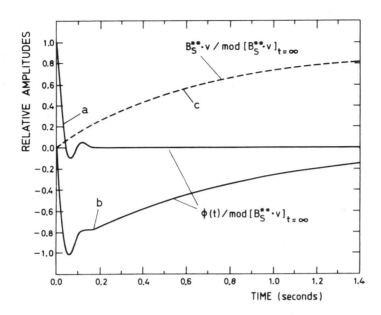

Fig. 7 Muscle spindle output response $\phi(t)$ to a step command (u+ B_S^{**}v) for filtering situation 8, $F_2 = k_2$, $k_2 = 0.04$, $k_S^* = 1.0$, $k_t^* = 0.05$ and (a) $F_1 = (s+b_s)$ (b) $F_1 = 1$. The waveform of the fusimotor command $B_S^{**} \cdot v(t)$ is a step function in case (a) and a slowly growing exponential (c) in case (b). The waveform amplitudes are relative to the limit for $t = \infty$ of modulus of $B_S^{**} \cdot v$.

the corresponding link, i.e., when F_1 is a simple scalar gain, the waveforms of $B_S^* \cdot v$ and of $\phi = A_S^* \cdot x_o + B_S^{**} \cdot v$ are those illustrated in Fig. 7(c) and (b) respectively.

The alphamotor pathway can provide further means for the conditioning of characteristics of the system. The scalar gain k_2 in $F_2(s) = k_2$ influences the amplitude level of both alpha and gamma efferent commands, mod (u) and mod ($B_S^{**} \cdot v$) respectively, which decrease with the increase in the value of k_2.

The compensation for the influence of pole $s = -\beta$ in GH could be achieved by inserting the compensating factor $(s+\beta)/\beta$ in F_2 instead of in F_3 and F_4. Such an alternative certainly represents a much more elegant solution for the filtering problem as in this case $E_3 = A_S^{*-1}$ and $E_4 = A_T^{*-1}$ are true matched filters. We shall call this the filtering situation 9. This situation only differs from situation 8 in the transmission gain $T(\omega) = G/(1+GH)$ due to the fact that pole $s = -\beta$ is now removed in G and not in H. As a consequence, with the exception of the 3db-bandwidth and the rise time, the two filtering situations share the same figures of merit and boundaries of stability. If, for example, we use the same valued of k_2, k_s and k_t as those used for the four cases of situation 8 described in Table 2, the bandwidth and the rise time will be, for all three cases, of the order of 120 rad/s and 25 ms respectively, i.e., four times greater and four times smaller than the corresponding values in the table. The step response displays a damped oscillation and an overshoot of the order of 1.4. The figures of merit for filtering situations 8 and 9 are reasonably similar and it was decided to consider that filtering situation 8 provides the best fit for the available experimental data. It should however be pointed out that the available experimental information is not sufficient to allow a clear choice between the models represented by filtering situations 8 and 9 and, further-more, that all the conclusions drawn for one of these filtering situations are also valid for the other. The choice of situation 8 to model the mechanoeffector unit implicitly corresponds to assume that the CNS accepts the basic dynamic characteristics of the plant it controls – the extrafusal fibres – because they are quite satis-factory for the needs of everyday life and that, in order to achieve the desired performance, it prefers to tune-up and optimize the sensory pathways.

Finally, attention is drawn to the fact that the existence of a finite series stiffness (K_{ss}) in cascade with the active muscle introduces an additional real valued pole in the open-loop transfer function G(s) of the system and degrades its performance. If this pole is removed, the behavior of the system suffers an alteration similar to that described for filtering situation 9; the system becoming faster and more prone to oscillation. It may instead be considered the inclusion in F_2 of an extra lead-lag filter, of the form $(s+a_3)/(s+p)$, to replace the pole $s = -a_3$ by a pole $s = -p$ and to use the value of p as a design parameter. The filtering situa-tion which results from situation 8 by introducing this filter in the corresponding efferent pathway is called situation 10. In this case the critical value of k_t^* is given by the expression $k_{tc}^* = 0.0029p$ and the stability boundaries have the same shape as for situation 8 but their size decreases with p. The system becomes more lively as p decreases with the tendency to display smaller position errors and rise times and larger bandwidths. This influ-ence of the value of p could provide the CNS with a device for improving the system characteristics when shorter reaction times are desired.

6. CONCLUDING REMARKS

The theoretical analysis presented in this chapter is based on three main assumptions: a) the mechanoeffector unit, defined in Fig. 1 and integrated at spinal cord levels, is the CNS basic mechanical peripheral assemblage, b) the force feedback from the tendon organ is positive, and c) the nervous circuitry which is responsible for the functional integration of the unit processes the afferent data from the sensors and the efferent commands to the muscle fibres through neural filters which lead to simpler and more efficient systems.

The first of these assumptions corresponds basically to putting together concepts which have been around in the literature for quite a while. The main criticisms the mechanoeffector unit presented here relates to its usefulness in modeling real muscles. Since real muscles are three dimensional bodies in which important transverse stresses — not considered in Fig. 1 — develop and since their motor units are territorially intermingled into complex structural arrangements the present model may not be fully adequate to represent them.

The choice of the positive sign for the tendon organ feedback connection is closely related to the question of whether the stretch-reflex servo controls the muscle length or its stiffness (21, 38-40). We have assumed that the latter is the basic variable the servo controls and adopted for both types of mechanoreceptors the connections which maximize their respective action. Indeed, the position error and the output elastance are two characteristics of the mechanoeffector unit which deserve close attention. In fact, the smaller they are the more precise and the less sensitive to mechanical loading respectively, are the movements of the mechanoeffector unit. Therefore, its response to the CNS commands is more consistent. It should be borne in mind that the only connection the brain has with the outside world is through its sensorial and mechanical peripherals which therefore must provide reliable channels for information gathering and for effector action, i.e., channels which respond, consistently, both to outside world stimuli and to the CNS commands; or else that world would seem totally chaotic and unmanageable. Hence, the CNS must be capable of guaranteeing adequate precision and stiffness from ts peripherals. Thus, the answer to the question of what the stretch-reflex servo controls, embodied in Eqns. 12, 15 and 16 is the following: the servo controls the variables which define the state of the mechanoeffector unit, namely, its output length x_0 and force y_0, as well as its sensitivity to the action of external forces (through Z_0). What is suggested in this chapter is that, by using properly designed filtering schemes, the CNS is able to control precision and stiffness simultaneously, but by two reasonably independent channels, viz., the spindle and the tendon organ feedback loops.

Another consequence to motor control of what has been said above is well worth our consideration: indeed, if a peripheral is sufficiently precise and stiff there will be, within reasonable limits of loading and velocity of operation, no need to command it in a closed-loop mode; on the contrary, its control in an open-loop mode will be faster and more efficient. From the point of view of the organization of motor control, therefore, it will be advantageous that the integration at segmental level is capable of transforming the neuromuscular peripherals into well behaved tools which can be controlled by the high CNS centres in an open-loop mode. With such a hierarchical organization, closed-loop servo operation involving higher CNS centres would be eminently confined to the learning of new skills and to the slow performance of new and unusual tasks which involve sensorial information of non-mechanical nature. On the other hand, it is reasonable to assume that open-loop control of the mechanical peripherals occurs in all the normal physiological functions which deal with routine loading. It should be pointed out however that this mode of operation may involve quite modest reflex controls gains (41): this will be the case when the loads are constant and predictable or when there is the possibility of resorting to an higher level of control involving other sensorial feedback pathways. On the extreme end of motor control, fast skilled movements such as those which occur in some artistic and sports practices and in fighting, provide good illustration of instances when the CNS needs extreme precision and stiffness from its peripherals and there is no room for an error-correcting feedback play by the high CNS centres or even, perhaps, by the spinal cord centres. In these instances, the CNS depends entirely on its exact knowledge of its peripherals characteristics and of the loads to be dealt with.

The CNS potentials for computation and information processing have long been acknowledged (42). Its role in the control of neuromuscular systems is obvious and there is sufficient evidence that the signal cord is capable of commanding the automatic performance of elaborated mechanical acts (43). The search for the filtering configurations used by the CNS in its role of the mechanoeffector unit control was not carried very far in this study since all the variables (such as the energy expenditure) which are involved in real neuromuscular systems were not considered. The only optimal criterion we used was to look for filtering schemes which minimized the analytical relationships describing the mechanoeffector unit performance while meeting the available experimental data on the neuromuscular performances. The major merit of our matched-filtering solution is thus the simplicity of the analytical description it leads to and which makes the corresponding mechanoeffector assemblage a very convenient device for modeling a large range of neuromuscular situations. Many other filtering schemes could possibly be devised to meet the available experimental data but they would be likely to lead to more complex models. It would be extremely difficult however, to distinguish between such models on a basis of experimental evidence. Other merits of match-filtering the transfer characteristics of the different mechanoeffector unit components (filtering situation 8)

are clearly shown by the present results: a) the transfer functions A_S^*, A_T^* and B_S^{**} are drastically simplified, b) the position
error is minimized and becomes highly sensitive to k_s^* while the
system assumes a very stable configuration, and c) the roles of the
muscle spindle and of the tendon organ come out quite distinctly,
viz., the spindle controls the speed of response and the position
error whereas the tendon organ is most effective in controlling the
output elastance and, through it, in making the mechanoeffector
unit less sensitive to load disturbances.   The separation of functional roles of the length and force sensors which is thus achieved
provides the CNS with two almost independent channels for the
control, via k_s and k_t, of the corresponding characteristics of the
system and this certainly should make for higher performance and
reliability.

The loop gains k_s and k_t cannot be measured experimentally
because the neuronal circuits which perform the summing of the
feedback signals are not clearly identified but some conclusions
can nevertheless be drawn with regards to these gains.   Firstly,
the large differences which exist in the values of k_s and k_t give
an indication of the reasons why, in the past, the allocation of a
functional role to the tendon organ has been so difficult.   Secondly, the high frequency response of the system is much more sensitive to k_t than to k_s and the system is easily made to oscillate by
the tendon organ.   This proneness to oscillate which is evidenced
in shivering or in pathological tremors could therefore be an
important attribute of the tendon organ feedback loop.

A few remarks about the mechanoeffector unit sensorial equipment are now in order.   Pressure transducers of the fast adaptive
type like the Pacinian corpuscles, have not been considered.   The
fact that they are normally associated with extramuscular tissues
and tissues which are capable of undergoing large movements (6, 44)
makes it reasonable to assume that they merely represent an adapta-
tion thanks to which the fragile nerve endings may be safely implanted in such tissues.   They would still be mechanical stress
transducers whose response characteristics, which reflect their
histological constitution, could be corrected by filtering − a
suitably adapted low pass filter would produce a transformed
response identical to that of a tendon organ − to let them perform
their role in the respective control assemblage.   Similar considerations also supply the rationale for the choice made in this
paper of the "single-efferent-single-afferent" model (26) to represent the muscle spindle sensor: any other form of spindle response
could be synthetized from it by an adequate neuronal processing.
As it turned out, the match-filtering of the spindle sensor characteristics proved to be a very important and necessary part of the
mechanoeffector unit model and it was therefore felt no need for
distinguishing between primary and secondary sensory endings.   The
possible role of the primary endings sensitiveness to velocity in

speeding-up the response of the loaded mechanoeffector unit to the CNS commands and in reducing overshoot, is satisfactorily played through the differential mechanism which the gamma-command to the intrafusal fibres mediates. A functional reason must therefore be found for the differentiation of the intrafusal fibres and for the differences in their innervation. According to experimental evidence (45-74), it is the mechanical characteristics of the intrafusal fibres which determine the dynamical behavior of the sensorial endings associated with them and so, the reason for the differentiation between the three types (slow and fast nuclear bag and nuclear chain) of intrafusal fibres is most likely one of a mechanical nature. The slow nuclear bag fibres do possibly possess a mechanical endurance which makes them suited for the monitoring of a sustained contraction of the extrafusal fibres whereas the fast nuclear chain fibres are the natural sensors for fast muscle movements. The fact that individual type I_a afferent fibres inner-vate simultaneously nuclear bag and nuclear chain intrafusal fibres (48) could be interpreted as meaning that such bag-chain fibre associations constitute sensorial assemblages which are capable of monitoring sustained movements as well as of providing the fast response needed for the efficient control of faster movements. The I_a nerve fibres which subserve the bag-chain assemblages have large diameters and are therefore capable of faster propagation veloci-ties and of supplying a large population of synapses in the spinal cord. These facts could perhaps indicate that the bag-chain assemblages are associated with more extensive nervous processing of the sensorial information. The type II afferent nerve fibres usually originate from a single chain fibre and are of a smaller diameter than the I_a fibres although they tend to be slightly more numerous than the latter. It thus seems reasonable to assume that type II fibres subserve the motor control of smaller and faster motor units.

Finally, the implications of postulating, as it has been done, an optimal mechanoeffector unit design which depends on the match-filtering of its sensorial equipment, should now be considered. Such a postulate in fact does mean that from an effector point of view the biological sensors are far too cumbersome to allow an efficient performance, and therefore, they need to be complemented by corrective filters. It does not mean however, that the full sensorial output has no functional role to play. On the contrary, what it seems to suggest is that the neuromuscular peripherals are integrated into two distinct, although complementary, functional spaces: an effector space which is essentially of a centrifugal nature and a sensorial space which is obviously of a centripetal nature and which, possibly, makes use of all the information the sensors are capable of generating.

REFERENCES

1. Stein, R.B., Physiol. Rev., 54(1)(1974), 215-243.
2. Chin, N.K., M. Cope & M. Pang, In: Symposium on Muscle Receptors, D. Barker, Ed. (Hong-Kong, Hong-Kong Univ. Press, 1962), 241-248.
3. Eldred, E., C.F. Bridgman, J.E. Swett & B. Eldred, In: Symposium on Muscle Receptors, D. Barker, Ed. (Hong-Kong, Hong-Kong Univ. Press, 1962), 207-213.
4. Botterman, B.R., M.D. Binder & D.G. Stuart, Amer. Zool., 18 (1978), 135-152.
5. Marchand, R., C.F. Bridgman, E. Schumpert & E. Eldred, Anat. Rec., 169 (1971), 23-32.
6. Wohlfart, G. & K.G. Henriksson, Acta Anat., 41 (1960), 192-204.
7. Eccles, J.C. & C.S. Sherrington, Proc. Roy. Soc., B106 (1930), 326-357.
8. Buchthal, F., Res. Publ. Ass. Res. Nerv. Ment. Disc., 38 (1961), 3-30.
9. Boyd, I.A. & M.R. Darvey, Composition of Peripheral Nerves (London, E. and Livingstone Publishers', 1968).
10. Burke, R.E., D.N. Levine, P. Tsairis & P.E. Zajac III, J. Physiol., 243(3)(1973), 723-748.
11. Houk, J.C. & E. Henneman, J. Neurophysiol., 30 (1967), 466-481.
12. Stuart, D.G., C.G. Mosher, R.L. Gerlach & R.M. Rinking, Exp. Brain Res., 14 (1972), 274-292.
13. Burke, R.E. & P. Tsairis, J. Physiol., 234 (1973), 749-765.
14. Clark, D.A., Am. J. Physiol., 96(2) (1930), 296-304.
15. Roberts, W.J., N.P. Rosenthal & C.A. Terzuolo, J. Neurophysiol., 34 (1971), 620-634.
16. Houk, J.C., J.J. Singer & M.R. Goldman, J. Neurophysiol., 33 (1970), 784-811.
17. Granit, R., J. Neurophysiol., 13 (1950), 351-372.
18. Laporte, Y. & D.P.C. Loyd, Am. J. Physiol., 169 (1952), 609-621.
19. Granit, R., J.O. Kellerth & A.J. Szumski, J. Physiol., 182 (1966), 488-503.
20. Houk, J.C. In: Biocybernetics IV, H. Drischell and P. Dettmar, Eds. (Jena, Fischer, 1972), 125-144.
21. Matthews, P.B.C., In: Myotatic, Kinesthetic and Vestibular Mechanisms, A.V.S. de Reuck and J. Knight, Eds., Ciba Foundation Symposium (London, J. and A. Churchill Ltd. Publishers, 1967), 40-50.
22. Pringle, J.W.S., Symp. Soc. Exp. Biol., 14 (1960), 41-68.
23. Alnaes, E., Acta Physiol. Scand., 70(1967), 176-187.
24. Houk, J.C. & E. Henneman, J. Neurophysiol., 30 (1967), 466-481.
25. Jansen, J.K.S. & T. Rudjord, Acta Physiol. Scand., 62 (1964), 364-379.

26. Gottlieb, G.L., G.C. Agarwal X.L. Stark, IEEE Trans. Man Machines Syst., MM2-10(1), (1969), 17-27.
27. Andersson, B.F., G. Lennerstrand & V. Thoden, Acta Physiol. Scand., 74 (1968), 301-381.
28. Crowe, A. & P.B.C. Matthews, J. Physiol., 174 (1964), 109-131.
29. Lippold, O.C.J., J. Nicholls & J.N.I. Redfearn, J. Physiol., 153 (1960), 209-217.
30. Matthews, P.B.C. & R.B. Stein, J. Physiol., 200 (1969), 723-724.
31. Wells, J.B., J. Physiol., 178 (1965), 252-269.
32. Bana, P., A. Mannard & R.B. Stein, Biol. Cybernetics, 22 (1976), 129-137.
33. Cooper, S. & J.C. Eccles, J. Physiol., 69 (1930), 377-385.
34. Bahler, A.S., J.T. Fales & K.L. Zierler, J. Gen. Physiol., 51 (1968), 369-384.
35. Jewel, B.R. & D.R. Wilkie, J. Physiol., 143 (1958), 515-540.
36. Durbin, F., Computer J., 17(4) (1974), 371-376.
37. Hammond, P.H., Proc. IEE. Third Int. Cont. Med. Electronics (1960), 190-199.
38. Houk, J.C., Ann. R. Physiol., 41 (1979), 99-114.
39. Houk, J.C., In: Posture and Movement, R.E. Talbot and D.R. Humphrey, Eds. (New York, Raven Press, 1979), 231-241.
40. Houk, J.C., P.E. Crago & W.Z. Rymer, In: Muscle Receptors and Movement, A. Taylor and A. Prochazka Eds. (London, MacMillan Publishers Ltd., 1981).
41. Bizzi, E., P. Dev, P. Morasso & A. Polit, J. Neurophysiol. 41 (1978), 542-557.
42. Harmond, L.D. & E.R. Lewis, Physiol. Rev., 46(3) (1966), 513-591.
43. Fuckson, O.I., M.B. Berkinblit & A.G. Feldman, Science, 209 (1980), 1261-1263.
44. Barker, D., In: Myotatic, kinesthetic and Vestibular Mechanisms, A.V.S. de Reuck and J. Knight, Eds., Ciba Foundation Symposium (London, J. and A. Churchill Ltd. Publisher, 1967), 3-19.
45. Boyd, I.A., Quart. J. Exp. Physiol., 61 (1976), 203-254.
46. Boyd, I.A., In: Progress in Brain Research, Vol. 44, Understanding the Stretch Reflex, S. Homma Ed. (Amsterdam, Elsevier/North Holland Biomedical Press, 1977), 33-50.
47. Boyd, I.A. & J. Ward, J. Physiol., 244 (1975), 83-112.
48. Granit, R., The Basis of Motor Behavior (New York, Academic Press, 1970).

ELECTROMECHANICAL PROPERTIES AND ELECTROMAGNETIC STIMULATION OF BONE

N. Güzelsu

Biomechanics Program, University of Medicine and Dentistry of New Jersey-NJSOM and Bioengineering Program, Rutgers University, P.O. Box 55, Piscataway, NJ 08854, U.S.A.

1. INTRODUCTION

The use of electromagnetic stimulation of tissues has been increasing in the clinical fields. It is mainly used in the clinical cases when the classical, well-known methods fail or in order to accelerate the recovery of healing. The non-unions of bone fractures are the best application area at this time for the electromagnetic stimulations. Analyzing the electro-mechanical feedback systems of the tissue leads the way for how one can use electromagnetic stimulation in order to duplicate natural bioelectric signals. Although different artificial electromagnetic stimulation techniques could be equally effective in the treatment of the same pathological cases, they would differ in their tissue culture and cellular level responses. That is, the overall response of the tissue (healing of a non-union) would be the same for different stimuli but their cellular level reactions would be different. The tissue culture experiments and well controlled in vivo experiments will illuminate this point in the near future by bridging the overall response of the tissue to cellular level activities.

2. ELECTRO-MECHANICAL PROPERTIES OF BONE

The piezoelectricity and streaming potentials have been suggested as the conversion mechanism of the mechanical stimuli to bio-electrical signals in bones (1-7). Early investigations on dry bone have suggested that the piezoelectricity is the main coupling mechanism between the mechanical and electrical fields. Later experiments showed that streaming potentials due to amphoteric behavior of the organic matrix of the wet bone tissue could be the main measurable quantity in in-vitro experiments and hence should be directly related to the bioelectric signals (4,8-11). The measurements of particle electrophoresis of compact bone tissue (12) showed that bone has an isoelectric point near pH=5 and that the overall electrophoretic mobility of the bone particles is similar to collagen particles obtained from human Achilles Tendon (13). The piezoelectric constant d_{33} of wet bone tissue was measured at different pH levels (14). This measurement showed that the constant (d_{33}) went through a minimum value of 2.2×10^{-8} c.g.s. units at pH=5. At pH=5.0 the main contribution of the electro-mechanical output of bone is coming from the piezoelectric output where the streaming potential effect is zero (isoelectric point).

Most of the organic compounds of the bone matrix have an amphoteric ionic structure attaining the highest degree of charge, both positive and negative, in the isoelectric pH range (15). The piezoelectric response in the bone tissue is mainly dipole polari-zation (16) due to (COO^- and NH_3^+) and it has the highest value at the isoelectric point. Moving from the isoelectric point would reduce the piezoelectric response because some of the COO^- or NH_3^+ groups loose their charges by accepting or donating protons (H^+) according to the pH level of the fluid. This can be shown in the following way: The simplified structure of isoelectric colla-gen is of the type $COO^- R. NH_3^+$. Therefore the proton transfer can be summarized as below (15).

$$COO^-.R. \; NH_3^+ + H^+ \rightarrow COOH.R. \; NH_3^+ \; \text{(in acid solution)}$$

$$COO^-.R. \; NH_3^+ - H^+ \rightarrow COO^-.R. \; NH_2 \; \text{(in alkaline solution)}$$

In the physiological range (pH 7.2-7.4) bone matrix has a net excess immobilized negative electrical charge and dipoles. Al-though the number of available dipoles are less than the isoelec-tric point, still they can cause local piezoelectric response to mechanical inputs.

Therefore, one can conclude that at the physiological pH ranges bone has streaming potentials and can exhibit piezoelectric response to mechanical inputs. The piezoelectric response signals in in-vitro experiments are usually buried under the streaming potential response, but they could be effective on the cellular level activities. Streaming potential responses last longer and they can be observed in in-vitro wet bone experiments (11).

Shamos and his co-workers (17) showed that the surface charges appearing on the stressed bone might control the bone formation, and that the local electrical field due to these surface charges

could effect the orientation and deposition of bone micro structure. Bassett (18) also pointed out that the negative charges
accumulating on the concave sides of a bent bone cause regeneration. Bone tissue is removed from the convex side and deposited on
the concave side. The electrical signals generated due to the
electromechanical properties of bone tissue and caused by the
external effects, carrying the necessary information to the bone
cells. These bio-electric signals regulate the biological functions of the bone cells, therefore the bone tissue can adjust its
density and micro structure orientations according to its various
physiological functions.

3. BONE REMODELING

Bone remodels itself under the external effect by using a
biological control systems. This system is related to the feedback
mechanism of bone tissue (6,19) as shown in Fig. 1.

Mechanical, electrical, thermal and chemical effects can cause
callus formation in bones (20). These different stimuli, which can
be obtained without fracture, are first converted to bioelectrical
signals through physical and chemical properties of the bone
tissue. The callus formation will take place according to the
electrical signals received.

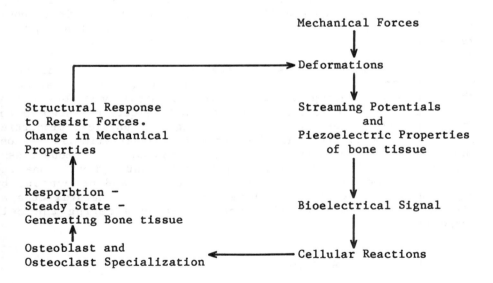

Fig. 1 Feedback system in bones due to the electromechanical
properties of bone tissue.

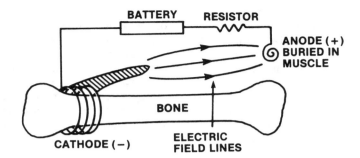

Fig. 2   Callus formation due to electrical stimulation of intact bone. The stainless steel electrode was wrapped around the femur of a rabbit, and the anode was placed in muscle (21).

Under an applied electric current one can control the orientation of the structural changes in bones (21,22). It has been shown that a stainless steel cathode electrode wrapped around a rabbit femur and carrying one microampere, can cause callus formation toward the anode which is placed in the muscle (21) (Fig. 2). The electric current across the limb at the fracture site can effect the callus formation and the direction of the trabecular orientation. This effect was observed in a rabbit radius. The high levels of current changed the trabecular orientation from longitudinal to transverse by overriding the natural tissue growth mechanism (22).

The remodeling process in living bone is the mechanism by which the bone changes its internal structure, due to changes in the functional loading. The electro—mechanical behavior of bone tissue converts the functional forces to bioelectrical signals for the bone cells. The cell reactions change the physical properties of living bone due to long—time applied external stimuli. If one knows exactly the nature of the feedback system of the bone tissue and how the cells are responding to different stimuli, one can accelerate the healing process of fractures and non—unions by applying more electrical stimulus similar to the natural ones at the "fracture" site of the bones, thereby altering the cell responses.

4.   ELECTRICAL STIMULATION

Different types of electromagnetic stimulation have been used for fracture healing in bones. Mainly, these are: direct current, pulsating current, capacitive electric fields and induced electric fields due to time dependent magnetic fields. Electric stimulation

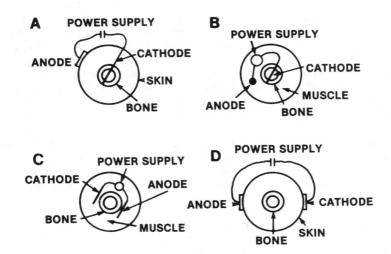

Fig. 3 Direct and alternating current stimulation techniques.
(a) Semi-invasive; stimulating electrode in fracture site (32),
(b) Invasive; stimulating electrode in fracture site, return electrode is buried in muscle, (c) Invasive; electrodes are away from
the fracture site, (d) Non-invasive; electrodes are direct contact
with skin across the fracture site (37).

by different devices, electrodes, current levels, potential levels
and frequency showed that in certain intervals of the physical
parameters the electrical stimulation can promote osteogenesis
(21,23-40).

4.1 Direct Currents

The electrical stimulation of bone fractures with direct
current can be obtained with different techniques. The stimulating
and the return electrodes can be placed in different configurations
with respect to the fracture site (Fig. 3). In the semi-invasive
technique, the cathode (stimulating electrode) is placed at the
fracture site and the anod (return electrode) is placed on the skin
(32). In the invasive technique, the cathode is again at the
target site and the anode is buried in the soft tissue away from
the fracture site (30). Also, in the invasive technique both
electrodes can be placed in the soft tissue or bone in such a way
that they create an electrical current across the fracture
site (41).

The non-invasive technique utilizes external electrodes placed
across the fracture site (22). All the above techniques either
apply the cathode at the fracture site, creating current between

the electrodes, or generating direct current across the fracture site. The experimental evidence strongly suggests that a cathodal current of ten to twenty micro amp at the fracture site with stainless steel electrodes promotes fracture healing (23,32,41).

Direct current is applied for osteogenesis with different current levels, electrode materials, power supplies, (22,23,30-32, 41-67) and even monophasic pulsed form. The mechanism which generates cellular osteogenic response to electrical stimulation could be different in each case. The current can cause direct effects on the cells (mesenchymal, osteoblast, osteocytes, fibrocytes) and also it can change the membrane charge configuration or change local ion concentration. Also, the current would indirectly effect the cells by altering the concentration of oxygen, enzymes and other species around the cell.

The effect of electrical stimulation in general on the cell can alter the cyclic-AMP and DNA synthesis by distributing the charge configuration at the membrane (68,69). The experiments on rabbits with pulsed current showed that the ATP concentration in healing callus was increased with respect to control ones hence suggesting that the increased cellular activity or energy production was caused by the electrical stimulation (70). One of the indirect effects of the direct current is the oxygen reduction. At a cathode surface, the reduction of molecular oxygen is the predominant reaction. The effect of oxygen tension in healing of bone defects has been investigated (71-77). In vivo and in vitro experiments or epiphyseal plate, the metaphysis and diaphysis indicated that an oxygen gradient exists corresponding to the morphological zones. The experiments on the oxygen tension indicate that a) very low oxygen tension is present in the callus within the first few days after fracture, b) it is lowest in hemotomo, low in newly formed cartilage and fiber bone, c) it is highest in fibrous tissue, and d) it stays low in callus until the healing of the medullary canal (75).

These observations on oxygen tension suggest that the direct current stimulation of cathode, which reduces oxygen tension in the fracture area and increases pH level depending on the voltage level, might be the main mechanism for osteogenesis due to D.C. current.

The experiments with D.C. current led to the following: The cathode stimulates osteogensis at the fracture site; cell necrosis could occur around the anode; active circuit must be used for maintaining the constant current; direct current is better or as good as low frequency alternating current or pulsed current.

Commercially, there are two electrical apparatus available for direct current stimulation which are used for the above observation. The first system is semi-invasive and uses four stainless

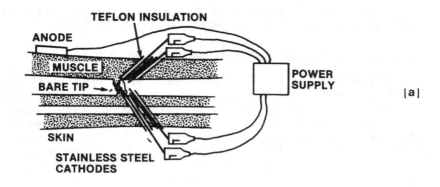

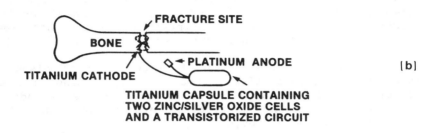

Fig. 4 (a) The direct current (semi-invasive) bone growth stimulator. The placement of stainless steel cathode electrodes to the fracture site (32). (b) Implantable bone growth stimulator. The cathode is threaded across the fracture site (30).

steel cathode electrodes and an anode made of self adherent tape which is placed on the skin (Fig. 4a). The circuit supplies constant current of twenty microamperes to all the cathode electrodes which are insulated with teflon except for the one centimeter-long bone tips.

The second system is invasive and contains batteries and a circuit in a titanium capsule (Fig. 4b). The titanium cathode is threaded across the fracture site or buried in it and the platinum anode buried in the soft tissue. Again the cathode is supplied by a twenty microamperes of constant current through 2 zinc/silver oxide cells and the transistorized circuit.

Clinically, the main difference between these two methods are that the first one uses stainless steel electrodes which can be administered externally to the fracture site and therefore it is semi-invasive. The second system is totally inplantable and uses titanium cathode electrodes.

The clinical results of the direct current stimulation have been reviewed and analyzed extensively (30-32,52,58).

4.2 Capacitive Fields and Alternating Currents

Capacitive electric fields have also been used for fracture healing (78-80,81). Static electric fields usually require high voltages to be applied across the electrodes. The electric fields are usually applied to bone fractures by insulated electrodes which are placed across the fracture site. The low voltage sinusoidal electric currents are applied on the skin for osteogensis (78) in order to eliminate the high voltage electric fields which are used in the capacitive method. The experiments showed that the capacitive field by itself is not a very good way for promoting osteogenesis. In order to improve the technique, Brighton and his co-workers (37,82,83) used conducting gel between the bare electrodes and skin. Now their non-invasive technique uses low voltage and 60 kHz alternating current across the fracture site.

Inhibition or prevention of osteoporosis of disuse has been tried by using capacitive methods (84,85). Also, the effect of electric fields on the tissue culture experiments indicated that the proliferative and functional capacity of connective tissue cells can be affected (86,87).

4.3 Callus Formation by Charged and Piezoelectric Polymers

Electrically charged and pizoelectric films have been used for promoting osteogenesis. Electrically charge films (electrets) have a permanent polarization in the direction of the thickness and are made of certain waxes, plastics and polymers (88,89). Electrets can be classified according to their charge composition: i) Dipolar electrets are produced by heating the material which reduces its internal viscosity so that the electric dipoles of the film are easy to rotate under an applied electric field. After sufficient time, the film is cooled while the field is still applied. The increased internal viscosity due to cooling holds the dipoles in a permanent orientation hence causes sustaining polarizaton in the electret. ii) Internal space charge electrets are produced from a matreial which has free charges. The internal viscosity of the material is lowered by heating, the free charges are separated by an electric field, and a permanent polarization is obtained by cooling. iii) Injected space charge electrets are obtained by transfering charges to the films from contacting electrodes. iv) Deposited charge electrets are produced by bombarding the film with a corona discharge in air or with an electron beam in vacuo. A charge one sign is deposited on the surface of the electret and is trapped at or close to the surface.

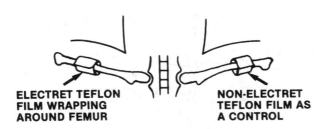

ELECTRET TEFLON FILM WRAPPING AROUND FEMUR

NON-ELECTRET TEFLON FILM AS A CONTROL

Fig. 5   The application of electret and non-electret teflon film around femurs of a rat.

Experiments on rabbit femurs showed that an electret which is placed on the surface of a bone causes a callus formation within two weeks after the operation (21,90).   Also, experiments on the rats with teflon films showed that the charged teflon films which were wrapped around the mid-femoral shaft showed callus formation and the control ones without charged teflon films showed no callus formation (91) (Fig. 5).

Piezoelectric films which are capable of converting the mechanical energy to electric energy are also used for promoting osteogenesis.   A strip of PMLG (Poly-γ-Methyl-L-Glutamate Film) was tied to the tendinous portion of the distal quadriceps in the supratellar area of the rat and the other end of the film was sutured to the femoral biceps of the rat proximmaly (61).   For the control side the PMLG film is left free.   The sutured site produced osteogenesis because motion of the animal produced piezoelectric output and hence osteogenesis.   The other group experiments (61) used one side with sutured PMLG and the other side with teflon electret.   Electret induced callus because maximum at the fifth week and then because atrophic because of the loss of induced charge in the teflon film.   On the other hand PMLG film-induced callus continued to grow because of continuous stimulation of the bone due to motion of the film.

4.4   Electromagnetic Fields

The first non-invasive method for clinical use is developed by using time dependent magnetic fields.   The externally applied time-dependent magnetic field can produce an induced electric field (92) in the body.   The external magnetic field is produced either by Helmholtz-aiding coils (33,93-100) (Fig. 6a), or by an electro-magnet (34,101-104) (Fig. 6b).   The wave shape and the amplitude of the induced electric field is non-union, or fracture sites, depend upon the current fed to the coils or electromagnets.   The main difference between the two systems is that the Helmholtz coils

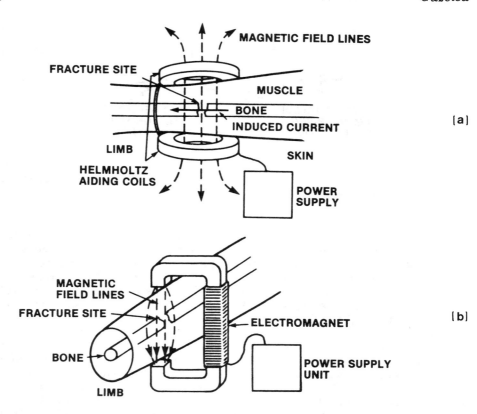

Fig. 6 (a) The Helmholtz-aiding coils produce time dependent magnetic field in the limb at the fracture site. This time dependent magnetic field induces electric field hence current at the fracture site (33). (b) Electromagnet generates the time dependent magnetic field, hence, the induced electric field is generated at the fracture site (34).

developed by Bassett and his co-workers generate high frequency and low magnetic flux density, whereas, Watson and his co-workers' electromagnet generates high magnetic flux density and low frequency. Utilizing electro-magnetic fields for fracture healing provides a non-invasive method for the physician. On the other hand, the patient has to be immobilized for the duration of the treatment. Direct current and capacitively coupled electric current apparatuses provide more freedom for patients. In order to overcome immobilization of the patient, Watson's group introduced a light weight magnet and battery operated power pack (102). Also, Bassett's group's wave form is duplicated with a portable unit (American Med. Elect. Inc.-Physio-Stim).

Now, portable, non-invasive techniques are available for patient management. Another apparatus, which has been developed by Kraus and Lechner (35,105,106) consists of an electromagnet which produces a pulsating magnetic field with a frequency range of 2-3 Hz, a receiver buried near the fracture site which receives the magnetic energy from the electromagnet and transforms that energy to desired electrical potential and semi insulated screws which produce current at the fracture site due to electric output from the receiver.

Also, they developed an electro-nail which contains a receiver and two surface electrodes which produces an electrical field perpendicular to the bone axis in the marrow cavity. This method is invasive and also requires the immobilization of the patient during the treatment.

5. CONCLUSIONS

Electrical stimulation of bones has been shown to be effective in certain groups of patients. Non-unions and other disorders can be treated effectively by electrical stimulation as an alternative means to other methods. Up to this time the electrical stimulation has been shown to be safe and it has no observable adverse effects. The experiments on the tissue culture have not been close to results which can lead to general conclusions such as how the cells react to different stimuli what kind of physiological reactions they show and so on. The long term more comprehensive study in the cellular level eventually will lead the way to better understanding the mechanism of electrical stimulation in bones. The research on the feedback mechanism due to electro-mechanical properties of bone and the cellular level experiments will give physicians a good guide for predicting the reaction of the bone tissue to different mechanical and electrical stimulation in their treatment.

REFERENCES

1. Yasuda, I. Piezoelectricity of Living Bone. J. Kysto Pref. Univ. Med 53 (1953) 325.
2. Fukada, E. and I. Yasuda. On the Piezoelectric Effect of Bone. J. Phys. Soc. Japan. 12 (1957) 1158-1162.
3. Bassett, C.A.L. Biophysical Principles Affecting Bone Structure, in The Biochemistry and Physiology of Bone, edited by G.H. Bourne, Second Ed., Vol. III (Academic Press, New York, 1971) pp. 1-76.
4. Eriksson, C. Electrical Properties of Bone, in The Biochemistry and Physiology of Bone, edited by G.H. Bourne,

Second Ed., Vol. IV, (Academic Press, New York, 1976) pp. 329-384.

5. Guzelsu, N. and H. Demiray. Electromechanical Properties and Related Models of Bone Tissues. Int. J. Engng. Sci. 12 (1979) 813-851.

6. Guzelsu, N. Mechanoelectrical Effects in Biological Systems, in Electronic Conduction and Mechanoelectrical Transduction in Biological Materials, Edited by B. Lipinski (Marcel Dekker, Inc., New York, 1982) pp. 201-280.

7. Williams, W.S. Sources of Piezoelectricity in Tendon and Bone, in Critical Reviews in Bioengineering, edited by D. Fleming, Vol. 2 (CRC Press, Baco Raton, Florida, 1974) pp. 95-118.

8. Cignitti, M., F. Figura, M. Marchetti and A. Salleo. Electrokinetic Effects in Mechanoelectrical Phenomenology of the Bone, Arch Fisol. 68 (1970/71) 232-249.

9. Johnson, M.W., D.A. Chakkalakal, R.A. Harper and J.L. Katz. Comparison of the Electromechanical Effects in Wet and Dry Bone. J. Biomechanics 13 (1980) 437-442.

10. Williams, W.S. Piezoelectric Effects in Biological Materials. Ferro-electrics 41 (1982) 225-246.

11. Pienkowski, D. and S.R. Pollack. The Origin of Stress-Generated Potentials in Fluid-Saturated Bone. J. Orthopaedic Resch. 1 (1983) 13-41.

12. Guzelsu, N. and J. Donofrio. Particle Electrophoresis of Compact Bone Tissue. J. Bioelectricity. 2 (1983), 187-196.

13. Anderson, J.C. and Eriksson, C. Electrical Properties of Wet Collagen, Nature. 218 (1968) 166-168.

14. Anderson, J.C. and Eriksson, C. Piezoelectric Properties of Dry and Wet Bone. Nature, 127 (1970) 491-492.

15. Gustavson, K.H. The Chemistry and Reactivity of Collagen (Academic Press, New York, 1956).

16. Hastings, G.W., M.A. ElMessiery and S. Rakowski. Mechano-electrical Properties of Bone. Biomaterials, 2 (1981) 225-233.

17. Shamos, M.H., L.S. Lavine and M.I. Shamos. Piezoelectric Effect in Bone. Nature, 197 (1963) 81.

18. Bassett, C.A.L. Electrical Effects in Bone. Scientific American. 213 (1965) 18-25.

19. Guzelsu, N. A Piezoelectric Model for Dry Bone Tissue. J. Biomechanics 11 (1978) 257-267.

20. Yasuda, I., Fundamental Aspects of Fracture Treatment. Clin. Orthop. Related Research, 124 (1977) 5-8.

21. Yasuda, I. Electrical Callus and Callus Formation by Electret. Clin. Orthop. Related Research, 124 (1977) 53-56.

22. Piekarski, K., D. Demetriades and A. Mackenzie. Osteogentic Stimulation by Externally Applied D.C. Current. Acta. Orthop. Scand. 49 (1978) 113-120.

23. Friedenberg, Z.B., B.I. Smolenski, B.W. Pearl and C.T. Brighton. Bone Reaction to Varying Amounts of Direct Current. Surg. Gynec. and Obstet. 131 (1970) 894-899.

24. Liboff, A.R. and R.A. Rinaldi. Electrically Mediated Growth Mechanism in Living Systems. Annals New York Acad. Sci., Vol. 238 (1974).
25. Burny, F., E. Herbst, and M. Hinsenkamp. Electric Stimulation of Bone Growth and Repair (Springer-Verlag, Berlin, 1978).
26. Brighton, C.T., Bioelectric Effects on Bone and Cartilage. (Guest Ed.) Clinic Orthop. Related Res. 124 (1977).
27. Brighton, C.T., J. Black and S. Pollack. Electrical Properties of Bone and Cartilage (Editors) (Grune and Stratton, New York, 1979).
28. Watson, J. The Electrical Stimulation of Bone Healing. Proceeding IEEE 67 (1979) 1339-1352.
29. Spadaro, J.A. Electrically Stimulated Bone Growth in Animals and Man Clin. Orthop. Related Res., 122 (1977) 325-332.
30. Paterson, D.C., G.N. Lewis and C.A. Cass. Treatment of Delayed Union and Non-union with an Implanted Direct Current Stimulator. Clin. Orthop. Related Res., 148 (1980) 117-128.
31. Paterson, D.C., G.N. Lewis and C.A. Cass. Treatment of Congenital Pseudarthrosis of the Tibia with Direct Current Stimulation. Clin. Orthop. Related Research. 148 (1980) 129-135.
32. Brighton, C.T., J. Black, Z.B. Friedenberg, J.L. Esterhai, L.J. Day and J.F. Connolly. A Multicenter Study of the Treatment of Non-Union with Constant Direct Current. J. Bone Joint Surgery. 63-A (1981) 2-13.
33. Bassett, C.A.L., S.N. Mitchell and S.R. Gaston. Treatment of Ununited Tibial Diaphyseal Fractures with Pulsing Electromagnetic Fields. J. Bone Joint Surgery. 63-A, (1981) 511-523.
34. Watson, J. and E.M. Downes. The Application of Pulsed Magnetic Fields to the Stimulation of Bone Healing in Humans. Japanese J. Applied Physics. 17 (1978) 215-217.
35. Kraus Von, W. and F. Lechner. Die Heilung von Pseudarthrosen und Spontanfrakturen durch strukturbildende Electro dynamische Potentiale. Munch med. Wschr. 114 (1972) 1814-1819.
36. Connolly, J.F. Clinical Applications of Bioelectrical Effects (Guest Ed) Clin. Orthop. Related Research 161 (1981).
37. Brighton, C.T., G.B. Pfeffer and S.R. Pollack. In vivo Growth Plate Stimulation in Various Capacitively Coupled Electrical Fields. J. Orthopaedic Research. 1 (1983) 42-49.
38. Yasuda, I. Mechanical and Electrical Callus. Annals. New York Acad. Sci. 238 (1974) 457-465.
39. Spadaro, J.A. Bioelectric Stimulation of Bone Formation: Methods, Models and Mechanism. J. Bioelectricity. 1 (1982) 99-128.
40. Herbst, E., Electrical Stimulation Bone Growth and Repair in F. Burny, E. Herbst and M. Hinsenkamp, ed., Electric Stimulation of Bone Growth and Repair. (Springer-Verlag, Berlin, 1978) p. 1-13.
41. Friedenberg, Z.B., P.G. Roberts, N.H. Didizian and C.T. Brighton. Stimulation of Fracture Healing by Direct Current in the Rabbit Fibula. J. Bone Joint Surgery. 53-A (1971) 1400-1408.

42. Bassett, C.A.L., R.J. Pawluk and R.O. Becker. Effects of
     Electric Currents on Bone in vivo. Nature, 204 (1964) 652-654.
43. Minkin, C., B.R. Poulton and W.H. Hoover. The Effect of
     Direct Current on Bone. Clin. Orthop. Related Research., 57
     (1968) 303-309.
44. Lavine, L.S., I. Lustrin and M.H. Shamos. Experimental Model
     for Studying the Effect of Electric Current on Bone in vivo.
     Nature (1969) 1112-1113.
45. O'Connor, B.T., H.M. Charton, J.D. Currey, D.R.S. Kirby and S.
     Woods. Effects of Electric Current on Bone in vivo. Nature,
     222 (1969) 162-163.
46. Lavine, L.S., I. Lustrin, M.H. Shamos and M.L. Mass. The
     Influence of Electric Current on Bone Regeneration in vivo.
     Acta. Orthop. Scandinav. 42 (1971) 305-314.
47. Friedenberg, Z.B., M.C. Harlow and C.T. Brighton. Healing of
     Nonunion of the Medial Mallolus by Means of Direct Current. A
     Case Report. J. Trauma 11 (1971) 883-885.
48. Friedenberg, Z.B. and C.T. Brighton. Electrical Fracture
     Healing. Annals New York Acad. Sci., 238 (1974) 564-574.
49. Klapper, L. and R.E. Stallard. Mechanism of Electric Stimula-
     tion of Bone Formation. Annals New York Acad. Sci., 238 (1974)
     530-542.
50. Friedenberg, Z.B., L.M. Zemsky, R.P. Pollis and C.T. Brighton.
     The Response of Non-Traumatized Bone to Direct Current. J.
     Bone Joint Surgery. 56-A (1974) 1023-1030.
51. Connolly, J.F., J. Ortiz, R.R. Price and R.J. Bayuzick. The
     Effect of Electrical Simulation on the Biophysical Properties
     of Fracture Healing. Annals New York Acad. Sci., 238 (1974)
     519-529.
52. Brighton, C.T, Z.B. Friedenberg, L.M. Zemsky and P.R. Pollis.
     Direct-Current Stimulation of Non-Union and Congenital Pseud-
     arthrosis. J. Bone Joint Surgery. 57-A (1975) 368-377.
53. Harris, W.H., B.J.L. Mayen, E.L. Thrasher, L.A. Davis, R.H.
     Cobolen, D.A. MacKenzie and J.K. Cywinski. Differential
     Response to Electrical Stimulation. Clin. Orthop. Related Res.
     124 (1977) 31-40.
54. Weigert, M. and C. Werhahn. The Influence of Electric Poten-
     tials on Plated Bones. Clin. Orthop. Related Res., 124 (1977)
     20-30.
55. Jacobs, J.D. and L.A. Norton. Electrical Stimulation of
     Osteogenesis in Periodontal Defects. Clin. Orthop. Related
     Res. 124 (1977) 41-52.
56. Stan, S., J.C. Mulier, W. Sansen and P. DeWaele. Effect of
     Direct Current on the Healing of Fractures, in Electric Stimu-
     lation of Bone Growth and Repair, edited by F. Burny, H.
     Herbst and M. Hinsenkamp (Springer-Verlag, Berlin, 1978) pp.
     47-54.
57. vonSatzger, G. and E. Herbst. Electrical Stimulation of
     Osteogenesis, in Electric Stimulation of Bone Growth and
     Repair, edited by F. Burny, H. Herbst and M. Hinsenkamp
     (Springer-Verlag, Berlin, 1978) pp. 55-60.

58. Brighton, C.T., Z.B. Friedenberg and J. Black. Evaluation of the use of Constant Direct Current in the Treatment of Non-union, in Electrical Properties of Bone and Cartilage, edited by C.T. Brighton, J. Black and S.R. Pollack (Grune-Stratton, New York, 1979) pp. 519-547.

59. Hassler, C.R., K.D. Cummings, L.C. Clark, E.F. Rybicki and R.B. Diegle. Augmentation of Bone Healing via Electrical Stimuli, in Electrical Properties of Bone and Cartilage, edited by C.T. Brighton, J. Black and S.R. Pollack, (Grune-Stratton, New York, 1979) pp. 155-168.

60. Kenner, G.H., J.W. Precup, E.W. Gabrielson, W.S. Williams and J.B. Park. Electrical Modification of Disue Osteoporosis Using Constant and Pulsed Stimulation, in Electrical Properties of Bone and Cartilage, edited by C.T. Brighton, J. Black and S.R. Pollack (Grune-Stratton, New York, 1979) pp. 181-187.

61. Inoue, S., T. Ohashi, E. Fukada and T. Ashihara. Electric Stimulation of Osteogenesis in the Rat: Amperage of Three Different Stimulation Methods, in Electrical Properties of Bone and Cartilage, edited by C.T. Brighton, J. Black and S.R. Pollack (Grune-Stratton, New York, 1979) pp. 199-213.

62. Treharne, R.W., C.T. Brighton, E. Korostoff and S.R. Pollack. Application of Direct, Pulsed and SGP-Shaped Currents to in-vitro fetal Rat Tibiae, in Electrical Properties of Bone and Cartilage, edited by C.T. Brighton, J. Black and S.R. Pollack (Grune-Stratton, New York, 1979) pp. 169-180.

63. Zichner, L. Repair of Nonunions by Electrically Pulsed Current Stimulation. Clinical Orthop. Related Res. 161 (1981) 115-121.

64. Brighton, C.T., Z.B. Friedenberg, J. Black, J.L. Esterhai, J.E. Mitchell and F. Montique. Electrically Induced Osteogenesis: Relationship between Charge, Current Density and the Amount of Bone Formed. Clinical Orthop. Related Res. 161 (1981) 122-132.

65. Jacobs, R.R., U. Luethi, R.T. Duelard and S.M. Perren. Electrical Stimulation of Experimental Nonunions. Clin. Orthop. Related Res. 161 (1981) 146-153.

66. Spadaro, J.A. Electrically Enhanced Osteogenesis at Various Metal Cathodes. J. Biomedical Mat. Re. 16 (1982) 861-873.

67. Jorgensen, T.E. The Effect of Electric Current on the Healing Time of Crural Fractures. Acta Orthop. Scandinav. 43 (1972) 421-437.

68. Norton, L.A., C.A. Rodan and L.A. Bourret. Cyclic AMP Fluctuation in Bone Growth in Electrical Fields. J. Dent. Res., 55B (1976) 215.

69. Rodan, G.A., L.A. Bourret and L.A. Norton. DNA Synthesis in Cartilage Cells is Stimulated by Electric Fields. Science, 199 (1978) 690-692.

70. Landa, V.A. and B.K. Baranow. On the Effect of Impulse Electrical Current on Reparative Regeneration of the Bone Tissue. Orthop. Tram. Protest. No. 10, (1976) 55-59.

71. Bassett, C.A.L. and I. Herrmann. Influence of Oxygen Concentration and Mechanical Factors on Differentiation of Connective Tissues in vitro, Nature, 190 (1961) 460-461.

72. Coulson, D.B., A.B. Ferguson and R.C. Diehl. Effect of Hyperbaric Oxygen on the Healing Femur of the Rat. Orthop. Surgery. 17 (1966) 449-450.

73. Brighton, C.T., R.D. Ray, L.W. Sable and K.E. Kuettner. In vitro Epiphyseal-Plate Growth in Various Oxygen Tensions. J. Bone Joint Surgery. 51-A (1969) 1383-1396.

74. Brighton, C.T. and R.B. Heppenstall. Oxygen Tension in Zones of the Epiphyseal Plate the Metaphysis and Diaphysis. J. Bone Joint Surgery, 53-A (1971) 719-728.

75. Brighton, C.T. and A.G. Krebs. Oxygen Tension of Healing Fractures in the Rabbit. J. Bone Joint Surgery, 54-A (1972) 323-332.

76. Heppenstall, R.B., G. Grislis and T.K. Hunt. Tissue Gas Tensions and Oxygen Consumption in Healing Bone Defects. Clin. Orthop. Related Research. 106 (1975) 357-365.

77. Brighton, C.T., S. Adler, J. Black, N. Itada and Z.B. Friedenbrg. Cathodic Oxygen Consumption and Electrically Induced Osteogenesis. Clin. Orthop. Related Research. 107 (1975) 277-282.

78. Brighton, C.T., S.R. Pollack and R.E. Windsor. Stimulation of Fracture Healing by a Capacitively Coupled Electric Field in the Rabbit Figula. Transaction-27th Annual Meeting Orthop. Resch. Soc. 6 (1981) 93.

79. Norton, L.A. In vivo Bone Growth in a Controlled Electric Field. Annals New York Acad. Sci., 238 (1979) 466-477.

80. Norton, L.A., G.A. Rodan and L.A. Bourret. Epiphyseal Cartilage cAMP Changes Produced by Electrical and Mechanical Perturbations. Clin. Orthop. Related Research. 124 (1977) 59-68.

81. Marino, A.A., J.M. Cullen, M. Reichmanis and R.O. Becker. Fracture Healing in Rats Exposed to Extremely Low Frequency Electric Fields. Clin. Orthop. Related Research. 145 (1979) 239-244.

82. Brighton, C.T. and S.R. Pollack. Treatment of Non-Union with a Capacitively Coupled Electrical Field: Preliminary Findings. Transactions of the Third Annual Meeting of BRAGS, Vol. III (1983).

83. Brighton, C.T., W.J. Hozack and S.R. Pollack. Fracture Healing in Response to a Time-Varying Capacitively Coupled Electrical Field in the Rabbit Fibula. Transactions Third Annual Meeting of BRAGS. Vol. III, (1983) 46.

84. McElhaney, J.H., R. Stalnaker and R. Bullard. Electric Fields and Bone Loss of Disuse. J. Biomechanics, 1 (1968) 47-52.

85. Martin, R.B. and W. Gutman. The Effect of Electric Fields on Osteoporosis of Disuse. Calcif. Tiss. Res. 25 (1978), 23-27.

86. Bassett, C.A.L. and I. Herrmann. The Effect of Electrostatic Fields on Macromolecular Synthesis by Fibroblasts in vitro. J. Cell Biology, 39 (1968) 9A.

87. Rodan, G.A., L.A. Bourret, and L.A. Norton. DNA Synthesis in Cartilage Cells is Stimulated by Oscillating Electric Fields, Science, 199 (1978) 690-692.
88. Perlman, M.M. Electrets Charge Storage and Transport in Dielectrics (The Electrochemical Soc., Princeton, NJ, 1973).
89. Sessler, G.M. (Ed.) Electrets. Topics in Applied Physics. Vol. 33 (Springer-Verlag, Berlin, 1980).
90. Fukada, E., T. Takamatsu and I. Yasuda. Callus Formation by Electret, Japan J. Appl. Phys., 14 (1975) 2079-2080.
91. Inoue, S., T. Ohashi, I. Yasuda and E. Fukada. Electret Induced Callus Formation in the Rat. Clin. Orthop. Related Research. 124 (1977) 57-58.
92. Wangsness, R.K. Electromagnetic Fields (John Wiley and Sons, New York, 1979). p. 297.
93. Bassett, C.A.L., R.J. Pawluk and A.A. Pilla. Augmentation of Bone Repair by Inductively Coupled Electromagnetic Fields. Science, 184 (1974) 575-577.
94. Bassett, C.A.L., R.J. Pawluk and A.A. Pilla. Acceleration of Fracture Repair by Electromagnetic Fields. A surgically Non-invasive Method. Annals New York Acad. Sci., 238 (1974) 242-262.
95. Bassett, C.A.L., A.A. Pilla and R.J. Pawluk. A Non-Operating Salvage of Surgically-Resistant Pseudarthroses and Non-unions by Pulsing Electromagnetic Fields: A Preliminary Report. Clin. Orthop. Related Res. 124 (1977) 128-143.
96. Bassett, C.A.L., A.A. Pilla, S.N. Mitchell and L. Norton. Repair of non-unions by pulsing electromagnetic fields. Acta Orthopedic Belgica. 44 (1978) 706-724.
97. Bassett, C.A.L. Pulsing Electromagnetic Fields – A New Method to Modify Cell Behavior in Calcified and Non-calcified Tissues. Calcif. Tissue Int. 34 (1982) 1-8.
98. Bassett, L.S., G. Tzitzikalakis, R.J. Pawluck and C.A.L. Bassett. Prevention of Disuse Osteoporosis in the Rat by Means of Pulsing Electromagnetic Fields in Electrical Properties of Bone and Cartilage, edited by C.T. Brighton, J. Black and S.R. Pollack (Grune-Stratton, New York, 1979) pp. 311-332.
99. Mulier, J.C. and F. Spaas. Out-Patient Treatment of Surgically Resistant Non-unions by induced Pulsing Current-Clinical Results. Arch. Orthop. Traumat. Surg., 97 (1980) 293-297.
100. Heckman, J.D., A.J. Ingram, R.D. Loyd, J.V. Luck and P.W. Mayer. Nonunion Treatment with Pulsed Electromagnetic Fields. Clin. Orthop. Related Res. 161 (1981) 58-66.
101. Watson, J. and E.M. Downes. Clinical Aspects of the Stimulation of Bone Healing Using Electrical Phenomena, Med. and Biol. Eng. and Comput. 17 (1979) 161-169.
102. Watson, J. and E.M. Downes. Light-Weight Battery-Operable Orthopaedic Stimulator for the Treatment of Long-bone Non-unions Using Pulsed Magnetic Fields. Med. and Biol. Eng. and Comput. 21 (1983) 509-510.

103. Watson, J. and E. M. Downes. A Battery-operated portable Orthopaedic Stimulator. Transactions Third Annual Meeting of BRAGS III, (1983) 55.

104. DeHaas, W.G., M.A. Lazarovici and D.M. Morrison. The Effect of Low Frequency Magnetic Fields on the Healing of the Osteotomized Rabbit Radius. Clin. Orthop. Related Research. 145 (1979) 245-251.

105. Lechner, F. Die Behandlung von Knochenbruchheilungsstorungen mit Electromagnetischen Potentialen, Mschr. Unfallheilk, 77 (1974) 245-251.

106. Lechner, F. and R. Ascherl. Experiences and Results of the Electrodynamic Fields Treatment in uses of Pseudarthroses and Delayed Bone Repair. Acta Orthop. Belgica, 44 (1978) 699-705.

BIOMATERIALS

P. Lawes

Howmedica International, Inc.,
Limerick, Ireland

1.   INTRODUCTION

The subject of biomaterials is vast. The bibliography at the
end of this chapter shows a large number of lengthy texts, some of
which are good summaries of the subject while others go into
selected aspects (for example biocompatibility) in great depth.

Figure 1 shows a scatter diagram in which the reader should
start at the middle with the general concept of "Biomaterials In
Joint Replacement" and work outwards through the various headings
and subheadings under which the total subject may be discussed.

It is the objective of this chapter to cover all the aspects
of biomaterials shown in the scatter diagram: some at a very
cursory level and others in greater detail.

To avoid confusion, there is no unique logic about the
structure of the diagram of Fig. 1.   The subheadings are by no
means independent. Some of the materials which will be treated as
futuristic here (e.g. tantalum) appear in the history of
orthopedics; and a topic such as corrosion fatigue could be
discussed either under the heading of Corrosion Resistance or
Mechanical Properties. The scatter diagram should be seen as a
substitute contents list which gives some structure to a test that
might otherwise appear to be rambling from topic to topic.

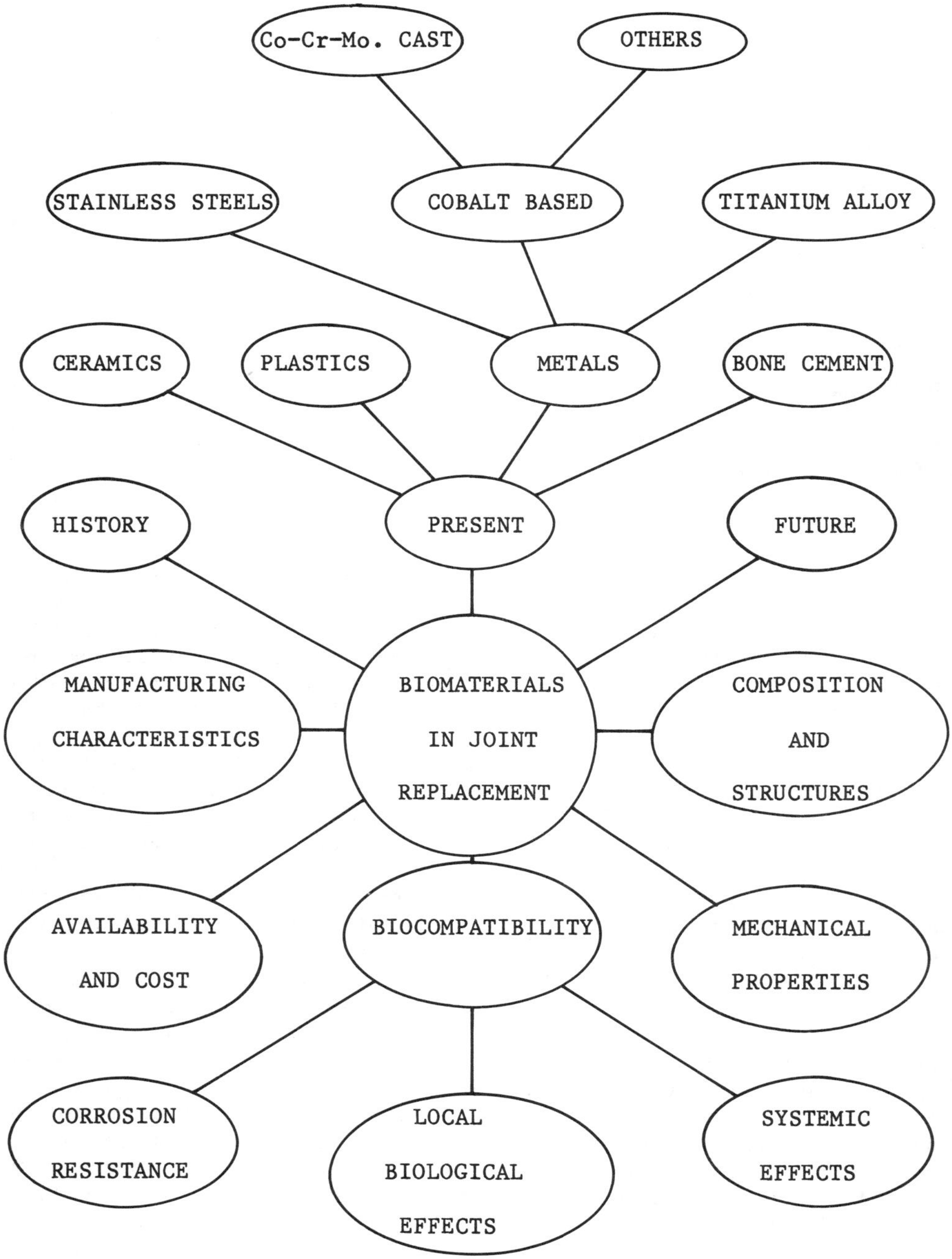

Fig. 1 Biomaterials in Joint replacement.

2. HISTORY

There have been three major periods of biomaterials' progress this century. The first was the development of stainless steels, the second was the discovery of the special biocompatibility characteristics of cobalt-chromium-molybdenum alloy and the third was the simultaneous introduction of polymethylmethacrylate bone cement and high-density, ultra-high molecular weight polyethylene. All these materials have continued to see further developments and improvements since their introduction.

Prior to this century, many different materials had been tried in clinical use. There are records of gold plates used during the 16th century by one Petronius. Suture wires made in bronze, gold and iron were used in the 17th century. Silver was also used to hold together bone fragments in trauma surgery in New York about 150 years ago.

In joint replacement and bone fracture fixation a wide variety of materials has been used, particularly throughout the 19th century and into the early part of the 20th century:

gold foil	silver	lead
platinum	ivory	glass
Bakelite®	Cellophane®	Pyrex glass
zinc foil	wood	high-carbon steel
nickel-plated steel	brass	copper
aluminum	gold-plated steel	magnesium

The names associated with early biomaterials' development are several. Lane, designed and used a high-carbon steel bone plate around the year 1900. Albin and Elie Lambotte of Brussels, used and evaluated a variety of bone-fracture fixation devices in several materials and eventually recommended nickel-plated steel around 1913. Sherman of Pittsburgh also chose nickel-plated steel for his own design of bone plate around 1912 which was a modification of the Lane plate, eliminating many of the stress-raising features. For reasons of strength and ductility, Sherman turned to using vanadium steel for his plates.

The steels remained the orthopedic materials of choice through to the 1920s when the inadequacies (corrosion, tissue staining, implant loosening) became well known and clinically established. It was necessary to look for better materials.

The cobalt-based Stellite alloy was recommended by Zierold in 1924 after an evaluation of many materials, including all the then-orthopedic metals, but this recommendation was ignored. The concept of a stainless (or corrosion resistant) steel was also introduced about the same time, but, within the hostile environment of the body, it was found not to be so corrosion resistant. A 3% molybdenum stainless steel was available from 1926 but was not accepted as an orthopedic material. (The molybdenum stabilizes the austenitic structure, thereby improving corrosion resistance).

In 1928, a company called Austenal Laboratories was formed to introduce a new alloy, cobalt-chromium-molybdenum alloy, into dentistry. It took until 1936 and its discovery by Venable and Stuck for it to be introduced into orthopedics.

In 1938 tantalum was found to have many good properties which suited it to implantation, but it failed to gain popularity.

In France, in the 1940s, the Judet brothers designed and implanted many hip prostheses which were made of acrylic (polymethylmethacrylate thermoplastic) alone in the original design, but later reinforced with stainless steel. In its own right, this device was not a success, but the acceptance of this thermoplastic material within the body was an important discovery for later developments. The design failed for reasons of high wear rates, broken implants and ineffective sterilization techniques.

3.   PRESENT DAY

Referring back to the scatter diagram of Fig. 1, the most popular joint replacement arthroplasties involve metal components in one of three materials (American Standard 316 stainless steel, cobalt-chromium-molybdenum alloy, and titanium-6% aluminum-4% vanadium alloy) plastic components usually made from ultra-high-molecular weight polyethylene, although polyacetal homopolymer is also used to a lesser extent, and finally, self-curing polymethylmethacrylate bone cement.

Polypropylene, silicone rubber and polyethylene terephthalate are also in present-day use, notably in finger joint protheses, but these will not receive further mention.

Alumina ceramics have achieved some popularity in the last five years and will be briefly described.

3.1 Stainless Steels

From the early surgical steels already introduced came the later developments of the 18% chromium, 8% nickel, 3% molybdenum stainless steels to the present specifications shown in Table 1.

The improvements offered were in both mechanical and biocompatibility properties.

	BRITISH STANDARD EN58J	AMERICAN STANDARD 316	AMERICAN STANDARD 316L	AMERICAN STANDARD 316 LVM	REX 734	THYSSEN MEDICAL GRADE
CARBON	0.12 Max	0.08 Max	0.03 Max	.03 Max	.03 Max	.028 Max
MANGANESE	2 Max	2 Max	2 Max	2 Max	0.5 - 2	1.4 - 2
PHOSPHORUS	0.4 Max	0.03 Max	0.03 Max	.025 Max	.03 Max	.02 Max
SULPHUR	0.03 Max	0.03 Max	0.03 Max	.01 Max	.02 Max	.01 Max
SILICON	1 Max	0.75 Max	0.75 Max	0.75 Max	0.25 - 0.75	0.2 - 0.5
CHROMIUM	16.5 - 19.5	17-20	17-20	17-20	16.5 - 17.5	17.4 - 18.2
NICKEL	10 - 15	12-14	12-14	10-14	13-14	13.4 - 14.2
MOLYBDENUM	2.5 - 3.5	2-4	2-4	2-4	2.5 - 3	2.6 - 3
IRON	Balance	Balance	Balance	Balance	Balance	Balance

Table 1 Composition of Surgical Stainless Steels (% of Weight)

Current surgical stainless steels are all of the austenitic type as they have better resistance to corrosion. However, within the body, stainless steels are not perfectly corrosion resistant and carbon content is one factor influencing this. The 316 grade was refined to the tighter specification of 316 L (L signifies low carbon). A further refinement to 316 LVM created a grade containing fewer impurities likely to cause corrosion. The purification of the alloy is obtained through vacuum melting the original low-carbon grade, hence the designation LVM.

Very recently, a further improved specification has been introduced commercially into orthopedics. Two examples of this low cost new stainless steel are REX 734 (Firth Brown Ltd., U.K.) and Thyssen Medical Grade (Thyssen, Germany).

These new steels are all 316 austenitic steels but within the general specification they contain less carbon, phosphorus, sulphur, and silicon and more nitrogen (0.39%). They appear to be great improvements on the earlier 316 grades in that corrosion resistance and fatigue strength are markedly improved. However, all 316 steels pose the prosthesis designer with a difficult decision. Austenitic stainless steels cannot be hardened by heat treatment, but it is possible to double the tensile strength and decimate ductility by cold working or forging them. Unfortunately, such processes significantly reduce resistance to corrosion. Of the stainless steel prostheses currently available, some manufacturers have chosen to optimize the mechanical properties, others have chosen corrosion resistance and yet others have compromised both.

The molybdenum content is important. Below 2.5%, the resistance to crevice and pitting corrosion increases. Some maintain that it should not be allowed to fall below 3%.

3.2   Cast Cobalt-Chromium-Molybdenum Alloys

In 1936, Venable and Stuck caused cobalt-chromium alloy to be introduced into orthopedics and, as it appeared to be the long-awaited answer to the problem of corrosion, it rapidly monopolized the business. Competing brands, to similar chemical compositions, later became available, and local national specifications were written to include the range of compositions locally available.

The nickel, iron, manganese, and silicon are thought to be undesirable. They occur as trace impurities within the major constituents of the alloy and it becomes expensive to reduce their presence. The molybdenum increases the alloy's strength by reducing the grain size.

	BRITISH STANDARD 3531 (1968)	AMERICAN STANDARD F75 - 74	FRENCH STANDARD NFS90 - 402
CARBON	0.2 - 0.35	0.35 (Max)	0.15 - 0.35
CHROMIUM	27 - 30	27 - 30	27 - 30
MOLYBDENUM	5 - 7	5 - 7	4.5 - 7
SILICON	1 (Max)	1 (Max)	1 (Max)
MANGANESE	1 (Max)	1 (Max)	1 (Max)
NICKEL	2.5 (Max)	2.5 (Max)	2.5 (Max)
IRON	0.75 (Max)	0.75 (Max)	1 (Max)
COBALT	Balance	Balance	Balance

Table 2   Composition of Cast Co-Cr-Mo Alloy (% by weight).

The differences between the competing brands of cast cobalt-chromium-molybdenum alloys lie in the levels of undesirable elements, the quality of casting (inclusions, gas porosity, shrinkage voids) whether or not they have been heat treated to change the as-cast grain structure and the associated carbide distribution and also in the use of such processes as vacuum-cast-vacuum-melt versus air-cast-air-melt, or hot isostatic pressing to reduce the level of shrinkage voids.

Apart from the corrosion resistance and mechanical strength differences between the steels and cobalt-chromium (see Table 3) the latter had another important advantage: two polished surfaces could articulate against each other in total joint replacement well enough to be clinically acceptable at least until Charnley, in 1966, developed and established a prosthetic bearing of improved performance (friction torque, and generation of wear particles).

Even today, there are significant numbers of total knee and total hip prostheses being implanted which use designs made entirely of cobalt-chromium alloy.

The heat treatment of the alloy reduces its ultimate tensile strength but improves fatigue strength and ductility. This is a result of removing the as-cast structure, creating smaller grains with a more uniform grain structure and precipitating the majority of the carbides out into the grain boundaries.

3.3 Other Cobalt-Based Alloys

The difference between a good casting and a bad casting is partially determined by the level of voids and porosity. No

	TENSILE STRENGTH (MPa)	YIELD STRENGTH (0.2% proof)	FATIGUE STRENGTH, 10 cycles (MPa)	ELONGATION AT FRACTURE percent
Co-Cr-Mo (AS CAST)	660-830	450-580	260	8
Co-Cr-Mo (HEAT TREATED)	650-760	450-500	380	17
STAINLESS STEEL (COLD WORKED)	850-1000	680-880	320	12
STAINLESS STEEL (ANNEALED)	500-550	220-260	260	40

Table 3   A Comparison of Mechanical Characteristics - Cobalt-Chromium and Steels (316).

	PERCENT BY WEIGHT
CARBON	0.025 Max
CHROMIUM	18 - 21
IRON	1 Max
MANGANESE	0.15
MOLYBDENUM	8.5 - 10.5
NICKEL	33 - 37
SILICON	0.15
TITANIUM	0.65 - 1
COBALT	Balance

Table 4   Composition of MP35N®.

casting is defect free, although good castings do have a good record of clinical success. In an effort to produce an alloy with the same biocompatibility and corrosion resistance as the cast cobalt-chromium material but with improved mechanical character-istics, a hot-forging, multi-phase, cobalt-nickel-chromium-molybdenum alloy (MP35N®) was first introduced around 1970, followed, around 1978, by forging and sintering cobalt-chromium alloys to the same specification as shown in Table 2.

	TENSILE STRENGTH (MPa)	YIELD STRENGTH (0.2% proof)	FATIGUE STRENGTH, 10 cycles (MPa)	ELONGATION AT FRACTURE percent
REX734® (COLDWORKED)	790	550	700	16-22
FORGED/SINTERED Co-Cr-Mo	1400-1500	900-1000	793-966	28
MP35N®	850-1200	650-1000	540-600	35-55
TITANIUM-6AL-4V	880-990	810-920	400-450	10-15

Table 5   A Comparison of Strengths of the New High Strength Orthopedic Metals.

The multi-phase alloy is easier to forge than those made to the original cobalt-chromium specification.   These materials are used in designs with highly-stressed intramedullary stems, and particularly in hip joints.   The MP35N® femoral stems of hip joints usually utilize cast cobalt-chromium bearing surfaces at the femoral head to utilize the established and clinically acceptable performance of the older alloy at the articulation.   The high nickel level in MP35N® and the potential for galvanic corrosion where the dissimilar materials of the head and stem join have not been shown to be clinical problems.

3.4   Titanium Alloy

Pure titanium was tried in orthopedic implants in the 1950s. At that time total joint replacement designs all involved metal articulating against metal and titanium performs very badly in such circumstances.   It did not even achieve popularity in single-component applications or multi-component, non-articulating applications, probably because surgeons were satisfied with their clinical experience of stainless steels and cast cobalt-chromium. At 260 MPa the fatigue strength or pure titanium is relatively low and this could have contributed to its lack of success.

Titanium alloy incorporating 6% aluminum and 4% vanadium appeared in the 1960s as an improvement on pure titanium.   By then, Charnley's metal-plastic articulation concept also opened up opportunities for this new alloy which, like pure titanium, could not articulate against itself in a clinically acceptable manner.

	SPECIFIC GRAVITY	YOUNG'S MODULUS (GPa)
TITANIUM-6AL-4V	4.5	120x
STAINLESS STEEL (316)	7.9	210x
COBALT CHROMIUM	8.3	210x
MP35N®	8.3	230x
REX 734®	7.9	210x

Table 6   Density and Modulus of Orthopedic Alloys.

The advantages of titanium and its alloys are:
a) inertness in the body (i.e. better corrosion resistance than either stainless steels or cobalt-chromium)
b) low density (a marginal advantage for most implant applications) and
c) low modulus of elasticity (the significance of modulus will be considered in the chapter on Design).

Where titanium alloy bears against a plastic bearing surface, there has been some evidence of tissue staining.

This has caused some designers to place a cobalt-chromium femoral head onto a titanium intramedullary stem. Like the similar design concept using MP35N®, galvanic corrosion between the dissimilar materials has not been clinically established.

There are several femoral stems totally manufactured of titanium alloy and some of these are very recently introduced.

3.5 Ceramics

The only ceramic material which is in present-day commercial use and has several years of clinical experience is alumina - high purity aluminum oxide Al_2O_3.

Alumina in orthopedic implants is most commonly available as the spherical femoral head of a total hip prosthesis fitted to a stem made of cobalt-chromium, or titanium alloy or MP35N®. Acetabular cups made from alumina are also fairly common. However, complete joint replacements are rare for two reasons: the tensile strength of alumina is poor and very dependent on grain size; and the special inertness of the material is only of primary importance at the bearing surfaces where the products of wear are generated.

Knee prostheses in alumina have been made but are not generally available.

Alumina probably gives an improved wear rate compared to stainless steels or cobalt-chromium when bearing against poly-ethylene. Alumina bearing against alumina in laboratory tests has shown excellent wear rates. However, in certain clinical cases where a few abrasive particles (perhaps chips of bone or bone cement or loose particles of alumina) have been trapped between the bearing surfaces, there have been reports of highly accelerated wear rates. It is claimed that in such cases, massive amounts of debris are well stored in the body and have not caused any adverse reaction or inflammation: however, the prostheses were necessarily revised.

Alumina is also a brittle material and there have been reported cases of acetabular cups and prosthetic heads breaking.

For orthopedic applications of alumina, the grain size is typically less than 5 microns, the purity greater than 99.5% and as high as 99.9% (magnesium oxide forming the remainder), and the specific gravity is very high (about 4).

The compressive strength at 5000 MPa is literally decimated in tension: the bending strength of alumina being about 500 MPa. It has a high modulus at 380 GPa.

Alumina bearing against alumina can have a self-polishing effect (provided particles are not allowed to enter the bearing area) which will produce surface finishes of less than 0.1 microns and reduce the wear rate to immeasurably low values.

Table 7 shows a comparison of coefficients of friction. It is presented only as a guide. Depending on the method used to measure friction and the chosen magnitudes for sliding velocities and loads, the selected lubrication system and the surface finish of the harder of the two materials, it is possible to effect con-siderable change in the calculated coefficient.

Furthermore, a frictional coefficient of 0.1 coupled with a head size of 22 mm gives only a slightly larger friction-torque value than an alumina coefficient of 0.05 coupled with a head diameter of 32 mm or 35 mm. (There are no 22 mm diameter ceramic heads commercially available).

The wear rates of Table 7 must also not be considered in isolation. Cobalt-chromium bearing against cobalt-chromium gives the best (i.e. lowest) rate of wear in a hip prosthesis, but for particular patients, the products of wear can be undesirable. The alumina-alumina combination compromises wear rate in comparison to

	COEFFICENT OF FRICTION (IN SYNOVIAL FLUID)	COEFFICIENT OF FRICTION (DRY)	HIP WEAR RATE (mm/year)
METAL (Co-Cr, or STAINLESS STEEL) vs. POLYETHYLENE	0.1	0.3	0.1 - 0.2
ALUMINA vs ALUMINA	0.05	-	0.015
CAST Co-Cr vs CAST Co-Cr	0.15	0.4	0.001

Table 7   A Comparison of Hip Joint Friction.

cobalt-chromium to obtain the advantage of more biologically toler-
ated wear debris.   More will be said about this aspect of biocompatibility later.   As an aside, Charnley quotes the coefficient of
friction in an animal joint as 0.01 or less.

3.6 Plastics

      In 1966, the Charnley total hip incorporating a femoral stem
made of EN58J stainless steel and an acetabular cup made of ultra-
high-molecular-weight polyethylene was generally released.   Since
that time this particular type of polyethylene has dominated the
joint replacement business.

      Charnley tried several plastics during the course of develop-
ing his new prosthesis.   The most notable of these was PTFE (poly-
tetraflourethylene)   which   had   excellent   frictional   properties
(stainless steel against PTFE gave a coefficient of friction of
around 0.01 - 0.02) but a rate of wear causing the femoral ball to
penetrate the socket 500 - 1000 times faster than polyethylene.
Hence, PTFE and filled PTFE were abandoned and the search continued
until high-density, UHMW polyethylene was discovered.

      The only plastic used in joint replacement before Charnley was
Plexiglas in the acrylic Judet prothesis already mentioned under
Historical Materials.

      Since Charnley, in an effort to look for wear rates better
than 0.1 mm per year or to reduce the cost of manufacture, other
plastics have been tried.   Polyethylene terephthalate (a polyester)
has been used both for acetabular cups and for plastic-femoral
head/metal-acetabular cup design configurations.   A polyacetal

homopolymer has also been used in different joint designs and continues to perform successfully in the Christiansen trunnion-bearing total hip. Carbon-filled, UHMW polyethylene has also been tried and continues in service.

The original material chosen by Charnley is clinically very successful. Its disadvantages are that it does creep under stress unless the complete prosthesis design constrains it from doing so; it distorts at around 100 $^{\circ}$C and so cannot be steam sterilized; it is difficult or expensive to form during manufacture by molding; the wear rate of 0.1 mm per year for young patients makes an eventual revision operation highly likely.

Of these, the most significant problem is that of cold flow or creep. Sterilization is now conventionally performed by irradiation (either gamma rays or electron beam) and the components are supplied in a presterilized package. The wear rate has been reported to be even less than 0.1 mm per year on average by some clinicians and at such a rate, it is only of significance to a very small percentage of the total patient population. Modern machining methods and the development of molding technology can both now produce sophisticated shapes cost effectively.

The polyester, polyethylene terephthalate, was both stronger and more creep resistant than UHMW polyethylene. However, clinical trials showed that wear debris caused bone resorption. This may have been because the design configuration chosen for clinical evaluation involved the Weber-Huggler hip prosthesis which incorporated a plastic femoral head articulating against a metal acetabular cup (spherical bearing) and a metal femoral stem (trunnion bearing). This type of design gave rise to high wear rates as probably would also have happened had the Charnley material been used. There is also evidence that large quantities of debris of many materials, including UHMW polyethylene will cause bone resorption. It is a historical fact that the occurrence of resorption caused this polyester to be abandoned. It is not clear whether one can conclude that polyethylene terephthalate is an unsuitable replacement for UHME polyethylene.

Polyacetal homopolymer continues in clinical use, although Scales in Britain has reported high wear rates with this material. The same has not been found in many thousands of Delrin® acetabular cups used in the Christiansen hip. The clinical suitability of this material remains unresolved.

The structure of UHMW polyethylene comprises long chains of ethylene CH_2:

```
      H     H     H     H
      |     |     |     |
  —  C  —  C  —  C  —  C  —
      |     |     |     |
      H     H     H     H
```

The structure of polyacetal homopolymer also comprises long chains of molecules:

```
      H           H           H
      |           |           |
  —  C  —  O  —  C  —  O  —  C  —
      |           |           |
      H           H           H
```

Of the five materials shown in Table 8 only two (high-density polyethylene and polyacetal homopolymer) continue to be implanted. Peak stresses in the acetabular cup in the hip of an active subject will often exceed 10 MPa and occasionally climb past 20 MPa. In the knee joint where contact areas can, by design, be very small, instantaneous peak surface stresses can be even larger. Hence, Table 8 shows that high-density polyethylene is being permanently loaded near the limit of its capability and that the polyacetal homopolymer can offer improved characteristics. The widely

	YOUNG'S MODULUS (TENSILE) (MPa)	ULTIMATE TENSILE STRENGTH (MPa)	BENDING STRENGTH (MPa)	ELONGATION percent
POLYETHYLENE (HIGH DENSITY 0.95 – 0.965	500	20 – 46	15 – 20	Up to 800
POLYETHYLENE (LOW DENSITY 0.918 – 0.94)	150	7 – 17	No Break	Up to 650
POLYETHYLENE TEREPHTHALATE	3000	30	90	Up to 300
POLYACETAL HOMOPOLYMER (Sp.Gr. = 1.41)	2800	65	90	Up to 100
POLYACETAL COPOLYMER (Sp.Gr. = 1.45)	3000	70	100	Up to 75

Table 8   The Mechanical Properties of Plastics (from Ref. 1).

differing clinical findings of polyacetal homopolymer need to be resolved.

To illustrate the creep behavior of UHMW polyethylene, Hoechst have published technical data for their material (Hostalen® RCH 1000). At 50 °C and 12 MPa a sample was put under compression. The compression load was removed and one minute later 5.4% of deformation was measured: 24 hours later this had reduced to 3.5%.

3.7   Bone Cement

In 1958, Charnley began using pink dental acrylic cement in him program to develop a new total hip arthroplasty. Shortly afterwards, McKee and Farrar used it with their own prosthesis.

Prior to this, acrylic resins were known in dentistry, (the pink palate plates in partial dentures) and in the Judet hip prosthesis introduced in 1946. In 1951, a femoral head liner made of acrylic was cemented to the femoral head using acrylic resin and Haboush also used the resin to fix a femoral implant in place. Nevertheless, while Charnley probably benefited from prior knowledge of the orthopedic application of polymethylmethacrylate (acrylic) he can claim to have fathered its successful introduction. By now, acrylic bone cement has probably been used in well over a million human joint reconstructive operations worldwide.

The basic bone cement available specifically for orthopedic use is a little different from the dental variety: the differences are, particle size, molecular weight and modified chemistry to give handling properties more suited to joint replacement. The basic variety has undergone development over the last 20 years: the introduction of sterilization of the powder; the addition of radiopaque components; and the inclusion of antibiotic premixed with the cement.

All these cements are supplied as ampoules of 20 ml of liquid and 40 gm of powder. By volume, the liquid consists of 97.4% of methyl methacrylate (monomer), 2% - 2.6% N, N-dimethyl-p-toluidine (DPT) the agent which initiates polymerization, and 0.006% - 0.01% hydroquinone which inhibits spontaneous polymerization. The structure of the monomer is:

$$CH_2 = C - COOCH_3$$

(methylmethacrylate monomer)

$$CH_3$$

The composition of the powder mixture varies depending on what type of cement is being used. The original, basic or plain variety typically comprises 82.9% (by weight) of methylmethacrylate –

styrene copolymer, 16.6% of polymethylmethacrylate, 0.5% - 2.5% of an activator (benzoyl peroxide). This 5:1 mix is also used for the radiopaque variety but 10% by weight of barium sulphate (U.S.P.) is added.

There are alternatives to the above compositions. Zirconium dioxide is also used as a radio-contrast component which may occupy 15% by weight of the 40 gm sachet. Pigments are sometimes added typically 0.02%) to distinguish the normally-bone-coloured cement from the bone itself.

Different manufacturers add various antibiotics to the powder pack: Penicillin[TM] and Erythromycin[TM], Gentamycin[TM], Neomycin[TM] and Bacitracin[TM], Erythromycin[TM] and Colistin[TM]. The proportions vary between 0.5% and 2% by weight.

The structure of the cement after it has set is long chains of polymethylmethacrylate:

$$- - - \overset{\overset{\textstyle CH_3}{|}}{\underset{\underset{\textstyle COOCH_3}{|}}{C}} - CH_2 - \overset{\overset{\textstyle CH_3}{|}}{\underset{\underset{\textstyle COOCH_3}{|}}{C}} - - -$$

polymethylmethacrylate - "polymer")

This polymerization occurs when the liquid is added to the powder. The activator (benzoyl peroxide) decomposes rapidly when mixed with the accelerator (DPT). This decomposition causes free radicals (unpaired electrons) to be generated which, in turn, cause the monomer molecules to link together in chains, i.e., the polymerization process.

Without the addition of the DPT accelerator, this process could happen very slowly within the ampoule, particularly in the presence of light or heat. The inhibitor hydroquinone is added to prevent this. On mixing the DPT (in the liquid) with the benzoyl peroxide (in the powder) the small quantity of hydroquinone is unable to prevent the peroxide decomposition.

Table 9 shows a wide variation in the mechanical properties of polymethylmethacrylate. The table is a summary of many reported values and the differences are a consequence of the several test methods used.

Within the operating room, it is certainly possible to change the eventual properties of the bone cement. One of the major advances in joint replacement has been improvements in the management of implant fixation using acrylic resin. Bone preparation

BENDING STRENGTH	(MPa)	100 - 120
FATIGUE LIMIT	(MPa)	48
YIELD STRENGTH	(MPa)	55
COMPRESSIVE STRENGTH	(MPa)	63 - 97
TENSILE STRENGTH	(MPa)	25 - 70
SHEAR STRENGTH	(MPa)	40 - 49
MODULUS OF ELASTICITY	(MPa)	1600 - 3000
ELONGATION TO FAILURE	(percent)	1.2 - 5
IMPACT STRENGTH	(J/M Notch)	16.5 - 27.5

Table 9   Mechanical Properties of Acrylic Bone Cements.

preferably leaves rough bone surfaces (grooves, drill holes, notches) and open cancellous bone trabeculae (i.e., not filled with bone debris generated by reaming and drilling) into which the cement can key. Hence, bone brushes, water jets and bone drying devices are now in frequent use.

Intramedullary plugs are used to prevent the cement from being forced down the marrow cavity and thus they cause the pressure generated upon insertion of the prosthesis to force the cement into a more intimate contact with the bone. Several new designs of prostheses and instruments are available which promote the same phenomenon.

Acrylic bone cement is called "cold curing" because no heat is applied to cause polymerization. However, the reaction is exothemic and temperatures as high as 80 °C - 90 °C have been quoted, although Reckling et al and Jefferiss et al show that it is not helpful to quote such absolute numbers: it is possible that temperatues are much lower than this (less than 48 °C). Charnley admits to an 0.5 mm layer of dead bone in contact with the cement but says that in the short term it causes no problems for the patient and in the longer term the dead bone is replaced. Vernon-Roberts and Freeman report up to 1.5 mm of fibrous tissue at the bone/cement interface(2). Charnley agrees that the acrylic cement technique is not recommended for use in 45 year old patients, but says that he has not found the same results as Vernon-Roberts and Freeman in post mortem cases up to 12 years after implantation.

Whatever doubts there may be over the long-term success of polymethylmethacrylate cements, there are some short-term hazards of which the surgeon is warned. Inhalation of very large doses of monomer vapor can cause respiratory arrest at worst and irritation (to eyes or respiratory tract), drowsiness, headaches, and hypotension at best.

The ·monomer will rapidly dissolve in water and be removed from the patient's body. (The residual level is typically 3% - 4%). There have been no reported cases of chronic toxicity from these low levels of exposure.

The monomer can also cause contact dermatitis if those who handle it are allergic to it. It may penetrate rubber surgical gloves.

Infrequently, cardiac arrest of the patient has occurred after joint replacement with acrylic cements. It is not clear whether this is a consequence of the monomer entering the blood-stream or the result of fatty embolism after forcing or releasing the contents of the bone and medullary canal into the blood-stream.

The frequency of in-theatre complications is very small and in the short term (up to 12 years) the biomechanical success of acrylic bone cement is impressive, particularly with modern cement handling and contact methods.

Several competing brands of bone cement are available. Apart from differences of antibiotics, claims are also made for the non-antiobiotic types. Setting time, viscosity and mechanical properties form the bases for comparison. Some surgeons prefer setting times as short as 3 to 4 minutes while others, not wanting to be put under time pressure, prefer 10 to 12 minutes. Where a cement gun is used, the cement must be injected before it becomes too viscous to pass through the long narrow nozzle of the gun. Hence, low viscosity cements have been marketed. Even when a gun is not used, some surgeons prefer to insert the cement in a very liquid form (even though the free monomer level can be relatively high in this state) so that it more readily fills bone trabeculae, grooves and holes.

4.   FUTURE JOINT REPLACEMENT BIOMATERIALS

After twenty years and more of experience with cobalt-chromium alloys, stainless steel, high-density, UHMW polyethylene and acrylic bone cements, (generally good), and substantial experience (though less than twenty years) with titanium and cobalt-nickel-chromium alloys, there is widescale satisfaction with current biomaterials.

New materials are sought for a variety of reasons:
a) To improve wear rates in order to gain longer service lives and reduce the risk of adverse reaction to wear debris.
b) To achieve greater inertness, thereby reducing adverse body reactions to the implant itself, wear debris, or released ions and particles.

c) To improve the mechanical properties: higher strength and lower stiffness.

d) To improve the effectiveness of implant fixation.

e) To introduce materials which are cheaper or more readily available or easier to form.

Biodegradable implant materials are currently receiving much interest. However, the primary orthopedic applications being investigated are bone or ligament repair (as healing occurs the function or material of the implant disappears) and will not be considered further here other than to mention them by name. They may in the future become useful as devices for initiating bone in-growth into permanent implants, perhaps by being added to the implant as a coating.

Almost a century ago it was noted that if a hole in bone was filled with calcium sulphate (Plaster of Paris) it was resorbed and replaced by bone. Calcium and phosphorus are common constituents of bone and hence calcium phosphate (in particular hydroxyapatite and tricalcium phosphate) has been well analyzed. Other materials include calcium carbonate, calcium flourapetite, calcium aluminate and calcium phosphate magnesium aluminate. The reader is referred to "Biocompatibility of Clinical Implant Materials"(3).

The same reference includes a chapter on biodegradable polymers, e.g. polyvinyl alcohol used in resorbable sutures.

The use of high-purity, high-density alumina for improved wear rate and inertness of wear debris has already been discussed. Ceramic bearing surface coatings (onto conventional metal implants) are being investigated to overcome the tensile weakness of alumina components.

Bioglass coatings of implants (see Fundamental Aspects of Biocompatibility) which prevent the formation of the fibrous layer between bone and conventional implants by causing bone growth and direct bone attachment seem to offer a promising opportunity. Bioglass, reinforced with ductile metal wires, is being investigated in an attempt to make the coating less prone to cracking.

New metals being tested include the shape-memory metal, nitinol (nickel-titanium alloy), niobium and tantalum, also for fracture treatment. The special property of nitinol is that it can first be implanted and then, under application of heat, will return to its original (or "remembered") form. Thus, it can impose compression on a fracture site or straighten, say, a spinal deformity.

The attractive property of tantalum and niobium is their inertness in the body. It remains to be seen whether this advantage will bring about their popular introduction into bone fracture fixation devices which are currently being tried. In particular, tantalum has been used in surgery since 1938, mainly in plastic and neurosurgery, but also in orthopedic surgery. Both tantalum and niobium have a very stable oxide passive layer which gives them inertness. Like other metals, they can be used in a heavily cold-worked state or fully annealed. In the annealed state, their tensile strengths are less than half that when cold worked (300 - 1000 MPa), but, in the cold-worked state, their elongation at fracture is less than 1%. The modulus of tantalum is very similar to cast cobalt-chromium, whereas niobium is about half the value (115 GPa).

Their performance as implanted bearing surfaces does not appear to have been reported, even though joint replacement clinical trials have been conducted. One interesting characteristic of tantalum is that while its ultimate tensile strength is less than stainless steel, the fatigue strength is very close at around 380 MPa.

Carbon, in various forms, looks to offer some exciting opportunities in joint replacement. Glassy carbon is hard wearing, very biocompatible and may prove to be effective for bearing surfaces. Its modulus, at 15 GPa, is closer to that of cortical bone (at 10 GPa) than all metals.

Carbon fiber reinforced carbon has a much higher modulus than cortical bone (14 x) but its flexural strength at 800 MPa is 6 times higher than the glassy carbon.

Thermoplastics and epoxy resins reinforced with fibers (glass or carbon) also show promising characteristics. The fibers may be short and randomly oriented or they can be controlled (e.g. lying along the length of the device - unidirectional, or layered and lying in two or more directions - bidirectional, multi-directional) thereby enabling the designer to choose particular mechanical characteristics for tension, shear, bending and torsion.

Carbon seems to be an attractive material for future prosthetic applications due to its good tissue compatibility and range of mechanical characteristics.

Carbon filled polyethylene has been intrduced as a replacement for plain high-density, UHMW polyethylene. It is claimed that its creep resistance and wear properties are double those of the plain material and that tissue tolerance to both materials is equivalent.

Conventional metal stems or surface replacement prostheses with porous surfaces made of the same material as the parent metal have been introduced over the last ten years. Only recently have

PRESENT	FUTURE POSSIBILITIES
METAL INTRAMEDULLARY STEMS (Co-Cr, TITANIUM ALLOY, STAINLESS STEEL)	CERAMICS FIBER REINFORCED PLASTICS TANTALUM AND NIOBIUM
METAL BEARING SURFACES (Co-Cr, TITANIUM ALLOY, STAINLESS STEEL)	ALUMINA CARBON
POLYETHYLENE BEARING SURFACES	ALUMINA REINFORCED POLYETHYLENE
METAL SUPPORTS FOR PLASTIC BEARING SURFACES	FIBER REINFORCED PLASTICS
ACRYLIC BONE CEMENT	NEW CEMENTS OR ELIMINATE BONE CEMENT, e.g.: — BIOGLASS COATING ON METAL — CARBON COATING ON METAL — POROUS METAL SURFACE

Table 10   Possible New Biomaterials in Bone Joint Replacement.

they become popular. Their objective is to eliminate the need for bone cement.

Table 10 summarizes the possible changes which will be seen in joint replacement biomaterials.

5.   AVAILABILITY AND COST

Of the materials in common prosthetic implant manufacture, several suffer from availability problems. Cobalt and chromium come from such countries as Angola, Zimbabwe, Zaire and Zambia. The main source of titanium is Russia. Political instability can interrupt supply.

Furthermore, the three metals already named are well used in aircraft, aero-engine and weapon construction. Thus, the same political disturbance which interrupts supply might increase demand for the metals for military defense purposes.

In 1969, there was a nickel shortage which caused prices to rise. The same happened to cobalt in 1977, and titanium shortly after.

There is no shortage of the raw materials used in manufacturing polyethylene and acrylic bone cement. The major costs here are in forming and processing.

Approximate costs of the basic metals are:

surgical stainless steels – $10,000 – $15,000 per ton
cobalt-chromium alloy – $40,000 – $80,000 per ton
titanium alloy – $15,000 – $30,000 per ton

Over the last ten years, prices have fluctuated remarkably, particularly in times of shortage.

6. MANUFACTURING

More details of manufacturing are given in a separate chapter, but the following Table 11 will summarize the suitable and unsuitable manufacturing techniques of biomaterials in common present-day use.

	FORGE	CAST	SINTER	MACHINE	GRIND	WELD
STEEL	Yes	No	No	Yes	Yes	Not Advised
TITANIUM	Yes	Rare	No	Difficult	Yes	Yes
Co-Cr	Yes	Yes	Yes	Difficult	Yes	Yes
MP35N	Yes	No	No	Yes	Yes	Yes

	COMPRESSION MOLD	INJECTION MOLD	MACHINE
POLYETHYLENE	Yes	Difficult	Yes
POLYACETAL	No	Yes	Yes

Table 11 Manufacturing Techniques Used at Present.

7. BIOCOMPATIBILITY

The environment in which a joint replacement prosthesis exists can be highly corrosive to the implant and it may be the implant which is responsible for creating this corrosive environment.

Body fluids are usually very slightly alkaline, with a pH of around 7.4. The presence of an infection can make it much more alkaline and drive the pH value up to 9. The effect of the implant or the implantation, particularly where the flow of body fluids is impaired, can cause a local concentration of acids and a pH of 5.

It is important that the material chosen for an implant is able to resist such acidic and alkaline conditions, but it is equally important that the implant does not create them. The biocompatibility of implants should therefore be assessed under two headings: body tolerance of the device, and implant tolerance of the body. The first of these two headings can usefully be divided into two subheadings: local body tolerance and systemic tolerance. Local changes would include bone resorption, fibrous tissue generation, bone regeneration, and alterations in the chemistry of body fluids all in the immediate vicinity of the implant. Systemic tolerance would extend the analysis of the effects of the implant to all body organs, for example carcinogenesis or cardiac arrest.

7.1 Implant Tolerance of the Body

All metals corrode through chemical action, given the right conditions. With orthopedic metals, corrosion is resisted when they surround themselves with a passive layer. As this layer is broken, corrosion will take place. The passive layer may be broken by mechanical action or electrical action and the metal will endeavor to restore the integrity of the layer.

Metal orthopedic implants can be compared in terms of the ease with which the passive layer is broken and the speed with which it is rebuilt.

There are many corrosion mechanisms which cause breakdown of the passive layer. Surface irregularities (crevices, pits, scratches) and inclusions will create weaknesses in the layer and thus make it more liable to breakdown.

When two dissimilar metals are in electrical contact in a conductive liquid, a galvanic cell can be created which causes the removal of metal ions. This is galvanic corrosion. Unfortunately, the presence of inclusions or the same metal in two different states (cold worked/annealed or slightly different chemical compositions) might also be enough to cause galvanic corrosion.

For cobalt-chromium alloy, the potential required to cause breakdown is almost 1 volt, which signifies that in normal bodily conditions, breakdown should not occur. Pitting and crevice corrosion have not been reported clinically and Bolton et al show that crevices would need to be as deep as 1 mm to propagate fatigue cracks. (It is the chloride ions in the slightly alkaline body fluids which, coupled with metallurgical defects, can aggressively promote fatigue failure).

The passive layer in stainless steels is not strong. The breakdown potential is only 0.4 volts for general 316 types, but increases to around 1 volt for the new grades (e.g. REX 734®).

Pitting corrosion in 316 steels is well reported, as is crevice corrosion, although this is more commonly found in multi-component applications, and corrosion fatigue is well established in saline solutions.

Titanium forms a very thick passive layer and a breakdown potential of 9 volts is required to disturb it. Titanium can be combined with cobalt-chromium and yet not cause galvanic corrosion. The fatigue strength of titanium does decrease slightly in a saline environment, but this has not been shown to have caused clinical failure.

Polymers can also degrade in service. They can lose their strength; become brittle. The chains of molecules can lose some of their cross-linking and chain length can reduce. Polymethylmethacrylate can depolymerize, releasing large amounts of monomer with a reduction in molecular weight. Polyethylene can also degrade but to a much lesser degree than the bone cement.

7.2 Local Body Tolerance of Implant Materials

All-metal intramedullary stems, whatever metal used, have shown cortical thickening around the tip of the stem. This is Wolff's law in action and is a direct consequence of the stiffness of the metal stem relative to the flexibility of the cortical bone. Titanium alloy, having a much lower modulus of elasticity than steel and cobalt-chromium, would be expected to cause less cortical thickening for similar stem geometry, but this has not yet been established clinically.

Vernon-Roberts and Freeman have reported a fibrous layer forming between the acrylic cement and the bone(2).

Charnley identified giant cells caused by the implants or their debris, but did not see this as a problem.

It has already been stated that acrylic cement typically causes 0.5 mm of dead bone at the interface and that Charnley believes that this, in time, is replaced with good bone.

Where large quantities of particles of bone cement, polyethylene, or metals are produced, it is probable that they cause bone necrosis which, in turn, can cause implant loosening.

It is claimed that large quantities of alumina wear debris are contained locally within soft tissues and cause no adverse reaction.

7.3 Systemic Reactions to Implants

Dobbs and Minski (in Biomaterials 1980) measured high levels of cobalt and chromium in the lungs, liver, kidneys, spleen, urine and hair in an 81 year old patient who died fourteen years after an all-cobalt-chromium total hip had been implanted. In some instances they found 50 x normal levels of these elements. However, they draw no conclusions from this and comment on how little information is available on the pathological effects of such metal-ion levels.

Pedley et al (in Fundamental Aspects of Biocompatibility) show that metals and plastics can induce malignant neoplasms (tumors) in laboratory animals, but they state why it may not be reasonable to extrapolate these findings to cover implants in humans. Williams, in the same book, states that there is very little data on the relationship between the potential for metal-ion toxicity and the tissue response.

In the absence of much conclusive information on the systemic effects of common implant materials, the designers and manufacturers are obliged to base implant specifications on long experience of apparently adequate clinical service and on optimizing the characteristics of new materials, even if this involves unnecessary effort in search of properties far above what is clinically necessary. Until it can be established what the threshold of adequacy is (assuming it exists), it is right to follow a conservative approach.

REFERENCES

1. Williams, D.F. and R.Roaf. Implants in Surgery, W. B. Saunders Co., Ltd., 1973.
2. Vernon-Roberts, B. and M.A.R. Freeman. The Tissue Response to Total Joint Replacement Protheses. In S.A.V. Swanson and

M.A.R. Freeman ed., Scientific Basis of Joint Replacement, Pitman Medical, 1977.
3.   Williams, D.F.   Biocompatibility of Clinical Implant Materials, vols. I and II, CRC Press, 1981.

BIBLIOGRAPHY

1.   Artificial Hip and Knee Joint Technology. Schaldach and Hohmann Eds. (Springer-Verlag, 1976).
2.   Biomaterials 1980. Winter, Gibbons, Plenk, Eds. (John Wiley and Sons, 1982).
3.   Bolton, J.D,, Hayden, J., Humphreys, M. A Study of Corrosion Fatigue in Cast Cobalt-Chrome-Molybdenum Alloys. Engineering in Medicine (1982).
4.   Charnley, J. Acrylic Cement in Orthopedic Surgery (Churchill Livingstone, 1972).
5.   Charnley, J. Low Friction Arthroplasty of the Hip (Springer-Verlag, 1979).
6.   Dumbleton, J.H. and Black, J. An Introduction to Orthopedic Materials (Charles C. Thomas Publisher, 1975).
7.   Harms, J., Mausle, E., Mittelmeier, H. The Biocompatibility of Alumina Ceramics (Edizioni Minerva Medica, 1979).
8.   Hostalen™ RCH 1000. Technical Publication, Hoechst A.G.
9.   Jefferiss, C.D., Lee, A.J.C., Ling, R.S.M. Thermal Aspects of Self-Curing Polymethylmethacrylate. Journal of Bone and Joint Surgery, vol. 57-B, No. 4 (November 1975).
10. Lee, A.J.C. Exeter Cement Security System. Technical Monograph, Howmedica, Inc.
11. Micro-grain™ Zimaloy®. Zimmer USA Technical Publication.
12. Molded poly two™. Zimmer USA Technical Publication.
13. Palacos® R with Gentamycin. Technical Publication, Kirby-Warrick Pharmaceuticals Ltd.
14. Reckling, F.W. and Dillon, W.L. The Bone-Cement Interface Temperature During Total Joint Replacement. Journal of Bone and Joint Surgery, 59A (1980).
15. Scales, J. Informal meeting on Delrin®, London, June 23rd, 1981. To be published in Journal of Bone and Joint Surgery.
16. Semlitsch, M. Technical Progress in Artificial Hip Joints. Sulzer Technical Review (4/1974).
17. Surgical Simplex® P. Bone Cement. Technical Monograph, Howmedica, Inc.
18. Thackray Ortron™ 90. C.F. Thackray Ltd., Technical Publication.
19. Vitallium® FHS®. Technical Monograph, Howmedica, Inc.
20. The Vitallium® Story. Howmedica Int., Inc., Technical Publication.

21. Walker, P.S.   Human Joints and Their Artificial Replacements (Charles C. Thomas Publisher, 1977).

22. Williams, D.F.   Fundamental Aspects of Biocompatibility, vols. I and II (CRC Press, 1981).

DESIGN, MANUFACTURE AND TESTING OF PROSTHETIC DÉVICES

P. Lawes

Howmedica International, Inc.,
Limerick, Ireland

1.   INTRODUCTION

The scatter diagram shown as Fig. 1 illustrates how the subjects of manufacturing, testing and design are interlinked and how they can be reduced into many subheadings for the purposes of analysis and discussion. Regulatory affairs, which is an administrative aspect of manufacturing, places significant demands on testing, design and quality control and thus will be described. Marketing is shown on the scatter diagram, as much product testing and all product design are conducted in order to satisfy marketing objectives, namely, to expand or maintain the usage of a product. In this sense, the product could be, very specifically, a certain design or knee replacement or it could be the general product group of total-knee prostheses. Testing is performed to gain confidence in designs, new or old. The results may be used to promote the use of an implant or to satisfy regulatory requirements that it is suitable for, say, introduction into limited clinical trials.

Testing is also performed to maintain confidence in manufacture. A design may be well established and well tested, but the variations which can occur during manufacture demand that quality assurance tests are conducted. Thus, testing forms a part of the design process and a part of manufacturing (through quality assurance) and this chapter will treat it that way and not as an activity in its own right.

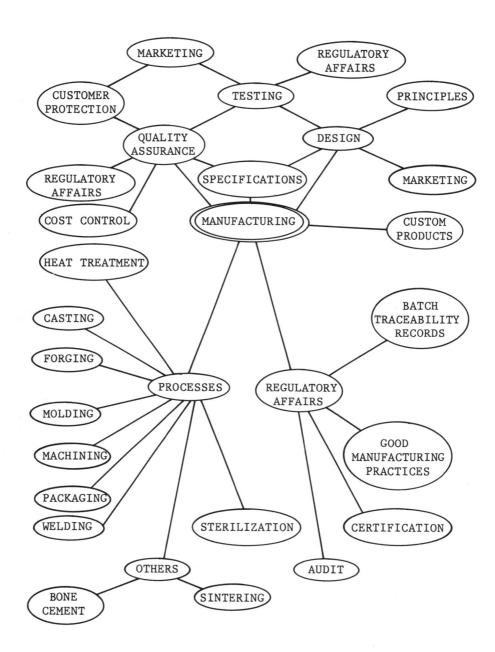

Fig. 1   Scatter Diagram: Manufacturing, Design and Testing.

2.　THE DESIGN PROCESS

The engineering design of an orthopedic device is important, not in its own right, but in the context of the total arthoplasty design:

    a)　Indications and contraindications (matching the arthroplasty to the patient and his or her circumstances).
    b)　Pre-operative preparation of the patient.
    c)　The device to be used.
    d)　The surgical operation.
    e)　Post-operative rehabilitation.
    f)　Limitations on in-service use.

In the mid-1970s, reports of fatigue failures of total-hip, intramedullary stems appeared.　The reaction was to redesign the stems, increasing section geometry and reducing the head-offset, thereby making the stems stiffer, the cement wall thinner and reducing the applied bending moments.　The consequences of these changes for the bone cement, the bone and the patient were considered later.

Cement management techniques have since improved through the introduction of new bone reamers and cutters, bone brushes, water sprays, cement introduucers and pressurizers and intramedullary bone plugs.

The stiffness of hip stems is also receiving more consideration.　Fatigue life can be improved without resorting to stem enlargement and stiffening.　Elimination of stress-raising features (sharp edges, notches, grooves), improvements in material quality and surface finish and optimizing the material properties (modulus and fatigue limit) thereby also optimizing stem flexibility, are all aspects of good intramedullary stem design.

Reaction to the problem of fatigue fractures caused stem sections to be increased and femoral head-offsets to be reduced. Since then, stem sections have again been reducing and head-offsets increasing (reducing the femoral head-offset makes the total femoral component much straighter and the biomechanical effect of this has been found to increase the risk of dislocation of the ball-and-socket joint).　While each of the devices can be said to have been designed, this process of attending to one or two design parameters as problems occur or as opportunities are sought, is more appropriately described as a development process.　To a large extent this is inevitable as it is partially through the development of implants that we learn about how human joints function.　It is difficult to design a device without knowledge of the in-service conditions.　Nevertheless, the application of good design principles and, in particular, total design principles, should help to reduce the number of development stages and increase the rate of progress toward more effective solutions.

There are several published definitions of design. One is: "Engineering design is a purposeful activity directed towards the goal of fulfilling human needs, particularly those which can be met by the technological factors of our culture"--Morris Asimow(1). Another: "Total design is a process of thoughtful compromise and snythesis ....involves a large measure of approximation and personal choice"--Ratcliffe(2). The first defines Engineering Design and reasonably concentrates on technology. The second defines Total Design and is more helpful in that it includes those aspects of design which cannot be quantified and yet are critical to its success. A third example, the one adopted by this author, also defines the problem of Engineering Design: "Devise, subject to certain problem-solving constraints, a component, system or process to accomplish a specified task optimally subject to certain solution constraints"--Dixon(3).

In designing a total hip arthroplasty, (and considering the complete system), problem-solving constraints would include suitable biomaterials and the available biomechanical knowledge of the prosthetic and pathological hip joint. Solution constraints would include the physical bone dimensions, their ranges of variation and the need for ease of implantation. Research and Development assists the designer by removing problem-solving constraints and allowing him to concentrate on the solution constraints.

The key stages of the design process are:

a) Goal Recognition
b) Task Specification
c) Planning and Communication
d) Concept Forming (Creative Phase)
e) Analysis
f) Specification of Solution
g) Monitor (Production - Distribution - Sales - Service).

As the designer monitors the new product, so new opportunities will be sought and the cycle recommences with the identification of a new goal.

Goal recognition describes the end objective of the project in broad terms and must refer to the totality of the design problem. Task specification gives more detail to the goal and quantifies performance characteristics and design variables without unnecessarily constraining the range of possible design solutions. It is easy for the task specification stage to hinder creativity and this must be avoided. There are many very useful techniques in creativity, well researched, including brainstorming morphological studies, synectics, analogy, empathy and fantasy. All have their place and are recommended. Edward de Bono has much to offer the designer in seeking new solutions to old problems(4-7).

Analysis can be theoretical (stress analysis, cost analysis, estimating the time and complexity of implantation) or can involve testing (laboratory testing, production trials, clinical trials). Testing can check the adequacy of an idea, optimize a design variable, generate promotional information or satisfy the requirements of regulatory authorities that the design has been scientifically analyzed.

Analysis might be used merely to reduce the number of potential solutions which result from the creativity stage. Further analysis could involve experimentation with the remaining preferred solutions. "Specification of solution: presumes some decision-making process takes place to choose which ideas the designer is going to commit himself to. Kepner and Trego(8) devised the system of "Musts and Wants." If a patient is known to be nickel-sensitive, the surgeon in making his implant choice, might rule out the use of stainless steel, regardless of how much he favors a particular steel device, because the expected outcome would probably be a clinical failure. Thus, biocompatibility is a "Must" in arthroplasty design. However, features such as weight and price qualify as "Wants": it is desirable that they are both low, but where a particular solution offers significant merits in other characteristics (long-service life, ease of implantation) its weight and price might be considered less important. When evaluating designs all the "Musts" and "Wants" are listed. The "Wants" must be weighted in terms of their relative importance. All the "Musts" have to be satisfied, otherwise the solution is immediately discarded.

For a design to be successful, it must satisfy all the "Must" objectives and optimize its performance against the "Wants." The designer is often faced with compromise to achieve this optimization. The final implant and arthroplasty might be scored against design for production, design for surgical implantation, design for in-service function, design for patentable features and marketing claims, design for storage and distribution (the packaging is often an important part of the total design, particularly when presterilized supply of implants is required).

The relative weighting of the "Wants" criteria is very subjective. Choosing this weighting is essentially a marketing function: the choice is made through understanding the surgeons' views which predominate at the time; promotion of the design will seek to convince the customer that the chosen weighting is correct and that any competing product has sought to optimize characteristics of less importance. Of modern designs of surface-replacement knee prostheses, some have maximized bearing-contact area in order to minimize wear rates. Others have avoided high loads on the implants which can cause loosening by reducing the bearing-contact areas, allowing some relative sliding movement at the bearing surfaces and leaving the soft tissues to transfer more of the horizontal forces directly from the tibia to the femur. The promotion of the first type of design endeavors to convince the customer that wear rate is most important, while the second emphasizes loosening.

Charnley made friction torque the most important feature of his total hip design. Muller increased the Charnley femoral head diameter of 22 mm to 32 mm and thus sacrificed friction torque in the belief that 32 mm would improve the wear.

It is interesting to review the evolution of the hip and knee joint prostheses as illustrations of the design process in action. Some of the redesigns have obviously considered the problem as treating human joints, while others only see the detail design of implantable hardware.

3. THE EVOLUTION OF HIP JOINT REPLACEMENTS

The history of hip joint implants used for the purpose of treating degenerated natural bearing surfaces (i.e. excluding fracture fixation appliances) contains several notable events:

1891: Theophilus Gluck implanted ivory prostheses in the hip. The devices had intramedullary stems and he used some bone cement.

1895: Jones used gold foil as an interposition arthroplasty.

1923: Smith-Petersen placed hip molds of glass and later (1933) Pyrex® between the two bony bearing surfaces as a means of encouraging redevelopment of good natural bearing surfaces. The problem was fracture of the implant materials.

1926: Hey-Groves used an ivory femoral head prosthesis. This articulated against the natural acetabulum.

1934: Rehn and Harmon added spikes to a steel Smith-Petersen type cup to fix it into the acetabulum.

1937: Smith-Petersen turned to Vitallium® alloy for his hip molds and had greater success. This device was commercially released (see Fig. 2).

1938: Wiles designed and implanted six, all-stainless steel total hips. The acetabular cups were held in place with bone

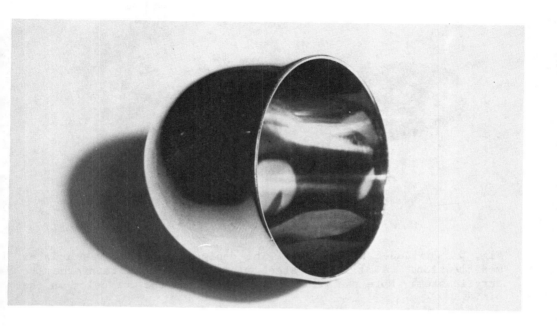

Fig. 2   The Smith Petersen interposition hip arthroplasty implant.
1937.

screws and the femoral component was a shell covering the femoral
head and supported by a pin-and-plate device similar to those used
for femoral neck and intertrochanteric fractures. After loosening
and fatigue failures, the device was redesigned in 1957 and bone
resorption and loosening followed.

1939:   Bohlman implanted a femor head replacement with a
trifin spike for fixation. After loosening occurred he added a
collar to bear against the cut bone face.

1946:   The Judet brothers commenced a long series of acrylic
femoral-head-replacement prostheses. Large quantities of these
implants were used by many surgeons. Unlike the devices of
Smith-Petersen and Wiles, this design was not a shell covering the
femoral head but was a solid, three-quarter sphere, i.e., the
natural femoral head was necessarily resected. The support stem
was a short acrylic peg (later reinforced with a stainless steel
core pin) which passed along the center of the femoral neck to the
lateral cortex of the greater trochanter (see Fig. 3).

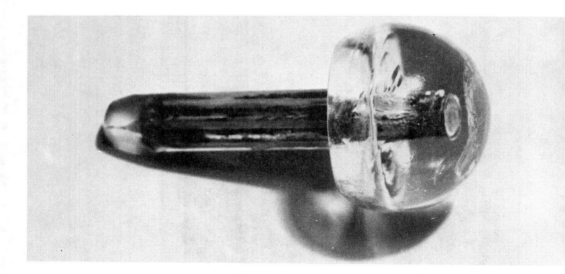

Fig. 3   The Judet hip.   1946.   The design shown here was a later
modification.   A stainless steel pin was added to reinforce the
acrylic stem.   Note the wear on the sphere and the corrosion on the
pin.

     1950:   McKee metal-metal total hip.   (Stainless steel
initially).   This used a small diameter ball-and-socket joint.   The
acetabular cup was screwed into the pelvis and then bone screws
were added to prevent it backing out.   The femoral component was
similar in form to the Judet design.   The stem, which supported the
prosthesis head passed along the femoral neck.   The ball-and-socket
joint was captive to prevent dislocation in service.   The square-
threaded end to the stem engaged with a bone plate which was fitted
to the lateral femoral cortex (see Fig. 4).

     1951/1952:   Thompson femoral head replacement.   This was
mounted on a stem which was not straight.   Instead, it was curved
to pass along the femoral neck and down the intramedullary canal
(see Fig. 5).

     1951/1952:   Austin Moore femoral head replacement.   This was
similar to the Thompson design.   However, the stem section was
rectangular and two large fenestrations were included in the large
proximal stem section.   These fenestrations were often packed with
bone chips to cause the formation of a bony bridge which held the
implant in place (see Fig. 5).

     1956:   McKee modified his metal-metal total hip.   The acetab-
ular component remained similar to that shown in Fig. 4.   The

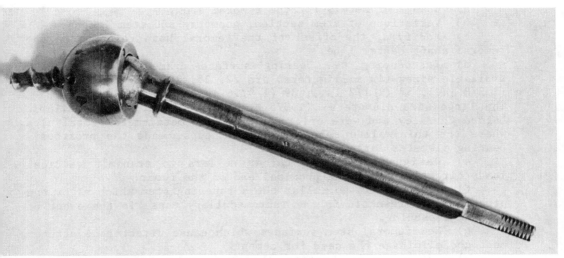

Fig. 4   McKee total hip.   The square threaded end to the stem
engaged with a bone plate not shown in this photograph.   The first
prototype was dated 1940 but the first implant was dated 1950.

femoral component was a modification of the Thompson stem with a
change in sphere diameter.   In 1960, the McKee-Farrar total hip
added the use of acrylic bone cement.   The femoral component hardly
changed; a larger head diameter, but the acetabular component was
very different (see Fig. 6).

1958/1966:   The development of the Charnley total hip introduced acrylic bone cement, a stainless steel femoral component with
a 22 mm diameter femoral head and intramedullary stem, an acetabular cup of high-density, ultra-high-molecular-weight (UHMW)
polyethylene and a new operative technique which improved access to
the hip by detaching the greater trochanter and reattaching it at
the end of the procedure.   The Charnley total hip was commercially
released in 1966 (see Fig. 7).

1974/1977:   Several designers returned to surface replacement
arthroplasty: eliminated the femoral intramedullary stem, relined
the femoral head with a metal shell and the acetabulum with a polyethylene liner.

With the exception of the development of the surface hip
replacement (which has lost much of its popularity now) modern
designs of total hip prostheses are all of the Charnley type.   The
modifications are of a detail design nature and, unlike the changes
from 1923 to 1966, do not challenge the total design concept.
Points of variation are:

a) Change of metals for the femoral stem.

b) Variations of stem section, geometry and stem lengths.

c) Modifying the offset of the femoral head relative to the femoral shaft center line.

d) Introducing new bearing surface diameters. Currently available sizes (in millimeters) are 22, 25, 26, 28, 29, 30, 32, 35 (1 3/8 in.), 38 (1 1/2 in.), 39 (1 9/16 in.) and 41 (1 5/8 in.). The large size diameters (1.375 in. to 1.625 in.) were available before Charnley and were originally used in metal-metal total hips where the thin-walled metal acetabular cups, made the prosthesis bearing diameter large.

e) Designs with large calcar collars to transmit vertical loads directly on the cut proximal end of the femur.

f) Designs with no collar but a tapering stem which allow the prosthesis to resettle in the intramedullary canal in the event of implant loosening.

g) New femoral stem surfaces which cause direct bone attachment and eliminate the need for cement.

h) Metal shells housing the UHMW polyethylene acetabular bearing surface. The shell may be present to allow for easy replacement of the liner (should it wear out). It may add rigidity

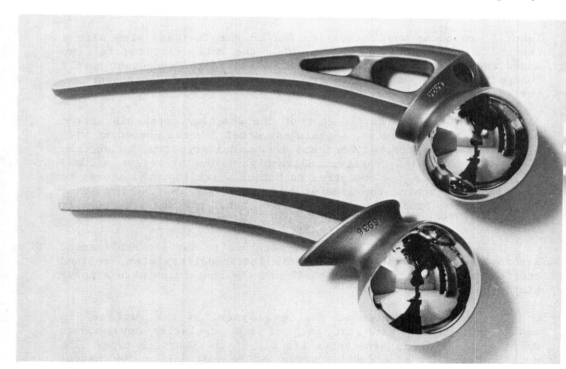

Fig. 5   The Austin Moore (top) and F R. Thompson designs of femoral head replacement. 1951/1952.

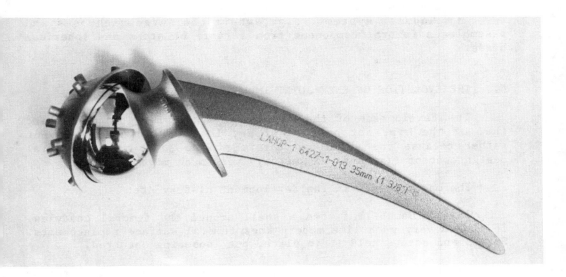

Fig. 6   The McKee-Farrar metal—metal total hip for use with acrylic
bone cement.   1960 onward.

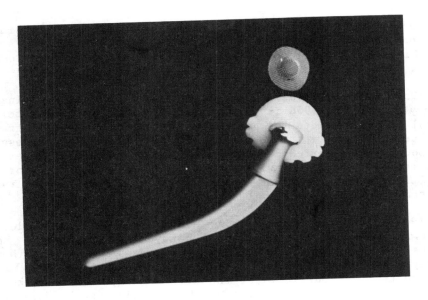

Fig. 7   The Charnley total hip.

to the acetabular component, thereby reducing the risk of cement fracture, or it may provide for direct bone attachment and eliminate the need for cement.

i) Modular systems, e.g., where the surgeon chooses and assembles a femoral component from a range of stems and spherical heads.

4.   THE EVOLUTION OF KNEE JOINT IMPLANT DESIGN

The development of the knee joint arthroplasty lagged behind that of the hip, not because of any lesser clinical need, but rather because the shape and nature of the joint made the total design concept (implant and surgery) very much more complex.

The major events in the development history are:

1940:   Campbell fitted a shell around the femoral condyles. It looked very much like modern knee femoral surface replacements. Spikes and screws held it in place, but loosening occurred.

1940/1942:   Smith-Petersen and Aufranc commenced mold arthroplasty at the knee following success with the hip mold since 1937. This was a bicondylar femoral liner with a fin which pressed into the bone for fixation. An intramedullary stem was later added.

1949:   Majnoni D'Intignano implanted a simple hinge knee made of acrylic.

1950:   Moeys used a simple all-metal hinge knee. Th simple hinge only allows flexion-extension of the knee. As will be seen, later hinge knees introduced other linear or rotary laxity into the design.

1951/1958:   Walldius developed a simple hinge knee, originally in acrylic, but by 1958 it was changed to Vitallium.® An anterior femoral flange provided for patellar articulation. Fins penetrated the bone to prevent rotation of the components within their respective bones. This device continues to be implanted today, albeit in small quantities. More recent modifications have provided for use with bone cement. Clinical problems include limited flexion range and stem loosening (see Fig. 8).

1952/1964:   Several surgeons designed metal tibial plateau against which the natural femoral condyles articulated. Most designs were unicondylar (MacIntosh and McKeever) although Townley's design covered both tibial bearing surfaces and had a large central cut out to clear the cruciate ligaments. Walker(9) does not give a date to the Townley design, although he does state that it came after a similar implant with only posterior cruciate

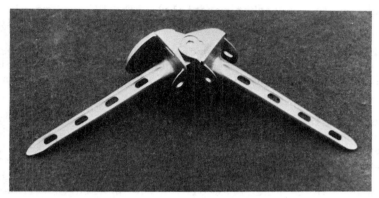

Fig. 8 The Walldius knee. The fins press into the bone. This was designed for use without bone cement.

ligament retention by Virgin and Carrell in 1941. The MacIntosh design was converted to Vitallium® in 1964 and is still in use. (see Fig. 9).

1953/1963: Several other surgeons designed their own simple hinge knee prostheses (Shiers, Young, MacAusland). The original Shiers' design was all stainless steel and suffered from intra-medullary stem breakage and infections.

1952: Walker reports the devices of Wilson, Scales and Lettin and again Kraft and Levinthal, which replaced not only the knee joint but large amounts of bony tumor along the bone shafts. They

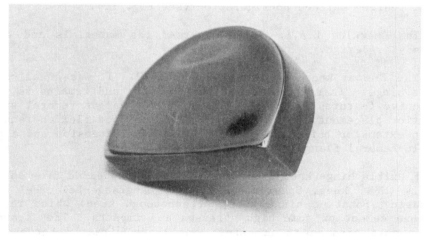

Fig. 9 The MacIntosh tibial plateau. The under surface, not seen in this photograph, is a roughened surface with no fins or keels.

both used acrylic (and other materials). The Wilson (et al) design employed flanges outside the bone and used screws for fixation.

1952/1959: The original concept of Campbell (1940), namely a metal shell placed over the femoral condyles was further developed by Finkelstein and Didinski in New York and later by Platt and Peppler in Britain.

1966: Following the success of the Charnley total hip in 1966, bone cement and UHMW polyethylene were soon applied to knee joint replacement. Gunston produced a unicondylar knee with a metal femoral condyle and plastic tibial plateau. The femoral component fitted into a deep and wide slot in the femoral condyle which could cause bone fracture. The bearing surfaces were analogous to a wheel (metal) running in a straight groove of semi-circular section (plastic). The metal femoral component was heavily constrained, both to orient itself and to move along the plastic tibial track.

From the Mayo Clinic came the Geometric knee (Coventry, Finerman, Riley, Turner, and Upshaw), in 1972. This was a bicondylar knee. The metal femoral component comprised two part-spherical bearing surfaces linked with a bridge. The tibial component was the same: the bearing surfaces being concave to match the convex femoral surfaces. The cruciate ligaments were retained. Loosening of the tibial component has been the major problem, although many surgeons are continuing to implant the device today with good results (see Fig. 10).

Many other designs of total knee surface replacement have since appeared, all using the metal femoral shell and polyethylene tibial bearing surface configuration (see Fig. 11).

The Charnley L.A.I.[®] knee reversed the materials and was a unicondylar design.

The Guepar knee was introduced in 1970. It was an all-metal simple hinge. It rapidly became very popular and remains so. The attractive features are: left and right $7°$ valgus femoral stems, posterior placement of the axle pin allowing good flexion range, a rubber extension buffer to prevent noisy hyperextension and a good patello-femoral flange.

Flexible hinge knee prostheses have also appeared from several centers (GSB[®] knee, Spherocentric[®] knee, Langrange-Letournel knee, Kinematic[®] rotating hinge knee, Attenborough knee) which relieve the bone cement of some high stresses and impacts. They leave it to the soft tissues to transfer some loads directly between the tibia and femur and allow them to act as shock absorbers.

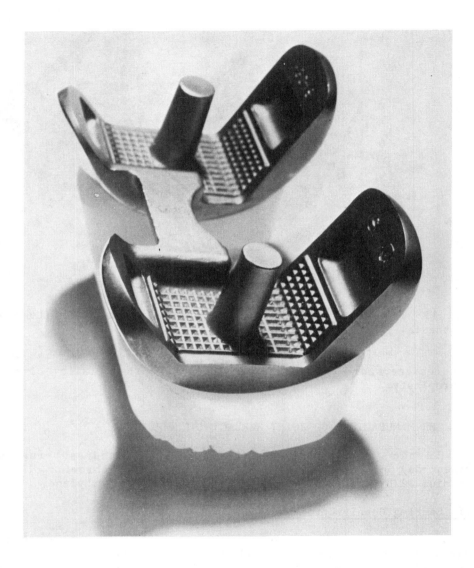

Fig. 10 The Geometric Knee from the Mayo Clinic.

The evolution of knee prostheses closes with the present period of greater attention to detail design, as is happening also to hip implants. Metal housings for plastic tibial bearing surfaces are appearing, as for acetabular cups. Cementable and noncementable knee designs are now available. Improved instrumentation shows

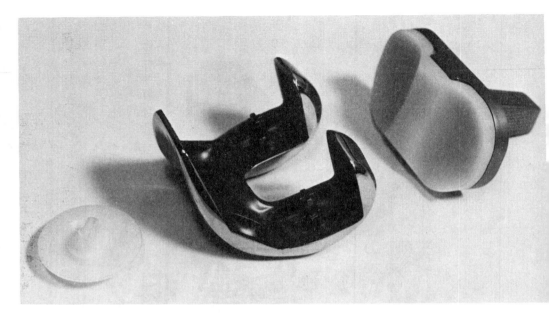

Fig. 11   A typical modern day surface replacement total-knee
prosthesis.   The Kinematic[TM] knee.

that designers are giving greater thought to the totality of the
arthroplasty.

5.   THE MANUFACTURE OF JOINT REPLACEMENT IMPLANTS

In the chapter on biomaterials, those listed as being in
present-day use were stainless steel, cast cobalt-chromium alloy,
titanium alloy, other cobalt-based alloys, UHMW polyethylene,

5.1   Casting Cobalt-Chromium Alloy

The so-called rough, or unfinished casting is produced by
pouring molten cobalt-chromium alloy into a ceramic mold or shell.
The cavity within the mold usually provides for several castings to
be produced and thus there is a network of feeders, runners and
risers to provide for metal flow and gas escape.   The molten alloy
can be produced by melting granules, chips or billets sized from
precast bar stock.   The melting temperature of cobalt chromium is
about 1350 - 1400 ^{o}C but it is poured at 1500 - 1650 ^{o}C into the
shell which is preheated to around 1000 - 1100 ^{o}C.   The precise
temperatures vary from product to product.   The shape of the cavity
to be filled, and the surface area (which affects cooling rate and

grain structure) influence the final choice of temperatures. Once established, the optimum mold and casting temperatures are carefully controlled. The casting flow can be induced by gravity, vacuum or centrifugal action. The model can be filled in atmospheric or vacuum conditions.

The ceramic mold is necessarily destroyed to reveal the solidified metal "tree" of castings attached to their metal feeder network. Destroying the ceramic and removing it from small recesses designed into the casting can be difficult. Pneumatic vibrators, water jets, sand blasters, leaching tanks, and an array of miscellaneous techniques can be used for this operation.

The castings are detached from the "tree" using thin, abrasive, rotary cutting discs, and the remaining stubs are ground down close to the required surface of the casting using abrasive belting machines. The metal in the discarded feeders can be reprocessed and then reused.

The resulting rough casting might be solution heat treated depending on the material characteristics required by the manufacturer.

The dimensions of the casting will usually be oversize compared to final design specifications to allow for subsequent finishing operations.

The casting process just described is entitled investment casting or the lost-wax process. For every casting required, one ceramic mold is made and destroyed. This mold is manufactured by first creating a wax "tree." This is made up of slightly oversize replicas of the eventual casting in a wax material, often based on beeswax or paraffin wax with several additives. Plastics such as polystyrene may also be used. The wax models are assembled to wax posts which define the metal feeder system. The "tree" of wax models with wax post is fitted to a ceramic pouring cup.

The complete assembly, the "tree", is then given several (typically 8) coats of a refractory slurry material. A fine layer of sand adheres to the outside of each slurry coat while it is still wet. The first coat is then allowed to dry. The second slurry coat, then applied, adheres to the fine sandy surface of the first coat.

The first coat might contain a proprietary nucleation inoculant to give a fine surface grain structure. The particle sizes in the first slurry coat and sand spray are very fine in order to give a good surface finish to the casting. In subsequent coats, particle sizes increase as the main function is to give strength to the shell.

The drying process for each coat must be well controlled. This necessitates frequent monitoring of the atmospheric conditions (humidity and temperature) and the slurry parameters (viscosity, density and drying time). After the last slurry coat is dry, the wax is melted out in an oven or steam autoclave leaving the mold with a good surface finish on the cavity wall. It then goes into the furnace in preparation for casting.

The wax models on which the ceramic mold is formed are usually made by injecting the wax into a metal mold. The temperature and pressure of this operation are important as the wax shrinks in the mold on solidification. Designing wax injection molds requires that dimensional allowances be made for finishing of the metal casting, shrinkage of the metal within the ceramic mold and shrinkage of the wax pattern within the wax mold.

Designing the mold also involves designing the gating system through which the metal will fill and feed the casting. The number, position, shape and orientation of the gates are critical to the eventual quality of the casting.

5.2 Forging

For orthopedic implants, only cobalt-chromium alloy is cast. However, all implant metals are forgable including cobalt-chromium. Forged cobalt-chromium has superior fatigue strength compared to the cast alloy. However, it is not an easy material to forge and this increases the cost of manufacture enough to leave a place in the market for both materials.

One further advantage of casting is that it offers much greater flexibility to the designer. Forgings must have simple shapes, otherwise, dies will break or wear out rapidly and the metal will not fill small surface features. With both casting and forging it is desirable that as much detail as possible is cast in or forged in. Leaving the creation of design features to the finishing operations can be expensive.

There are several variations of the forging process: hammer forging, drop forging, closed-die forging, and swaging. All are used in orthopedic implant manufacture. The variations between them are the cost and life of dies, the forging time per unit of production, the quality of the forging particularly in terms of the amount of finishing required, the material characteristics (some processes put more work into the forging than others), and the material usage per unit of production.

Forgings may be heat treated to improve corrosion resistance (particularly stainless steel) or to facilitate the finishing processes. Stainless steel is easy to forge hot and it may be done cold. Cobalt-chromium can only be forged hot.

Titanium forging temperatures must be well controlled to prevent oxidation, otherwise, it is not a difficult material to forge. MP35N was developed as a forging alloy.

5.3 Molding

Polyacetal homopolymer can be injection molded to form total hip prosthesis components. The molding parameters are established by the material supplier. The main manufacturing constraint in molding implants is that additives used in non-medical applications are avoided: release agents that ease removal of the product from the mold, lubricants, fillers and pigments. Also, for reasons of contamination control, the normal industrial practice of recycling the material in the sprues and in scrap components is not permitted.

UHMW polyethylene can also be injection molded, but it is difficult and rare. However, compression molding is more common. Injection molding fills a fixed cavity volume with molten plastic and holds the pressure in the cavity as the material solidifies. Compression molding commences with an accurately determined volume of which is introduced into one half of the heated mold. The other half of the mold is introduced and compresses the plastic material. As the two halves of the mold are a precise fit, the plastic cannot escape. The pressure and the temperature are controlled as the plastic solidifies, taking the form of the mold cavity. It is the volume of plastic material at the start of the cycle which determines the finished dimensions of the molded component.

Alumina forming can involve injection molding. Particles of alumina are mixed with a thermoplastic material. A molding is then produced which is fired to burn away the thermoplastic matrix material and the alumina is sintered, using a high-pressure, high-temperature fusing process. The initial molding is very much larger than the final sintered product, due to the loss of volume which occurs as the plastic is removed.

5.4 Welding

The major application of welding in orthopedics is in creating hollow femoral heads on hip prostheses. With all-titanium alloy components it is not necessary, as the forging process can produce large diameters without adverse material consequences and the low density does not cause adverse comment from surgeons concerning weight distribution. Some titanium alloy hips do have cobalt-

chromium femoral heads attached, either by mechanical means
(interference or shrink fitting) or by welding.

Stainless steel femoral heads on total hips can be forged
solid and there is no weight problem. The same is not true for
large diameter hemiendoprostheses which can be forged but suffer
from a weight distribution disadvantage. (This is probably of no
biomechanical significance but often gives rise to customer
resistance). The structure of stainless steels is very sensitive
to thermal treatments and inter-granular corrosion can result.
Williams and Roaf(10), in 1973, stated that no stainless steel
implant component was welded and the British Standard (3531)
advises against welding stainless steel for orthopedic implants.

With few exceptions, almost all femoral heads in cobalt-
chromium are welded to the stem. This may be done by T.I.G.
(tungsten inert gas) welding, or electron-beam welding.

Cast hips, with 22 mm head sizes, are all cast solid. Forged
cobalt-chromium heads can be and are sometimes forged solid, but
for reasons of supplying forged stems with a variety of head
diameters and satisfying a market preference for the long-
established cast cobalt-chromium bearing surface, the head and stem
are usually not integrally forged.

5.5 Machining and Finishing

Stainless steel is the easiest of present-day orthopedic
metals to machine and finish. Conventional turning and milling
operations, using relatively unsophisticated cutting materials, may
be used, particularly when the material is in the annealed state.
Spherical heads may be turned and polished. The material is
usually electro-polished to avoid crevice-corrosion problems,
although, to improve bone cement fixation, some stainless steel
devices do now have sand-blasted stems. It is essential that
stainless steel is passivated in nitric acid and then well washed.
This removes any iron particles from the finishing process which
could lead to corrosion and it also thickens the passive oxide
layer.

All orthopedic metals are suitable for electro-chemical
machining, spark erosion, and etching by electro-chemical or
laser-beam processes.

Finishing cobalt-chromium alloys is difficult, as they work
harden so rapidly. Thus metal is removed usually by grinding,
abrasive belting and stoning operations, all of which remove small
superficial positive or negative defects, flash lines and casting
gates. Spherical grinding of femoral heads and cam grinding of
femoral knee bearing surfaces are performed to achieve the

necessary precision. It is possible to machine the alloy, but diamond and tungsten carbide cutters have to be used. Cobalt-chromium is suited to sand-blasting which does not have adverse corrosion consequences. Shot peening is often used to improve fatigue strength. Nitric acid cleaning is recommended, primarily for the removal of iron particles which may be left on the surface from finishing operations.

Most conventional machining techniques can be used with titanium. As the material galls and seizes easily, the cutting tool must be very rigidly supported. If the material is allowed to become hot, it can become explosive. Slow machine speeds and feeds and good workpiece cooling are necessary. It is particularly difficult to obtain good sphericity and roundness on a titanium alloy femoral head.

UHMW polyethylene and polyacetal homopolymer are usually machine finished. Acetabular cup bearing surfaces may be turned using a form tool which plunges into the rotating cup. Single-point-profile turning is used and fly cutting, in which both tool and workpiece revolve on oblique axes to generate the spherical surface. External profiles can be machined using form-tool turning, profile turning and conventional grooving, drilling and milling operations. X-ray wires are attached by a variety of mechanical methods or by locally molding or welding the plastic material over the wire.

5.6 Packaging and Sterilization

More and more joint replacement prostheses are being supplied in a pre-sterilized state. It is essential for UHMW polyethylene as it cannot be autoclaved and ethylene oxide is not recommended, due to possible dimensional changes and the residual toxic vapor which can remain on the implant. Polyethylene is sterilized, either by electron beam or gamma irradiation. Conventionally, sterile products are supplied in a double sterile pack because this suits operating theatre practice and tradition. The entire contents of the outer pack, including its own inside surface, are sterile.

The same packaging technique is used for bone cement. Both the monomer and the powder are in a double pack. The monomer is in an ampoule contained in a polyethylene bag or blister pack. The powder is usually in a double polyethylene bag. The most important aspects of bone-cement manufacture are in the packaging, control of sterility and the quality control of the raw materials. The mixing of the components will not be discussed here.

To have confidence in the sterility of a product, it is important to control the maximum level of contamination of the product at the time of packaging (the bioburden). The configuration of products in the sterilization container must be consistent. Dose-mapping exercises to determine whether any radiation shadows exist, which could impair sterility, are conducted. Thereafter, as irradiation takes place routinely, sample dosimeters are placed in the containers at the established points of lowest intensity, so that the reading will show a minimum absorbed dose.

Many regulatory agencies demand that spore strips be included in the sterilization container. After irradiation, the spore strips and a sample of the product are tested while the full batch is held in quarantine. Only on negative results may the batch be released for distribution.

However, it is not enough to perform end-product sterility testing without establishing the effectiveness of the total process. Otherwise, one can never have confidence that the product samples and spore strips are representative of the batch.

To control the bioburden levels, which are defined in terms of bacteria densities and particulate densities for differing particle sizes, it is becoming common practice to use controlled environment areas, clean rooms and sterile rooms for packaging operations.

To maintain the sterility of the liquid monomer in bone cements is relatively easy as it is considered to be self sterilizing. The ampoules are cleaned and sterilized prior to filling. The containers and devices used to transfer the liquid into the bottle are also sterilized. The ampoule is filled and flame sealed. (As the monomer is explosive, this operation is very well controlled). The ampoule is put in a blister pack with a Tyvek® lid and is ethylene-oxide sterilized, which only affects the outside of the ampoule and the inside of the blister pack (the Tyvek® material is permeable to vapor but not penetrable by bacteria). The monomer may not be sterilized by heat or radiation as they would cause it to polymerize.

The powder can be gamma irradiated, although this does slow down the eventual setting process. It is also considered by many to be self-sterilizing. Some brands of cement place a formaldehyde vapor tablet between the two packs to sterilize only the packaging but not the contents. Charnley, in his monograph on cement, states his preference for non-irradiated cement powder(11).

In antibiotic bone cements, the powder may not be sterilized in any way once the antibiotic has been mixed. Therefore, the powder may be sterilized prior to mixing and thereafter it is processed in closely controlled sterile conditions.

6. QUALITY ASSURANCE AND REGULATORY AFFAIRS

Quality assurance is responsible for assuring that a company's products optimally satisfy customers' needs. But, within the context of this chapter, the technical role is limited to evaluation of the design (can the product perform adequately?) and evaluation of what is produced (does the product meet specification?).

Regulatory affairs agencies (notably the USA Food and Drug Administration) demand that adequate pre-market testing of a product is performed to support its introduction into the marketplace. They also demand that batch records are maintained to demonstrate that products were made according to specification and that all testing and critical operations (including inspection) were properly conducted at the appropriate time and by the appropriate people. The demands of these agencies also cover training, cleaning, maintenance, and many other aspects of manufacturing, but these will not be discussed here.

The testing required for a new design has briefly been mentioned earlier in the chapter. Depending on the nature of the novel features, appropriate tests have to be defined: toxicity tests, wear tests, fatigue tests, strength tests, etc. These will be conducted in laboratories, on animals or human beings, as appropriate.

Testing of products through manufacture involves:

a) Receiving inspection of bought-in raw materials, finished or semi-finished products and subcontracted operations on products.
b) Final inspection which releases the batch for sale.
c) Intermediate and in-process testing which monitors the manufacturing process.

It is frequently impractical to control quality only by testing the product. By ensuring that the process is performing correctly, not only will the incidence of scrapped products be controlled, but confidence in the quality of what is sold increases.

Technical tests, other than dimensional and visual inspection, which might be performed as part of the manufacturing process include: strength and ductility tests on material as received and on a sample of finished product, hardness tests (particularly for monitoring heat treatment), crack testing, X-ray testing, chemical analysis and sterility testing.

Fatigue testing, wear testing, and biocompatibility testing would only be performed as part of the design process. Once the specification is established, tests only need to check those features which can vary from batch to batch during manufacture.

REFERENCES

1.   Asimow, M.   Introduction to Design (Prentice Hall Publisher, 1964).

2.   Ratcliffe, W.E.   Designs and Plastics.   Plastics (Feb. 1967).

3.   Dixon, J.R.   Design Engineering (McGraw Hill, 1966).

4.   de Bono, E.   Children Solve Problems (Penquin Education, 1972).

5.   de Bono, E.   The Use of Lateral Thinking (Pelican Books, 1967).

6.   de Bono, E.   Practical Thinking: Four Ways to be Right; Five Ways to be Wrong; Five Ways to Understand (Pelican Books, 1971).

7.   de Bono, E.   Lateral Thinking (Pelican Books, 1977).

8.   Kepner, C.H. and Tregoe, B.B.   The Rational Manager (Kepner-Tregoe Inc., 1965).

9.   Walker, P.S.   Human Joints and Their Artificial Replacements (Charles C. Thomas Publisher, 1977).

10. Williams, D.F. and Roaf, R.   Implants in Surgery (W.B. Saunders Co., Ltd., 1973).

11. Charnley, J.   Acrylic Cement in Orthopaedic Surgery (Churchill Livingstone, 1972).

STRESS ANALYSIS AND FIXATION PROBLEMS IN JOINT REPLACEMENT

R. Huiskes

Biomechanics Section, Lab. Exp. Orthopaedics, University of Nijmegen, 6500 HB Nijmegen, The Netherlands

1. INTRODUCTION

Artificial joint replacement is a procedure performed relatively often in modern orthopaedic surgery. An estimated total of 65,000 patients annually in the U.S.A. (1), for example, and probably about an equal number in the rest of the world, receive total hip replacement (THR) for relief of pain and restoration of function. Most of these patients are over 60 years of age, and have severe osteoarthritis of the hip. Smaller groups suffer from post-traumatic conditions, rheumatoid arthritis or other disorders. Very few are younger than 50. THR represents major surgery, which is very successful as a treatment of severe disorders of the hip, both from the point of view of immediate post-operative pain relief and restoration of function, as well as its long-term results (1).

Less impressive in numbers, but following as a good second and increasing, is the amount of knee-joint replacements performed on a regular basis. Finger joints, too, are replaced quite frequently, for rheumatoid arthritis patients in particular. Other joints replaced less often are the shoulder, elbow and ankle. Whereas the clinical and engineering design problems in replacements of the various joints differ considerably, the most severe difficulties, those related to fixation of the implants to the bone, have a common denominator. Although this chapter will mainly focus on hip joint replacement, it must be kept in mind that the objectives and methods discussed here are applicable to joint replacement in general.

The success of joint replacement has followed major advances in surgical techniques and biomedical engineering during the last

20 years. Charnley (2), in 1960, introduced the use of acrylic cement as a space-filling fixation material and the concept of "low-friction" THR, replacing the acetabular component of the joint with a plastic cup and the femoral component with a metal endoprosthesis (Fig. 1.a). These concepts proved to be viable, and still today form the fundamentals on which many joint replacement procedures rest. Further improvements followed gradually, based on clinical and experimental research. In particular, the metals and plastics used for the prosthetic components became stronger, and the cementing technique matured through the application of cement syringes and pressurization.

Although joint replacement is successful, it is not without problems. Probably, the most severe long-term complication is aseptic loosening. Although the average life-span of the replacement system appears to be adequate in view of the age limitations usually applied to patients, it is certain that its integrity cannot be guaranteed forever. This is indicated by the increasing percentage of protheses that loosen in the course of post-operative time. Aseptic loosening is usually accompanied by failure of the cement mantle and the presence of a soft fibrous tissue layer between the cement mantle and the bone. Sometimes component fracture will occur in addition. Quite often massive bone resorption is seen at the proximal side of the femur after THR. These late complications are a particular threat to patients operated at young ages. However, the fibrous tissue liners at the cement-bone interface are also found to increase progressively in a relatively large number of patients with 5 to 10 years follow-up on post-operative X-rays (e.g. 3). Such liners are usually interpreted as a sign for forthcoming loosening.

The causes and mechanisms of late aseptic loosening are not well understood as yet. Obviously, (fatigue) fracture of prosthetic components is directly related to high stresses, as is fracture of the cement mantle. Massive bone resorption of the proximal femur is often thought to be related to reduction of stresses, when compared to those in the intact bone. Interface bone resorption and remodeling, which precedes the occurrence of fibrous tissue membranes, have been attributed to several causes. There is little dispute that in the initial stage, directly following implantation, a small layer of bone is necrotized and resorbed at the interface. This dead bone is a result of mechanical (vascular) damage during the bone preparation, leakage of cell-toxic monomer (monomethylmethacrylate) out of the acrylic cement mixture, and/or thermal damage due to heat generated within the curing cement (4, 5).

In a subsequent process of bone resorption and formation at the interface, stresses and strains probably play an important role to determine the eventual fixation strength. Whereas bone

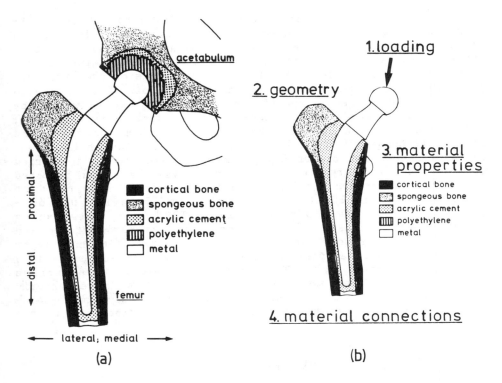

Fig. 1 (a) Schematic illustration of a (Charnley type) total hip replacement (THR); the metal and plastic components are fixated in the bone with a filling material, acrylic bone cement, a self-curing polymethylmethacrylate (PMMA); (b) the stress distribution within the materials and at their connections depends on four structural aspects, as indicated in the figure.

resorption and the formation of a soft fibrous tissue membrane between the implant and the bone can probably not be avoided altogether (2, 4-7), subsequent bone formation in that layer no doubt depends on local stresses and micromotions, and thus on joint loading (8).

It is obvious from the previous discussion that local stresses and strains play an important role in the chances for long-term survival of bone-prosthesis structures, in view of both structural strength and biological interface reactions. These stresses and strains are generated in the process of load transmission from the prosthesis to the bone, which is the most important function of the fixation structure (9).

The distribution of these stresses (Fig. 1.b), their magnitudes and orientations throughout the structure, depends on structural properties, i.e. loading characteristics, geometry, material properties and physical conditions at the interfaces. Hence, the stresses occurring within the materials of the structure and at their interfaces depend not only on the joint load, but also on the prosthetic design specifications and the way in which the components are placed into the bone. Optimal stress distributions, in other words, can only be obtained with optimal designs and fixation techniques. To evaluate stresses and study their dependency on structural properties, stress analyses must be carried out. A relatively large number of such analyses have been reported in the recent orthopaedic biomechanics literature, many of which aimed at shedding light on the mechanical behavior of bone-prosthesis structures, particularly in THR. Many interesting questions were addressed in these analyses, as for instance the effects on the stress distributions of acrylic cement layer thickness, implant material properties and design, joint loading, and fixation techniques. The aims and scopes of these stress analyses, and the three most commonly applied methods, i.e. experimental strain-gage techniques, analytical ("closed-form") solutions, and finite element methods, are briefly discussed in the following sections.

2. EXPERIMENTAL STRAIN-GAGE ANALYSIS

To understand the principles of experimental stress analysis, it must be appreciated that stresses cannot be determined directly, but only indirectly, by measuring their effects. The effects are deformations, represented by displacements between points, or strains. Of all strain measuring methods feasible (e.g. 10), strain-gage techniques have been applied most frequently in biomechanics (11).

Electrical strain-gages are based on the principle that the resistance of a material changes when stretched. The gage consists of a small electrical resistance which is glued to the surface of the structure, in a certain orientation. The change in voltage over the resistance is directly proportional to the relative change in its length. Thus, the strain registered is an average value over the length of the gage along its specific orientation. Strain gages are generally suitable to measure strains at free surfaces, where the strain state can be characterized by three variables, two principal strain magnitudes and the principal strain direction. These variables can be obtained by using strain rosettes with three elements, each registering strain in its specific direction. The stresses can subsequently be calculated from the measured strains, using Hooke's law of linear elasticity and the material properties (e.g. 11, 12).

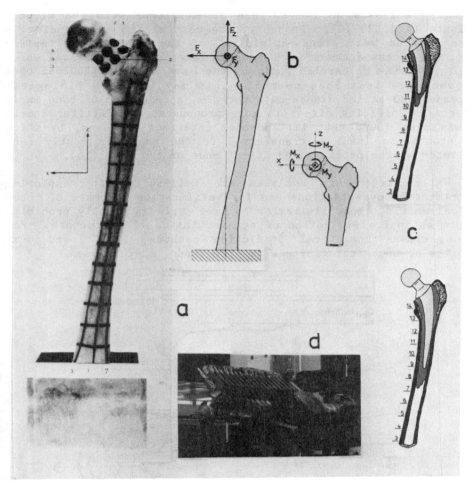

Fig. 2 Experimental strain gage analysis of a femur. Strain gages
were attached at the intersections of the black lines (a); forces
in 3 directions and moments in 3 planes were applied to the head
(b); measurements were performed on the intact femur and after
insertion of various hip prostheses (c); and (d) shows the
laboratory setting (reproduced from Ref. 19).

Strain gages have frequently been used in stress analyses of
bones, both in vivo (e.g. 13), and in vitro (e.g. 14). An example
of a laboratory setting of a human femur is shown in Fig. 2. In
this particular case, the strains on the femoral surface were
evaluated not only to study the mechanical behavior of the intact
bone under loading, but also to evaluate the influences of hip
replacement by intramedullary prostheses (14). Other studies of
this kind were also carried out by other investigators, all

comparing stresses on the surface of the femur with and without
implants (e.g. 15-18). Probably, the most significant finding in
these studies was "stress-shielding" of the bone by the implant
(Fig. 3). Because the prosthetic stem takes part of the load which
would otherwise be carried fully by the bone, the longitudinal bone
stresses are less than normal. This may induce a biological
process of so-called disuse-osteoporosis, a reduction of bone mass.
The stress-shielding effect is more pronounced with stiffer stems.
It was also found that implant-bone interface stresses, by which
the prosthetic load is transferred to the bone, is mostly con-
centrated at the proximal and distal ends of the stem (16).

While strain-gage analyses are well-suited for exploring
experimental investigations and for verification purposes of theoretical models, their limitation to free surfaces usually prohibits
a more extensive evaluation of strains inside the structure. For
this purpose theoretical prediction methods, as "closed-form"
theories or numerical finite element methods, must be used.

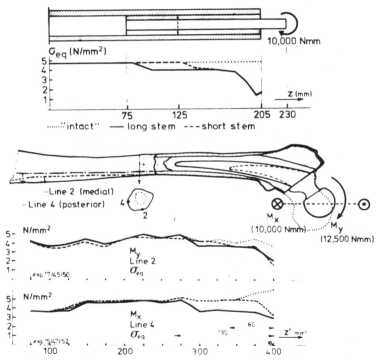

Fig. 3 Equivalent stresses at the outside surface of the femur,
intact and with two bending couples in different planes,
respectively. On the proximal side of the stem, the "stress-
shielding" effect of the stems with respect to the bone is easily
recognized, and again emphasized in a simplified, general model of
the intramedullary fixation structure (reproduced from Ref. 19).

3.   ANALYTICAL ("CLOSED-FORM") ANALYSIS

In experimental stress analysis a physical model is used, which for example can be a prototype. In theoretical analysis the model is mathematical, i.e. a set of equations. Theoretical methods can be divided into analytical and numerical ones. The former is used if the four structural aspects, discussed earlier, can be made to fit into a mechanics theory, for which "closed-form" solutions exist. In this case, the mathematical equations are solved directly, yielding formulas in which the stress magnitudes are directly related to the parameters describing the structural aspects. Numerical methods, including finite element methods, are based on the use of computers. The complex mathematical problem is reduced to a numerical procedure and the relationship between the resultant stress values and structural parameters is usually not obvious. Examples of closed form theories which are frequently applied in biomechanics are linear-elastic bar theory, beam theory and torsion shaft theory. All three are valid for slender, prismatic bodies whose length is much larger than the thickness, made out of linear elastic, isotropic and homogeneous materials, loaded in axial tension or compression, transverse forces or bending, and torsion, respectively. These theories are available for 2-D and 3-D structures, uniform and variable cross-sections, straight and curved bodies. Although, particularly in biomechanics, structures seldom behave exactly in accordance with these theories, approximative models can sometimes be developed. Prosthetic stems, bone pins and rods are good examples of structures that yield to these theories. Other examples include bone plates, although the holes present a complication, and diaphyses of long bones, by a rough approximation (14). Other simple closed-form theories used in hard tissue biomechanics are compound-beam theory (applied to bone-fixation plate and bone-prosthetic stem composites), beam-on-elastic-foundation theory (prosthetic stem and tibial plateau fixation), and plate and shell theories (skull).

Closed-form solutions are attractive for obtaining approximative solutions for certain problems. They often give a direct insight into relations between essential structural parameters and stress behavior. Their application is cheap, leads to results rapidly and they are therefore often used to obtain first-order reference solutions for more advanced experimental and numerical analyses.

As an example of an analytical analysis, which is relevant for the hip joint prosthesis-bone structure, consider a generalized intramedullary cemented stem structure with a uniform axisymmetric cross-section (Fig. 4). We limit ourselves to axial loading (N_o), other loading cases have been discussed elsewhere (9, 19). The question is how this load is transferred from the stem to the bone

through the cement layer, and in what way is the load-transferring
mechanism influenced by the structural parameters.

To fit this problem to a closed-form theory, it is assumed
that the stem and the bone, separately, behave according to bar
theory, i.e. that their cross-sections remain plane in deformed
state (e.g. 20). This implies that the axial stresses, (σ_z), in
a cross-section are distributed homogeneously (Fig. 4). We then
define the internal stem force, $N_s(z)$, and the internal bone force,
$N_b(z)$, according to

$$N_s = \sigma_{zs} A_s \qquad \text{and} \qquad N_b = \sigma_{zb} A_b \qquad (1)$$

where the subscripts s and b denote stem and bone respectively, and
A is the cross-sectional area. We further define the axial
rigidities

$$P_s = A_s E_s \qquad \text{and} \qquad P_b = A_b E_b \qquad (2)$$

where E is the Young's modulus of the material concerned.

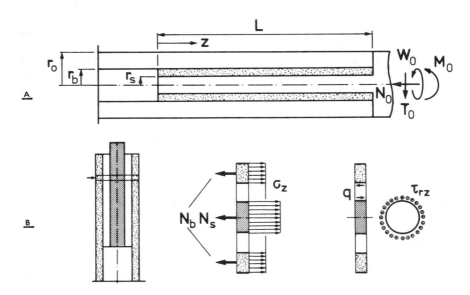

Fig. 4 (a) A general, axisymmetric model of an intramedullary
fixation structure; (b) when loaded by an axial force, the primary
bone and stem stresses are in the axial direction (σ_z) and can be
lumped into internal axial forces $N_b(z)$ and $N_s(z)$; the primary
stresses in the cement layer and at the interfaces are axial shear
stresses (τ_{rz}), which can be lumped into the internal axial shearing load $q(z)$.

We assume that the axial stresses in the cement layer are negligible when compared to those in the bone and the stem. The axial shear stress, τ_{rz}, in the cement layer and at the interfaces depends on the radius r (Fig. 4). However, from local equilibrium consideration it follows that $r\tau_{rz}$ is constant in a cross-section. The internal, distributed shearing load q(z) in the cement layer and at the interfaces is the local resultant of these shear stresses in a cross-section and is defined as

$$q(z) = 2\pi r \tau_{rz} \tag{3}$$

The stiffness of the cement layer against shear, C_n, can be defined as

$$q = C_n(w_b - w_s) \tag{4}$$

where $w_b(z)$ and $w_s(z)$ are the axial deflections of the bone and the stem, respectively. C_n can be approximated by

$$C_n \simeq - \pi E_c/(1 + \nu_c)l_n(r_s/r_b) \tag{5}$$

where E_c and ν_c are Young's modulus and Poisson's ratio of the cement, respectively (19).

Applying the differential equations for bar theory gives

$$P_s \frac{d^2 w_s}{dz^2} + q = 0 \quad \text{and} \quad Pb \frac{d^2 w_b}{dz^2} - q = 0 \tag{6}$$

which, together with Eqn. 4 and the appropriate boundary conditions gives solutions for $N_s(z)$, $N_b(z)$ and q(z) (19, 20).

In these solutions, two important lumped parameters appear,

the relative stem rigidity: $\quad \varepsilon_n = P_s/(P_s + P_b) \tag{7}$

the fixation exponent: $\quad \lambda_n = \sqrt{C_n(\frac{1}{P_s} + \frac{1}{P_b})} \tag{8}$

An example of results for specific parameter values is shown in Fig. 5, for the case that stem collar-bone contact is present, and for the case that the collar is not mechanically effective. These results clearly illustrate the load-transferring mechanism: at the proximal side the load, N_o, is fully carried by the stem. In the proximal load-transferring region, a part of this load is transferred to the bone, through the cement, which generates high cement and interface loading, q(z).

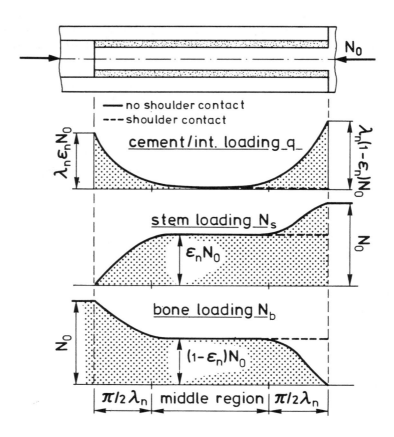

Fig. 5   Cement/Interface shearing load, q(z), stem axial internal
force, $N_s(z)$, and bone axial internal force, $N_b(z)$, as calculated
with the closed-form theory (see text).   If the stem is sufficiently long, the proximal and distal shear load concentrations in
the cement, the loading ratio between the stem and the bone, and
the lengths of the load transmission regions follow from simple
formulas, shown in the graphs, and depend on the fixation exponent
λ_n, the relative stem rigidity ε_n , and the external force N_o
(9, 19).

In the middle region the load is shared by the stem and the bone
depending on their stiffness ratios, indicating a "stress-shielding"
effect; and at the distal side the final portion of the stem load
is transferred to the bone, again through high cement and interface
loading, q(z).   The load-transferring mechanism occurs in this way
only if the stem is sufficiently long, i.e. if $L > \pi/\lambda_n$ (19).   In
this case, the most significant stress values can be directly

approximated in the structural parameters, as indicated in Fig. 5. For instance, using Eqn. 3 and the expressions in Fig. 5, the maximal cement stresses are,

on the proximal side: $\tau_{sp} = \lambda_n(1 - \varepsilon_n)N_o/2\pi r_s$ (9)

on the distal side: $\tau_{sd} = \lambda_n\varepsilon_n N_o/2\pi r_s$ (10)

In the process of developing this model, many simplifications were made. However, comparing the results of the formulas with those of more sophisticated finite element analysis of the same model, shown in Fig. 8, gives excellent agreement (19).

It is obvious that the model used in this case is a very simple one compared to the reality of hip prostheses fixated in bone. However, the results can be used in a qualitative way. For example, it can be seen from Eqns. 9 and 10 that reduction of λ_n without changing ε_n reduces the cement and interface stresses on both the proximal and distal sides. Referring to Eqn. 8, this implies reduction of C_n by reducing, for example, the cement Young's modulus E_c. Another significant finding relates to the length of the stem: lengthening the stem beyond $L \simeq \pi/\lambda_n$ only shifts the distal load-transfer region, and does not result in a stress reduction. Finally, it follows directly from Eqns. 9 and 10 that when $\varepsilon_n = 0.5$, the distal and proximal cement/interface stresses are equal. Reducing the stem stiffness, by reducing its modulus or thickness, reduces ε_n, hence increases the proximal stresses and reduces the distal ones. Increasing the stem stiffness has the opposite effect.

These and comparable qualitative effects can conveniently be assessed with simple analytical analyses of this kind (9, 19). In some cases a structure is such that predictions from these simple models can also have quantitative value, for example in intramedullary custom-fit prosthesis for tumor-resection patients (21). In most cases, however, more precise quantitative evaluations of internal stresses in bone-prosthesis structures will have to rely on numerical finite element methods.

4.   FINITE ELEMENT ANALYSIS

The Finite Element Method (FEM) was introduced in the orthopaedic literature in 1972 (22), about 15 years after it initiated a revolution in stress analysis of structures in engineering mechanics (23). The early applications concerned stress analysis of entire bones. Then, for the first time, the irregular structural features of human bones, both in geometry and in material properties, could be realistically included in the stress analysis.

The subsequent exponential growth of FEM applications in orthopaedic research, however, was not purely due to the interest in bone function, but mainly due to a need for realistic stress data on artificial joints and their mechanical interaction with the host bones.

The principles of the FEM are treated in depth by Zienkiewicz (23) and others, whereas a general description of its possibilities and limitations specifically in orthopaedic biomechanics were published elsewhere (11, 24). The following brief description, however, may help those who are not familiar with the FEM.

In using the method, a model of the structure to be analysed is defined first. This step entails the definition of external loads, geometry, material properties and material connections in a form which can be described in quantifiable terms, mathematically or numerically. This implies that certain assumptions and simplifications must be introduced. The nature of these simplifications determines whether the model, and hence the result, are realistic in a quantitative, or only in a qualitative sense. This model is then mathematically divided into a number of elements, connected at specific locations, called nodal points or nodes (Fig. 6). The connections and external loads are then defined numerically in boundary nodes. Every element is assigned one or more parameters, such as moduli of elasticity, which define its elastic behavior. The computer program calculates the stiffness characteristics of

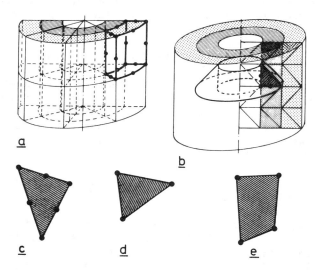

Fig. 6   A number of different element types, (a) 20-node isoparametric hexahedron for 3-D models, (b) 6-node axisymmetric ring element, (c) 6-node and (d) 3-node triangles, and (e) 4-node quadrilateral element for 2-D analysis (reproduced from Ref. 24).

each element and assembles the element mesh through mutual forces and displacements in each node. In fact, the FEM program solves a large number of equations that govern force equilibrium at element nodes. The computer time needed, and thus the cost of analysis, increase with the number of elements and nodes.

The solution obtained with this method is approximate in the sense that it converges to the exact solution for the model when the mesh density approximates infinity. Thus, the accuracy of a FEM model can be checked by refining the mesh and comparing the results obtained with the refined mesh to the original one. This is called the convergency test. In interpreting the FEM results we must differentiate between the validity of the model, i.e. the precision by which the entity of mathematical descriptions of structural properties mimic the real structure, and the accuracy of the model, which is the precision by which the FEM mesh can approximate the exact solution for that model. Only the accuracy can be checked with a convergency test, the validity must be assessed by experimental verification or other means.

A variety of element types are usually available for three-dimensional (3-D) and two-dimensional (2-D) structures in a FEM computer package (Fig. 6). The computer time required for 3-D element is many times more than that for 2-D elements. Because of its cost efficiency, mesh accuracy is easier to obtain in a 2-D model; however, 3-D models are often more realistic.

FEM programs are usually applied in combination with pre-processors and post-processors, which are computer programs that handle the element division, i.e. mesh creation, and graphical representation of the results, respectively.

The use of the FEM has been reported during the last decade in an increasing number of orthopaedic biomechanics publications, and include studies of stress related bone architecture and bone remodeling processes, design and optimization of artificial joints and fracture fixation devices, and mechanical analyses of tissues such as articular cartilage and intervertebral discs (24). The greater part of the FEM analyses was focused on joint replacement, in particular the total hip prosthesis. Early models of this structure were all 2-D ones (e.g. 25-27). A problem in 2-D models of the intramedullary hip joint fixation is to account for the 3-D structural integrity of the bone, which surrounds the implant. A solution can be found in attaching side plates to the 2-D model, thus using two superimposed element layers, an example of which is shown in Fig. 7. Another solution for simplified modeling is assuming the geometry to be axisymmetric, as illustrated in Fig. 8 (e.g. 19, 21). A more general description of the intramedullary fixation structure can be obtained in this way, which is suitable

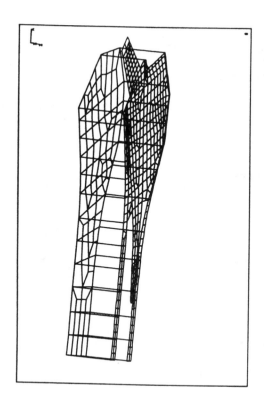

Fig. 7   A 2-D FEM model of a femoral THR structure, using a
sideplate to account for the 3-D integrity of the bone.

for extensive parametric analysis and used to establish the
principal concepts of the load transmission mechanism.

    "Anatomic" 3-D FEM models (e.g. 28-31), of course, are more
precise in their geometrical descriptions, but more tedious to
handle. Also, numerical accuracy is often difficult to obtain due
to computer time requirements and memory space limitations.   In
addition, these models are very costly, hence are more suited to
compare specific designs in a relative sense, than for parametric
analysis and design optimization.

    All these FEM analyses concerned prostheses fixated with
acrylic cement. Several questions regarding design and fixation of
these implants were addressed, and the results published certainly
led to a better understanding of their mechanical behavior, and the
development of more rational designs.   However, many important
questions remain unanswered, mainly because the short- and long-
term effects of stresses and strains on biological bone behavior at

the implant interfaces are essentially unknown.   In most models, linear elasticity, isotropy and homogeneity of bone were assumed.

A specific problem in analyses of bone-prosthesis structures is the description of the implant-bone connection.   Although these materials are usually not rigidly connected in reality, this is assumed to be the case in almost all models.   It was shown that this assumption leads to results which are not totally realistic, particularly for the stress distribution near these connections (19, 27, 32).

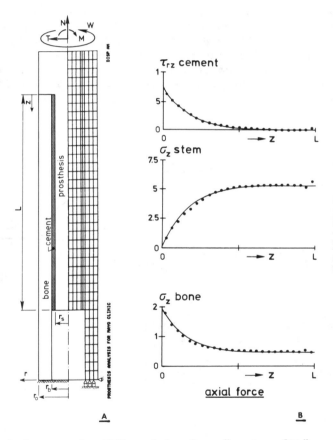

Fig. 8   (a) Axisymmetric FEM model of a "custom-fit" prosthesis fixation system (reproduced from Ref. 21); (b) some results obtained with this model for axial loading (assuming ideal collar-bone contact), stem-cement interface shear stresses (τ_{rz}), stem and bone axial direct stresses (σ_z), compared with analytical (closed-form) solutions (see Section 3, and Fig. 5).   With the FEM model, contrary to the analytical model, other stress components can be evaluated as well (19, 21).

FEM analyses of the acetabular component of total hip replacement have become popular only recently (e.g. 33, 34), probably due to the fact that complications of this part have become manifest in patient populations relatively late post-operatively. In addition, the pelvis and the acetabulum are difficult to model, due to their geometrical and material complexities.

Another hip replacement procedure that attracted interest from FEM analysts is the relatively new resurfacing prosthesis, which was studied with 2-D (35) and axisymmetric 3-D (36) models.

Other joints that received some attention include the knee and the finger joints. Artificial knee hinges were investigated using axisymmetric 3-D (37) and full 3-D (38) FEM models. The tibial plateau fixation of unconstrained knee prostheses were studied with 2-D models (39), axisymmetric models (40), and 3-D models (41, 42). A new finger joint prosthesis was evaluated with axisymmetric FEM models (43).

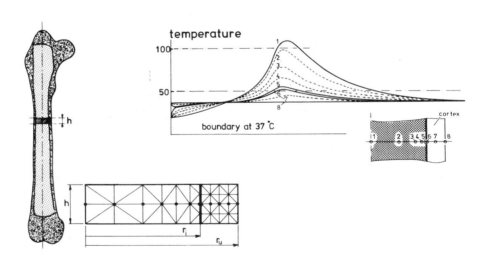

Fig. 9 FEM analysis of the transient heat generation and conduction process in and around acrylic bone cement in the curing phase. This particular model (left) is used to simulate an animal experiment in which cement is injected into rabbit femurs, and bone necrosis is studied histologically. The transient temperatures at several locations in the cement mass and in the bone cortex, calculated in the FEM analysis, are shown on the right; the peak temperature is reached in about 350 seconds (reproduced from Ref. 5).

Finally, a different type of biomechanics implant problem was also addressed with the FEM, using this method as a universal numerical tool to solve problems of heat and mass transfer in geometrically complex regions. An example of such a problem is the nonsteady heat generation and conduction that occurs in and around acrylic cement during its curing phase whle fixing an implant. The bone close to the cement rises in temperature and may undergo thermal necrosis. To investigate this process and evaluate the transient temperature distributions, the FEM was applied to simulate implant fixation in the femur and in the acetabulum (5, 44). An example of such a study is illustrated in Fig. 9.

5. DISCUSSION

Although the FEM has enhanced developments in orthopaedic biomechanics in general and artificial joint design in particular, its application in this area is still in an early stage. Several problems still hamper the use of stress analysis, the FEM in particular, to its full potential. Two aspects of bone-prosthesis structures specifically need attention in biomechanics research.

The first aspect is related to the complexity of the structures to be modeled and their individual variability, on the one hand, and limitations in computer capacities on the other. Even if the individual structural parameters, in terms of geometry and material properties, and loading histories of individual patient cases could be assessed with adequate precision, the costs of FEM would still prohibit individual case analysis, other than in exceptional circumstances. Hence, the objectives of investigations of this kind must be to provide general information on a relative basis. Even with this aim, the vagaries of the bone-prosthesis structure in general present numerous problems that have yet to be solved.

If we put the kind of information that can be obtained from stress analyses on a scale, ranging from general (qualitative, global) to specific (quantitative, local), it is evident that such a scale can be related to a scale of model sophistication, ranging from coarse to refined. Taking the THR structure as an example, we would find the strain-gage analysis and analytical ("closed-form") methods discussed previously on the coarse side, and 3-D, "anatomic" FEM models on the refined. Nevertheless, the information on the full scale must be compatible. Unfortunately, this is not always the case in the present state of the art, and further analyses of an experimental and theoretical nature, combined with clinical evaluations must be performed in order to fill the gaps in our knowledge.

Secondly, it is on the refined side of the scale in particular that we meet limitations of modeling feasibilities. These are not only related to limitations in computer capacities, which are progressively approached when 3-D mesh density is increased, but also to requirements of more precise descriptions of material properties and material connections, which are simply not available as yet. Hence, highly sophisticated experimental work is needed for the required data to supply the increasingly refined models, before progress in that direction can be made.

The second aspect concerns the reactions of bone to implants, and their presumed relations to stresses and strains. Any model, whether experimental, analytical or numerical, represents a particular bone-prosthesis structure at a particular point in time, e.g. immediately post-operative. Stresses and strains, determined for such a configuration have a significance for design purposes when they can be compared to stress-criteria, as the strength of bone, acrylic cement, and the implant materials. However, no such criteria exist for stresses or strains that would cause interface bone resorption or bone osteoporosis. In addition, these biological reactions would result in geometrical and/or material changes which, in turn affect the stresses and strains again. This biological feed-back loop in the structural behavior is illustrated in Fig. 10.a. It would be possible in principle to describe this loop mathematically (45), and incorporate it into FEM analysis to predict the eventual stress distribution. This, of course, would require experimental data on stress (strain) - bone remodeling relations which are not yet available.

The stresses in Fig. 10.a are called "global stresses". It is evident that the stresses predicted in a global FEM model of an entire bone-prosthesis configuration can only be considered as rough lumped internal loading variables for a small piece of bone material. However, it is probably based on the local stress state that bone reacts biologically. Hence, it is likely that stresses must be determined in detailed models which take local geometry and properties into account before a feed-back loop can be incorporated (Fig. 10.b). Although it is not realistic to assume that a FEM model can be realistic both on a global and a local level, a multiple model approach can be adopted to overcome this problem.

Despite the potential feasibilities of numerical methods, these techniques cannot be applied for objective stress and remodeling predictions until consistent quantitative experimental data on relations between stresses (strains) and bone remodeling are available. Nevertheless, analyses of this kind could certainly enhance developments in experimental work, in particular if the two approaches were combined in efforts of a truly multidisciplinary nature.

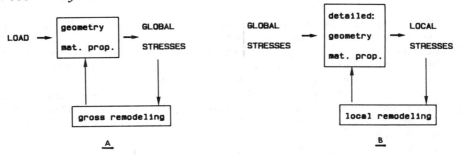

Fig. 10   Schemes for advanced stress analyses of bone-prosthesis structures, taking into account the biological feed-back loop. Because bone cells probably react to the local stress (strain) environment and FÉM models cannot be realistic and detailed on all levels, a multiple model approach can be adopted (a and b).

REFERENCES

1. Consensus Development Panel, NIH-Consensus Paper: Total Hip Joint Replacement, Bethesda, MD.   Partly published in JAMA, vol. 248, no. 15, (1982) p. 1817.
2. Charnley, J.   The Long-Term Results of Low Friction Arthroplasty of the Hip Performed as a Primary Intervention.   J. Bone Jt. Surg. 45-B (1972) p. 61.
3. Stauffer, R.N.   Ten-Year Follow-up Study of Total Hip Replacement.   J. Bone Jt. Surg. 64-A (1982) p. 1983.
4. Feith, R.   Side-Effects of Acrylic Cement, Implanted into Bone. Acta Orthop. Scand. Suppl. no. 161, 1975.
5. Huiskes, R.   Some Fundamental Aspects of Human Joint Replacement, Section II: Heat Generation and Conduction Analyses of Acrylic Bone Cement in Situ.   Acta Orthop. Scand. Suppl. no. 185 (Munskgaard, Copenhagen, 1979) p. 43.
6. Willert, H.G. and M. Semlitsch.   Problems Associated with the Cement Anchorage of Artificial Joints.   In: Advances in Artificial Hip and Knee Joint Technology (Edited by N. Schaldach and D. Hohmann, Springer Verlag, Berlin, Heidelberg, New York, 1976).
7. Freeman, M.A.R., G.W. Bradley, and P.A. Revell.   Observations upon the Interface between Bone and Polymethylmethacrylate Cement.   J. Bone Jt. Surg. 64-B (1982) p. 489.
8. Radin, E.L., C.T. Rubin, E.L. Trasher, L.E. Lanyon, A.M. Crugnola, A.S. Schiller, I.L. Paul, and R.M. Rose.   Changes in the Bone-Cement Interface after Total Hip Replacement.   J. Bone Jt. Surg. 64-A (1982) p. 1188.
9. Huiskes, R.   Design, Fixation and Stress Analysis of Permanent Orthopedic Implants: The Hip Joint.   In: Functional Behavior

of Orthopedic Materials (Edited by P. Ducheyne and G. Hastings, CRC-Press, Boca Raton, FL, vol. 2, ch. 5, 1983).

10. Durelli, A.J.   The Difficult Choice: Evaluation of Methods Used to Determine Experimentally Displacements, Strains and Stresses. App. Mech. Rev. 30, 9 (1977) p. 1167.

11. Huiskes, R.   Principles and Methods of Solid Biomechanics. In: Functional Behavior of Orthopedic Materials (Edited by P. Ducheyne and G. Hastings, CRC-Press, Boca Raton, FL, vol. 1, ch. 4, 1983).

12. Reilly, D.T. and A.H. Burstein.   The Elastic and Ultimate Properties of Compact Bone Tissue.   J. Biomechanics 8 (1975) p. 393.

13. Lanyon, L.E.   The Measurement and Biological Significance of Bone Strain in Vivo.   In: Mechanical Properties of Bone. (Edited by S.C. Cowin, AMD - vol. 45, ASME, New York, 1981) p. 93.

14. Huiskes, R., J.D. Janssen, and T.J. Slooff.   A Detailed Comparison of Experimental and Theoretical Stress Analyses of a Human Femur.   In: Mechanical Properties of Bone (Edited by S.C. Cowin, AMD - vol. 45, ASME, New York, 1981) p. 211.

15. Oh, I. and W.H. Harris.   Proximal Strain Distribution in the Loaded Femur. J. Bone Jt. Surg. 60-A (1978) p. 75.

16. Jacob, H.A.C. and A.H. Huggler.   An Investigation into Biomechanical Causes of Prosthesis Stem Loosening within the Proximal End of the Human Femur.   J. Biomechanics 13 (1980) p. 159.

17. Crowninshield, R.D., D.R. Pedersen, and R.A. Brand.   A Measurement of Proximal Femur Strain with Total Hip Arthroplasty.   J. Biomech. Engrg. 102 (1980) p. 230.

18. Rohlman, A., G. Bergmann, and R. Koelbel.   The Relevance of Stress Computation in the Femur with and without Endoprostheses.   In: Finite Elements in Biomechanics (Edited by R.H. Gallagher et al., John Wiley and Sons, New York, 1982) p. 361.

19. Huiskes, R.   Some Fundamental Aspects of Human Joint Replacement.   Part III: Stress Analyses of Intramedullary Fixation Systems.   Acta Orthop. Scand. Suppl. no. 185 (Munskgaard, Copenhagen, 1979) p. 109.

20. Timoshenko, S.P., and J.N. Goodier.   Theory of Elasticity (3rd ed.) (McGraw-Hill, Kogahuska, Tokyo, 1970).

21. Huiskes, R. and E.Y.S. Chao.   Optimal Stem Design in Tumor Prostheses.   In: Tumor Prosthesis for Bone and Joint Reconstruction (Edited by E.Y. Chao and J.C. Ivins, Thieme Stratton, New York, sect. 4, ch. 44, 1983) p. 367.

22. Brekelmans, W.A.M., H.W. Poort, and T.J.J.H. Slooff.   A New Method to Analyse the Mechanical Behavior of Skeletal parts. Acta Orthop. Scand. 43 (1972) p. 301.

23. Zienkiewicz, O.C.   The Finite Element Method (3rd ed.) (McGraw-Hill, London, 1977).

24. Huiskes, R. and E.Y.S. Chao.   A Survey of Finite Element Analysis in Orthopaedic Biomechanics: The First Decade. J. Biomechanics 16 (1983) p. 385.

25. McNeice, G.M., P. Eng and H.C. Amstutz. Finite Element Studies in Hip Reconstruction. In: Biomechanics V-A. (Edited by P.V. Komi, Univ. Park Press, Baltimore, MD, 1976) p. 394.
26. Andriacchi, T.P., J.O. Galante, T.B. Belytschko, and S. Hampton. A Stress Analysis of the Femoral Stem in Total Hip Prostheses. J. Bone Jt. Surg. 58-A (1976) p. 616.
27. Svensson, N.L., S. Valliappan, and R.D. Wood. Stress Analysis of Human Femur with Implanted Charnley Prostheses. J. Bio-mechanics 10 (19) p. 581.
28. Roehrle, H., R. Scholten, W. Sollbach, G. Ritter, and A. Gruenert. Der Kraftfluss bei Huftendoprothesen. Arch. Orthop. Unfall-Chir. 89 (1977) p. 49.
29. Hampton, S.J., T.P. Andriacchi, and J.O. Galante. Three-dimensional Stress Analysis of the Femoral Stem of a Total Hip Prosthesis. J. Biomechanics 13 (1980) p. 443.
30. Crowninshield, R.D., R.A. Brand, R.C. Johnston, and J.C. Milroy. An Analysis of Femoral Component Stem Design in Total Hip Arthroplasty. J. Bone Jt. Surg. 62-A (1980) p. 68.
31. Tarr, R.R., I.C. Clarke, T.A. Gruen, and A. Sarmiento. Pre-dictions of Cement-Bone Failure Criteria: Three-dimensional Finite Element Models versus Clinical Reality of Total Hip Replacement. In: Finite Elements in Biomechanics. (Edited by R. H. Gallagher et al., John Wiley and Sons, New York, 1982) p. 345.
32. Rohlmann, A., G. Bermann, and R. Koelbel. Aussagewert und Grenzen der Spannungsberechnung mit der Finiten-Element-Methode (FEM) bei Orhtopadischen Problemen. Z. Orthop. 118 (1980) p. 122.
33. Vasu, R., D.R. Carter, and W.H. Harris. Stress Distributions in the Acetabular Region-I. Before and After Total Joint Replacement. J. Biomechanics 15 (1982) p. 155.
34. Pedersen, D.R., R.D. Crowninshield, R.A. Brand, and R.C. Johnston. An Axisymmetric Model of Acetabular Components in Total Hip Arthroplasty. J. Biomechanics 15 (1982) p. 305.
35. Shybut, G.T., M.J. Askew, R.Y. Hori, and S.D. Stulberg. Theoretical and Experimental Studies of Femoral Stresses Following Surface Replacement Hip Arthroplasty. In: The Hip, chap. 10 (The C. V. Mosby Co., St. Louis, MO, 1980) p. 192.
36. Huiskes, R. and J. van Heck. Stresses in the Femoral Head-Neck Region after Surface Replacement, a Three-dimensional Finite Element Analysis. Proceedings 27th Annual Meeting Orthop. Res. Soc. (1981) p. 174.
37. Croon, H.W., D.H. van Campen, J. Klok, and R. Miehlke. Quasi Two-dimensional FEM Analysis and Experimental Investigations of the Tibial Part of Knee Endoprostheses with Intramedullary Stems. In: Biomechanics: Principles and Applications. (Edited by R. Huiskes et al., Martinus Nijhoff Publ., The Hague, Boston, London, 1982) p. 313.
38. Roehrle, H., W. Sollbach, and J. Gekeler. Stress Analysis in Artificial Knee Joints with Fixed and Movable Axis Using the

Finite Element Method. In: Biomechanics: Principles and Applications (Edited by R. Huiskes et al., Martinus Nijhoff Publ., The Hague, Boston, London, 1982) p. 305.

39. Askew, M.J. and J.L. Lewis. Analysis of Model Variables and Fixation Post Length Effects on Stresses around a Prosthesis in the Proximal Tibia. J. Biomech. Engng. 103 (1981) p. 239.

40. K. Murase, R.D. Crowninshield, D.R. Pedersen, and T.S. Chang. An Analysis of Tibial Component Design in Total Knee Arthroplasty. J. Biomechanics 16 (1982) p. 13.

41. Bartel, D.L., A.H. Burstein, E.A. Santavicca, and J.N. Insall. Performance of the Tibial Component in Total Knee Replacement. J. Bone Jt. Surg. 64-A (1982) p. 1026.

42. Lewis, J.L., M.J. Askew, and D.P. Jaycox. A Comparative Evaluation of Tibial Component Designs of Total Knee Prosthesis. J. Bone Jt. Surg. 64-A (1982) p. 129.

43. Huiskes, R., J. van Heck, P.S. Walker, D.J. Green, and D. Nunamaker. A Three-dimensional Stress Analysis of a New Finger-Joint Prosthesis Fixation System. In: Int. Conf. Proceedings on Finite Elements in Biomechanics (Edited by B.R. Simon, Univ. of Arizona Press, Tucson, AZ, 1980) p. 749.

44. Swenson, L.W., D.J. Schurman, and R.L. Piziali. Finite Element Temperature Analysis of a Total Hip Replacement and Measurement of PMMA Curing Temperatures. J. Biomed. Mat. Res. 15 (1981) p. 83.

45. Cowin, S.C. Continuum Models of Adaption of Bone to Stress. In: Mechanical Properties of Bone (Edited by S.C. Cowin, AMD-vol. 45, the Am. Soc. of Mech. Engrs., New York, 1981) p. 193.

STANDARDS FOR JOINT REPLACEMENTS

J. P. Paul

Bioengineering Unit, University of Strathclyde
Glasgow, Scotland, U.K.

There is currently activity in the International Standards Organization in particular with technical committee No. 150, whose remit is to look at surgical implants. One aspect of the work is joint replacement and the secretariat for this exercise is United Kingdom; participating members include West Germany, France, U.S.A., U.S.S.R. and several other countries; many other countries of the world are associated with this in the category of observer members. As other chapters in this book have indicated, selection of materials is particularly important for long-term surgical implants, and one of the early items of work of this committee was specification of the chemical composition, mechanical strength and other characteristics of metals and plastics and ceramics for use in orthopedic implants. Other matters currently under discussion, include marking and packaging of implants by the manufacturers to allow safe delivery, sterile where appropriate, with appropriate information to allow manufacturers to recall products of any batch of material if clinical use demonstrates that a fault may have arisen for any reason. Similarly there are guidelines for safe handling to avoid damage as well as sterilization procedures for those components which may be resterilized after the package is opened in the operating theatre, or for those components which are supplied in a non-sterile condition.

It is an interesting aspect of standards work that formal documents cannot be produced until precise terminology has been defined. One of the activities of ISO has been to formalize the terminology used in description of joint replacement and also to specify the way in which dimensions of prostheses should be reported.

No attempt is made however to standardize designs. In fact every encouragement is given to designers and manufacturers to introduce new shapes and designs of components; the only specification being related as far as possible to the safety of the patient who receives such an implant. Standards are however of advantage to the manufacturers in that the company wishing to export to another country derives a considerable advantage if they can certify that their product is in accordance with International Standards. Wasteful duplication of excessive ranges of sizes of components is usually avoided also by the specification of a preferred range of sizes.

In joint replacements the greatest progress and the most successful end result has been in the field of hip joint replacement, and the success in producing a consistently good product in this area has meant that it has been easier for standard writing to proceed rapidly. In the case of other joints where a widely accepted good result over a long period has been more difficult to find, then the criteria for the formulation of standards are obviously less definite and the standards are of a more rudimentary kind. With regard to hip joint replacements there are specifications for the surface finish and sphericity of the spherical end of the proximal femoral component, and consideration is currently being given to methods of mechanical test. The philosophy behind these two exercises is that rate of wear of the bearing surfaces is closely related to the surface finish. There has also been a history in a limited number of situations of fracture of the stem of the proximal femoral component. This occurs most frequently in patients of higher body mass associated with high activity level. The mechanism of failure appears to be that for uncertain reasons the bone around the section where the head and neck are detached from the femur may become reduced in strength due to resorbtion. Reasons for this are unclear, but two phenomena which have been cited are excessive contact pressure between the prostheses and the bone and reduction in the stress normally carried by the bone, corresponding to longitudinal load and bending moment, leading to 'disuse atrophy'. For whatever reason the resorbtion occurs, the result is that the implant is effectively not supported at its proximal end and the condition may arise where the implant is firmly fixed in a plug of cement at its distal end and loaded by the joint force. This gives a stress system, such as in a cantilever under bending, leading to a fatigue failure at a section situated at between 1/3 and 2/3 of the stem length from its tip. Wroblewski (1) quotes that the majority of these fatigue failures involve a fracture surface which is not perpendicular to the axis of the stem. This corresponds in fact to a combination of longitudinal bending and torsional loading and for this reason the test procedure proposed currently by the United Kingdom involves the proximal femoral component being held in a fixing medium, in such a way that a load applied to the head of the femur causes such a

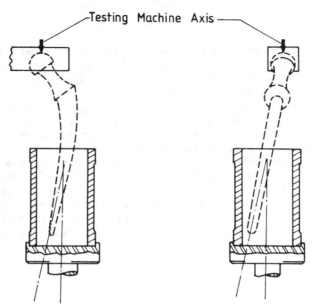

Fig. 1   Orientation proposed for fatigue testing of femoral component of total hip joint replacement prosthesis.

combination of stresses varying down the length of the stem. This is shown in Fig. 1.   Less significance is attached to this out of plane loading by other European countries and controversy appears likely to ensue.   All countries are however agreed that the corrosive effect of simulating the physiological environment in which the implant is situated must not be ignored, and for this reason it is usually specified that fatigue tests be conducted at 37 °C in a bath of Ringer's solution, whose chemical composition is maintained constant and which is maintained in an aerated condition while it is moved around over the surface of the prostheses.   There will probably be some new discussion before a uniform test procedure is agreed upon internationally, but the question is thought to be of such importance that strenuous efforts will no doubt be made.

Various countries have purchasing authorities responsible for the acquisition of implants from manufacturers and the distribution to appropriate hospitals.   An example of this is the National Health Service in the United Kingdom, and the Department of Health and Social Security itself has specifications for the characteristics of those implants which it will purchase, which may not always be in accord with international standards.   Similarly, the Food and Drug Administration in U.S.A. has its own standards in certain matters which will interact with the formulation of standards on an international basis in due course.

The provision of goods according to an international standard is a safeguard for the consumer, namely the patient who can expect to have the quality control and appropriate level of technical skill in the production of the device he receives. The surgeon similarly has the protection of knowing that the devices he delivers to the patient are of controlled quality. In the same way, the manufacturer has the protection of knowing that if he is delivering goods to a relevant current international specification, then he should be able to sell with confidence in his own country and overseas. Standardization appears to have benefits for all people concerned in the field, and it is only unfortunate that because of the extensive committee work involved, the effective adoption of agreed standards takes time periods from four years upwards between initiation of committee work and the production of the final document.

REFERENCE:

1.   Wroblewski, B.M.   Mechanism of Fracture of the Femoral Prosthesis in Total Hip Replacement. Int. Orthop. 3(2) (1979) 137-139.

SHORT CONTRIBUTIONS

1. RELATIONSHIPS AMONG OSTEOARTHROSIS,
   BONE MINERAL CONTENT, AGE AND SEX

R. Sumner*
Department of Anthropology, University of Arizona
Tucson, AZ 85721 USA

In recent years anthropology has begun to contribute to biomechanics. Anthropology emphasizes variability and explaining variability both within and among populations. The relationship between osteoarthrosis (OA) and bone mineral content (BMC) in femora of a prehistoric human population (Grasshopper Pueblo, Arizona) is examined. The age range of included individuals is 20 to 60. OA is scored on an ordinal scale by assessing the severity of (a) lipping around joint surfaces and (b) lesions on joint surfaces. BMC is measured with photon absorptiometry. Almost all individuals have some lipping. Lesions are most common on the condyles, followed by the patellar surface and the femoral head (e.g., 25%, 7%, 2%, respectively in males). Severity of OA increases with ages in both males and females. BMC decreases with age only in females. There is a negative correlation between severity of OA and BMC in females. No relationship between OA and BMC is discernible in males. These preliminary results agree with the conclusions of a similar study of the tibia (Burr et al., Am. J. Phys. Anthrop., 1983, 61:299-303) and a clinical study (Dequeker et al., JAMA, 1983, 249:1448-51). While OA and loss of BMC are both age-related phenomena, they appear to have different etiologies.

---

*Present address: Department of Orthopedic Surgery, Rush-Presbyterian-St. Lukes's Medical Center, 1753 West Congress Parkway, Chicago, Illinois 60612

2. INFLUENCE OF HIP ENDOPROSTHETIC DESIGN
    ON STRESS DISTRIBUTION

A. Rohlmann, U. Mossner and G. Bergmann
Department of Orthopedic Surgery, Free University in
Oskar-Helene-Heim, Biomechanics Laboratory
Clayallee 229, 1000, Berlin 33, West Germany

The stress distribution in a human femur with a hip endoprosthesis was determined. The finite element method was used for
a three-dimensional model with more than 15,000 degrees of freedom.
Geometrical and material data had been taken for this model from a
left femur with endoprosthesis. On the contralateral bone a strain
gage investigation was performed to validate the calculations.
Good agreement was achieved.

In a parameter study the influence of stem length, prosthetic
collar and stem material on the stresses in implant, cement and
bone surface has been analyzed. We could show that for the choosen
type of endoprosthesis a stem length greater than 100 mm has only a
minor effect on the stresses in the prosthetic stem/cement interface, and that from the mechanical point of view a prosthetic
collar is unimportant. The results are only valid for endoprosthesis with such structured stem surfaces as to allow transfer of
tensile and shear stresses.

3. THEORETICAL AND EXPERIMENTAL ANALYSES OF
    THE COUPLING OF ENDOPROSTHESIS AND FEMUR

M.M. Gola and A. Gugliotta
Department of Mechanical Engineering, Politecnico di Torino, Italy

The authors refer to their six years experience on the study
of the hip prosthesis/femur coupling and discuss it in the light of
the many results present in the literature. Experience includes
two dimensional and three dimensional numerical analysis and
experimental stress analysis: for the latter, three successive
types of transducer stems were designed and tested. The authors'

conclusion is that not always the cost and the intricacies of the finite element approach correspond to an adequate significance of the results and that experimental analysis is a more appropriate working- tool. In order to illustrate the shortcomings of the numerical approach, a theoretical statement of the problem is made singling out what may be considered new information from what could directly be obtained by qualitative reasoning. In particular the many uncertainties of the physical parameters into play are shown to form a striking contrast with the nominal accuracy of a refined finite element analysis. Realizing the importance of the experimental approach, the authors developed a special transducer stem with the idea of making a reusable device to be implanted in different bones in order to get statistical information, or directly in living animals. Three types of such transducers have been constructed since 1978. They were designed to overcome hysteresis and interfacial problems revealed during implantation and testing in dry and fresh bones. Results confirm previous findings on the distribution of load between stem and bone, or stem and cement.

4. GAIT ANALYSIS AS A DIAGNOSTIC TOOL

H. Ranu
Department of Biomedical Engineering, Louisiana Tech University, Ruston, Louisiana, 71272, U.S.A.

Normal and abnormal human gait has been studied extensively mainly using force platforms or walkways. Although these devices have led to a much better understanding of the gait cycle, yet they have made little impact on clinical evaluation of individual patient problems. In order to overcome this problem, Ranu et al (Proc. 26th Annual Meeting, Orthopedic Research Soc.--Orthopedic Trans. JBJS, 4(2), 1980, pp. 240-241) have developed a system which is capable of meeting the needs of individual patients by deter- mining load distribution under different regions of the foot during the stance phase.

A miniature triaxial load cell 14 mm thick x 19 x 19 mm in overall size has been developed. It consists of 4 loops of load bearing elements placed symmetrically around a 12.5 mm square which is located at the center of the load cell. There is no contact between the top and bottom square plates to allow load transfer through these loops. A total of 16 strain gages are used to achieve triaxial force output with minimal cross-talk. The load cells were attached to the shoe by means of a rigid backing plate (Fig. 1).

The initial concern was the correlation of shoe load cell data with those from a walkway force plate. However, the measured resultant force-time histories of the gait-cycle for the instrumented shoe and a conventional force plate in general only differed less than 2%.

Conclusions drawn from a number of tests using this system are: a) The transducer is a viable tool to assist in the rehabilitation of an amputee and other forms of pathological gait. b) The transducer can detect subtler differences between normal and abnormal gait. c) The transducer can help speed up the training of an amputee in use of a prosthesis. It is also possible to aid him in the development of a more normal gait. d) This method of analyzing gait is simple, accurate, non-invasive and has an enormous clinical potential in orthopedics and the rehabilitation of patients with lower extremity disabilities. e) The contribution of each load cell force-time history in different regions of the foot results in a normal gait-cycle, i.e., a "cumulative gait effect phenomenon". f) The transducer can aid in the design of suitable orthoses for polio patients.

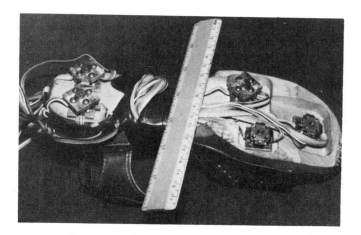

Fig. 1 Five triaxial load cells mounted under a shoe.

5. A SIMPLE FINITE ELEMENT MODEL OF THE MENISCUS

A.A.H.J. Sauren, A. Huson*, R.Y. Schouten, J.C. Nagtegaal
Department of Mechanical Engineering, Eindhoven University of
Technology; P. O. Box 513, 5600 MB; Eindhoven, The Netherlands
*Department of Anatomy and Embryology, University of Leiden
P. O. Box 9602, 2300 RC; Leiden, The Netherlands

    In order to obtain more insight into the mechanical function
of the meniscus, an axisymmetric finite element model has been
developed. The model comprises a plane tibia plateau, a spherical
femoral condyle (radius 30 mm) and a ring in between, representing
the miniscus (inner and outer radius 8 and 18 mm). The lower and
upper surfaces of the ring match the tibial and femoral surfaces
respectively. In the unloaded configuration there is tibial-
femoral contact. The most important characteristic of the model is
that it allows frictionless displacements of the meniscus with
respect to the tibial and the femur. This is achieved by the use
of especially developed gap elements. Both the bones and the
meniscus are assumed to be isotropic and linearly elastic. The
axial compression of the joint and the radially outward displacement of the meniscus are non-linear functions of the axial load
acting on the joint. In the configuration without meniscus, the

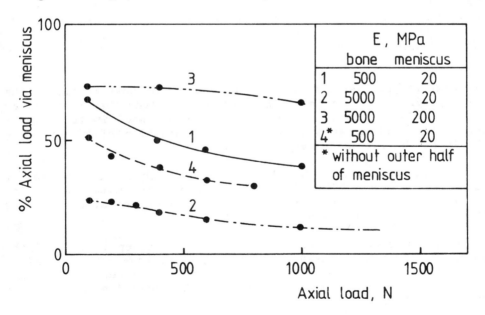

Fig. 2   Percent axial load transmitted by the meniscus (See text).

axial compression of the joint at a given load is larger than in the situation with meniscus. An increase of the Young's modulus of the bones or of both the meniscus and the bones yields a decrease of the axial compression of the joint and the radial displacement of the meniscus. Depending on the chosen combination of material properties of bone and meniscus, the contribution of the meniscus to the load transmission from femur to tibia amounts to 20 to 70% of the total axial load (Fig. 2). The inner half of the meniscus appears to contribute significantly more to load transmission than the outer half. Removal of the total meniscus results in an increase of the stress values in the tibial-femoral contact area of about 40%, whereas this increase amounts only to 5 to 15% upon removal of merely the outer half.

6.   EXPERIMENTAL STRESS ANALYSIS USING EPOXY MODELS
      OF THE HUMAN PELVIS AND FEMUR, BEFORE AND AFTER
      INSERTION OF A HIP PROSTHESIS

H.A.C. Jacob
Department of Orthopedic Surgery (Balgrist)
University of Zurich
Forchstrasse 340; Zurich, Switzerland

Experimental stress analysis on composite epoxy models of the human pelvis and femur have been employed to study the exact manner in which the proximal end of the bone is stressed in the physiological condition, as well as after implantation of a hip prosthesis of the intramedullarly anchored type.

Apart from the light thrown on the mechanical function of cortical and cancellous bone within the acetabulum and in the proximal region of the femur, a description of the stresses along the prosthesis stem has been obtained.

It has also been shown that a prosthetic replacement of the intramedullarly type could relax the cortical bone at the proximal end of the femur to such an extent that in some cases only about 40% of the natural stresses (i.e., in the physiologically intact state) may be present.

The presentation also included details pertaining to the justification of the use of such models and shows that the obtained results could be directly applied to bone.

7. EXPERIMENTAL VALGUS INSTABILITY OF THE KNEE

S. Nielsen, C. Kromann-Andersen and O. Rasmussen
The Biomechanics Laboratory, The Orthopaedic Hospital
Randersvej 1; Aarhus, Denmark

An apparatus was developed, which enables a continuous registration of the varus-valgus instability in the extension-flexion movement of the knee in the range of zero to 150 degrees during a well-defined, constant torque. By the use of osteo-ligamentous preparations, the importance of the medial collateral ligament and the anterior cruciate ligament of the knee in relation to valgus and varus instability was investigated. Mobility-patterns were drawn from ten preparations after successive transections of the structures. Cutting of the entire collateral medial ligament caused only slight valgus instability even when the knee was flexed. Further transection of the anterior cruciate ligament increased the instability considerably, but the knee remained stable in extension. The valgus instability after the transections was maximal at about 60 degrees of flexion.

8. FINITE AND INSTANTANEOUS HELICAL AXIS ESTIMATION FROM NOISY, DISCRETE LANDMARK MEASUREMENTS

H.J. Woltring
Laboratory for Experimental Orthopaedics, Faculty of Medicine and Dentistry, University of Nijmegen
P.O.B. 9101, NL - 6500 HB;
Nijmegen, The Netherlands

Recent advances in kinematic measuring equipment fostered the use of the helical- (or screw-) axis concept for quantitative and graphical representation of joint kinematics. Under this concept, movement of a body segment is described in terms of a translation along and of a rotation about a directed line in space. The parameters of this representation are typically derived from a discrete set of measured landmark coordinates in the body segments under investigation.

For finite movements, only the initial and terminal displacements are considered without regard to the trajectory along which the movements occur. For continuous movements, the continuous (or instantaneous) helical axis may be derived from the translational and rotational displacements and velocities.

The customary use of the finite helical axis, evaluated for sufficiently small movement steps, as an approximation of the true, continuous helical axis has been found to entail large measurement error sensitivities, particularly for the position and direction of the helical axis. A better approach is to fit the discrete landmark measurements or the rotation matrices and translation vectors calculated therefrom to a continuous movement model, e.g., as defined by a low-pass filtering operation. From the original data, smoothed displacements and velocities may be evaluated; hence the instantaneous helical axis is analytically derived. In this way, the noise sensitivity is substantially reduced, and the biases incurred by highly nonlinear transformations on noisy measurements are minimized.

9.   ON THE INITIATION OF SPONDYLOLYSIS
      THROUGH MECHANICAL FACTORS

H.A.C. Jacob and Y. Suezawa
Department of Orthopedic Surgery (Balgrist)
University of Zurich
Forchstrasse 340; Zurich, Switzerland

The etiology of spondylolysis has continued to remain obscure ever since the latter was described by Neugebauer in 1881. The cleavage in the interarticular portion of the lamina of the vertebral body (most often in the lower back region) is found in about 5% of the central European population. An alarmingly high percentage of spondylolysis occurs among top gymnasts; 30% have been reported to exhibit this structural discontinuity.

Although the hypothesis that mechanical overstressing could be the initiating factor has often been suggested, it has persistently eluded proving in in-vitro tests on cadaver specimens.

The present report describes a biomechanical investigation in which the manner of loading of the lumbar vertebrae has been determined in order to produce a fracture in the interarticular portion without causing damage to any other area of the vertebra. In-vitro tests with fresh cadaver specimens have given evidence that in some cases, an axial load of about 3 kN is sufficient to produce the fracture on condition the lumbar spine is in hyperextension.

10. INTRA-OPERATIVE MEASUREMENT OF CANCELLOUS BONE STRENGTH

I. Hvid
The Biomechanics Laboratory, The Orthopaedic Hospital
University of Aarhus
Randersvej 1; Aarhus, Denmark

An osteopenetrometer was developed to measure the resistance to penetration of cancellous bone at the knee. A mechanically powered 2.5 mm pointed needle is advanced at right angles to the resection surface into the bone. Simultaneous recording of needle load and depth of penetration is obtained on an X-Y recorder. The average penetration force over a selected depth interval is used as an expression of cancellous bone strength.

Osteopenetrometer measurements were compared to conventional tests in a materials testing machine by first measuring with the penetrometer and then removing a cyclindrical bone specimen with a 12 mm core drill around the mark left by the penetrometer-needle. The bone cylinders were tested to compressive failure. Comparison of penetration strength and ultimate strength in 18 specimens revealed a reasonably good and highly significant correlation (r=0.80, P< 0.001).

In another test series compression tests on machined cylinders (measurements: ultimate stress, elastic modulus, ultimate strain energy) and penetration tests in 8 and 4 knees respectively were related to the topography of the tibial condyles. Analysis of variance showed that the osteopenetrometer readings closely matched the pattern of ultimate strength, while the relation to elastic modulus and ultimate strain energy was less close.

A new instrument based on the same principle of measurement is presently used routinely during total knee replacement to obtain objective information on the quality of cancellous bone.

11. ON THE LOOSENING OF THE FEMORAL COMPONENT
     OF FREEMAN DOUBLE-CUP HIP PROSTHESES--
     A BIOMECHANICAL INVESTIGATION

H.A.C. Jacob and A. Schreiber
Department of Orthopedic Surgery (Balgrist)
University of Zurich
Forchstrasse 340; Zurich, Switzerland

The cancellous bone in the vicinity of the mouth of the femoral cup can be not only subjected to an axial load of about three times the value physiologically encountered, but the cup also tends to move transversally away from the medial bone margin in this area. Hence, fracture of the trabecular structure can occur, accompanied by cleavage and relative movement in this region. This leads to bone resorption and the development of a thick intermediate layer of fibrous connective tissue that spreads until eventually the whole cup becomes loosened. In the meantime the bone within the cup, further proximal, probably undergoes atrophy due to mechanical inactivity.

The purpose of this presentation was to expose the results of the biomechanical investigation which confirms our earlier presumption that the living bone was probably being subjected to unphysiological loads within the metal shell, thereby causing resorption of the bone, and hence loosening the device.

LIST OF PARTICIPANTS

Dr. J.M.C. Abrantes, Portugal
Dr. C. Agelidis, Greece
Dr. N. Akkas, Turkey
Dr. L.M. Alvim Serra, Portugal
Dr. C.B. Amado, Portugal
Dr. T.P. Andriacchi, U.S.A.
Dr. J.A.C. Antao, Portugal
Ms. M.J. Barreiros, Portugal
Prof. N. Berme, U.S.A.
Dr. A. Burssens, Belgium
Dr. T. Brown, U.K.
Dr. A. Cappozzo, Italy
Dr. K. Correia da Silva, Portugal
Dr. M.C.V. Duarte, Portugal
Ms. M.M.A. Durao, Portugal
Prof. J. Drukker, The Netherlands
Dr. G. Dumas, Canada
Mrs. A. Edwards, England
Prof. A.E. Engin, U.S.A.
Dr. J.H. Evans, U.K.
Mr. J.C.A. Fernandes, Portugal
Dr. S. Fioretti, Italy
Dr. E.A.P. Fonseca, Portugal
Ms. J.P. Fonseca, Portugal
Dr. M. Gugliotta, Italy
Dr. N. Guzelsu, U.S.A.
Ms. V. Harding, U.K.
Mr. G. Heydinger, U.S.A.
Dr. J. Hohne, West Germany
Dr. R. Huiskes, The Netherlands
Dr. L. Hvid, Denmark
Mr. H.A.C. Jacob, Switzerland
Dr. C. Jolliot, France
Dr. P. Lawes, Ireland
Ms. I.M. Machado, Portugal
Dr. L.P. Marques, Portugal
Ms. M.I. Melo, Portugal

Dr. A. Morais, Portugal
Prof. J.C. Mulier, Belgium
Dr. S. Nielsen, Denmark
Dr. J.E.M. Parra, Portugal
Prof. J.P. Paul, U.K.
Mr. K. Patel, U.K.
Prof. H.S. Ranu, U.S.A.
Dr. J.P. Renaudeaux, France
Dr. A. Rohlmann, West Germany
Dr. K.A. Sarafis, Greece
Dr. A.A.J. Sauren, The Netherlands
Dr. E. Sleeckx, Belgium
Mr. R. Sumner, U.S.A.
Dr. R. Van Audekercke, Belgium
Dr. O.M.V. Vasconcelos, Portugal
Dr. V.M.R. Vila Verde, Portugal
Dr. H. Woltring, The Netherlands

INDEX

.

DATE DUE

MAR 1 2 '89			
MAY 8 '89			
DEC 1 8 '89			
MAY 0 7 1998			
NOV 1 2 1998			
	261-2500		Printed in USA